Advances in IMMUNOLOGY

VOLUME 114

Synthetic Vaccines

ASSOCIATE EDITORS

Advances in **IMMUNOLOGY**

VOLUME 114

Synthetic Vaccines

Edited by

CORNELIS J. M. MELIEF

Department of Immunohematology,
Leiden University Medical Center,
Leiden, The Netherlands
Immune System Activation (ISA) Pharmaceuticals,
Leiden, The Netherlands

ELSEVIER

AMSTERDAM • BOSTON • HEIDELBERG • LONDON
NEW YORK • OXFORD • PARIS • SAN DIEGO
SAN FRANCISCO • SINGAPORE • SYDNEY • TOKYO
Academic Press is an imprint of Elsevier

Academic Press is an imprint of Elsevier
525 B Street, Suite 1900, San Diego, CA 92101-4495, USA
225 Wyman Street, Waltham, MA 02451, USA
32 Jamestown Road, London, NW1 7BY, UK
Radarweg 29, PO Box 211, 1000 AE Amsterdam, The Netherlands

First edition 2012

ISBN: 978-0-12-396548-6
ISSN: 0065-2776

For information on all Academic Press publications
visit our website at elsevierdirect.com

Printed and bound by CPI Group (UK) Ltd, Croydon, CR0 4YY

Transferred to Digital Print 2012

CONTENTS

CONTRIBUTORS

Numbers in parentheses indicate the pages on which the authors' contributions begin.

Myriam Arévalo-Herrera
Malaria Vaccine and Drug Development Center/Immunology Institute, Universidad del Valle, Cali, Colombia (*107*)

Ramon Arens
Department of Immunohematology and Blood Transfusion, Leiden University Medical Center, Albinusdreef 2, Leiden, The Netherlands (*217*)

Silvia Ariotti
Division of Immunology, The Netherlands Cancer Institute, Plesmanlaan, Amsterdam, The Netherlands (*203*)

Jaap W. Back
Pepscan Therapeutics, Lelystad, The Netherlands (*33*)

Winfried Barchet
Institute for Clinical Chemistry and Clinical Pharmacology, University Clinic Bonn, Bonn, Germany (*1*)

Nora Céspedes
Biochemstry Department, University of Lausanne, Epalinges, Switzerland; Malaria Vaccine and Drug Development Center/Immunology Institute, Universidad del Valle, Cali, Colombia (*107*)

Giampietro Corradin
Biochemstry Department, University of Lausanne, Epalinges, Switzerland (*107*)

Dmitri V. Filippov
Leiden Institute of Chemistry, Leiden University, Leiden, The Netherlands (*177*)

John B. Haanen
Division of Immunology, The Netherlands Cancer Institute, Plesmanlaan, Amsterdam, The Netherlands (*203*)

Gunther Hartmann
Institute for Clinical Chemistry and Clinical Pharmacology, University Clinic Bonn, Bonn, Germany (*1*)

Sócrates Herrera
Malaria Vaccine and Drug Development Center/Immunology Institute, Universidad del Valle, Cali, Colombia (*107*)

Andrey V. Kajava
CRBM, CNRS, University of Montpellier, Montpellier, France (*107*)

Selina Khan
Department of Immunohematology and Blood Transfusion, Leiden University Medical Centre, Leiden, The Netherlands (*177*)

Johannes P. M. Langedijk
Crucell, Innovation and Discovery Laboratory, Leiden, The Netherlands (*33*)

Cornelis J. M. Melief
Department of Immunohematology, Leiden University Medical Center and Immune System Activation (ISA) Pharmaceuticals, Leiden, The Netherlands (*77*)

Ferry Ossendorp
Department of Immunohematology and Blood Transfusion, Leiden University Medical Centre, Leiden, The Netherlands (*177*)

Esther D. Quakkelaar
Department of Immunohematology, Leiden University Medical Center, Leiden, The Netherlands (*77*)

Ton N. Schumacher
Division of Immunology, The Netherlands Cancer Institute, Plesmanlaan, Amsterdam, The Netherlands (*203*)

Jasper G. van den Boorn
Institute for Clinical Chemistry and Clinical Pharmacology, University Clinic Bonn, Bonn, Germany (*1*)

Sjoerd H. van der Burg
Department of Clinical Oncology, Experimental Cancer Immunology and Therapy, Leiden University Medical Center, Albinusdreef 2, Leiden, Netherlands (*51*)

Thorbald van Hall
Department of Clinical Oncology, Experimental Cancer Immunology and Therapy, Leiden University Medical Center, Albinusdreef 2, Leiden, Netherlands (*51*)

Antonio Verdini
Biochemstry Department, University of Lausanne, Epalinges, Switzerland (*107*)

Helen Y. Wang
Department of Pathology and Immunology, Center for Cell and Gene Therapy, Baylor College of Medicine, Houston, Texas, USA (*151*)

Rong-Fu Wang
Department of Pathology and Immunology, Center for Cell and Gene Therapy, Baylor College of Medicine, Houston, Texas, USA (*151*)

Gijs G. P. Zom
Department of Immunohematology and Blood Transfusion, Leiden University Medical Centre, Leiden, The Netherlands (*177*)

PREFACE

This volume of *Advances in Immunology* is entirely devoted to the science of synthetic vaccine development. While it is hard to exaggerate the public health importance of preventive vaccination, no fully effective preventive vaccines exist for many infectious diseases, with, as of this writing, the prominent examples of AIDS, tuberculosis, and malaria. Therapeutic vaccines are an even greater challenge, but as discussed in these chapters, some initial successes have been booked. It is my conviction that for further development of powerful vaccines, knowledge of the optimal chemical structure of immunogens needs to be combined with optimal insights into how the required innate and adaptive immunity can best be stimulated. This compilation of reviews constitutes a strong plea toward rational design of vaccines to address the unsolved vaccine challenges, away from empiric approaches with complicated poorly understood viral or bacterial vectors and away from live attenuated organisms. This approach requires detailed insights into how best to stimulate innate, as well as B and T cell responses and into regulation of these responses and delineates an excellent career path for a new generation of immunologists and vaccinologists. In Chapter 1, van den Boorn *et al.* elaborate in great detail the nature of pathogen-derived nucleic acids that stimulate innate and adaptive immune responses, illustrating lucidly how these well-defined sequences can be used as, e.g., adjuvants in synthetic vaccines and combinatorial immunotherapeutic approaches. In Chapter 2, Back and Langedijk discuss how detailed knowledge of the dynamic crystal structure of the HIV envelope provides novel insights that can lead to the development of a more efficient vaccine capable of inducing neutralizing antibodies against HIV. In Chapter 3, van Hall and van der Burg dissect the history of peptide vaccines to induce therapeutic T cell responses and discuss the importance of the presence of helper T cell epitopes, the necessity of uptake by professional antigen-presenting cells, biodistribution, influence of adjuvants, peptide length, peptide affinity, and mode of administration. In Chapter 4, Quakkelaar and Melief review the use of synthetic peptide vaccines in primates and in clinical trials. The combined evidence shows that synthetic long peptide vaccines are more effective than exact MHC class I binding peptide vaccines because the long peptides contain helper T cell epitopes and require processing by dendritic cells (DC), the prime initiators of immune responses. In Chapter 5, Corradin *et al.* discuss the history of peptide synthesis and provide a gripping overview of the current status of long peptide vaccines against malaria. In Chapter 6, Wang and Wang deliver arguments on how synthetic long peptide vaccines can be further improved by equipping them with cell-penetrating sequences, allowing prolonged DC antigen presentation. Another highly interesting efficiency-improving step can be achieved by covalent coupling the synthetic peptides to a TLR ligand, as illustrated in Chapter 7 by Zom *et al.* In Chapter 8, Ariotti *et al.* demonstrate the importance of the induction and persistence of tissue resident memory T cells. Surely vaccines need to induce such cells for long-term protection against potential invaders of these tissues. Last but not least, in Chapter 9, Arens draws an analogy between the immune evasion strategies operating in malignant tumors and those employed by persistent viruses and points out strategies to counteract these mechanisms. Together these chapters were a great joy to compile and to read. Undoubtedly, they will be a rich source of information and ideas that can help to develop a new generation of molecularly defined vaccines to address unsolved problems in preventive and therapeutic vaccination.

CHAPTER 1

Nucleic Acid Adjuvants: Toward an Educated Vaccine

Jasper G. van den Boorn, Winfried Barchet, and **Gunther Hartmann**

Contents

Institute for Clinical Chemistry and Clinical Pharmacology, University Clinic Bonn, Bonn, Germany

Advances in Immunology, Volume 114
ISSN 0065-2776, DOI: 10.1016/B978-0-12-396548-6.00001-9

Abstract

Two striking facts surround the practice of vaccination: It is the sole medical approach to have fully annihilated a disease, yet the development of most effective vaccines took place without considering the intricate cellular processes they wish to effectuate. While extremely potent vaccines have been developed that can protect practically a lifetime after a single dose, numerous other vaccines have utterly failed or provide only marginal protection. Here, we aim to illustrate why this difference in efficacy exists, and underline why specific cytotoxic T cell-inducing vaccines could combat persistent major diseases. Moreover, we discuss how the combinatorial use of nucleic acid adjuvants in vaccines could aid the development of the latter and move vaccine design from the empirical stage into an era of "educated design."

1. A SHORT VACCINATION HISTORY

The basic understanding that the burden of infectious disease brings with it a form of protection from reinfection, already dates back to several centuries B.C. when people noticed that they rarely acquired the same disease twice, at least not to the same extent of morbidity (Plotkin and Plotkin, 2008). It took some time before mankind actively exploited this "memory" phenomenon. The classical view states that it was not until 1796 that Edward Jenner pioneered and carried out his famous smallpox vaccinations, using the cowpox virus as inoculum (Jenner, 1798). Thereby he allegedly carried out the first human vaccinations. While these were indeed the first "vaccinations," a term coined by Jenner himself to identify the bovine origin of his inoculum, he basically optimized a method of immunization that had already been known for centuries.

The trail of active human immunization, in particular against smallpox, leads back well beyond the dark ages. It is highly likely that Jenner was inspired by the practices of the Dutch cattle trader Geert Reinders, who managed to stop the spread of cowpox in his region around 1774 by deliberately reinfecting cows that recovered from cowpox with scabs from recently infected animals. Reinders performed impressive fundamental work. In his age he documented that cows previously infected with cowpox produced offspring that were temporarily protected from this disease. Additionally, he described that deliberate reinfection of these "maternally protected" animals, or otherwise previously cowpox-diseased animals, actually protected his cattle from cowpox for a lifetime. Thereby he was the first to document maternal inherited immunity as well as functional booster immunizations.

Deliberate infection to confer protection against smallpox actually has its roots in religious rites. Practices to thereby protect against the disease were already carried out in India in 1500 B.C. While these early days of immunization remain obscure, the practice of supplying fresh smallpox scab-material to healthy individuals to induce immunity (a process called variolation), started to become more common in sixth century China. People ground dried smallpox-scabs from lightly diseased people and applied these in wet cloths to the noses of healthy individuals to induce protection. While other practices coexisted, like sleeping next to diseased people and wearing their used clothing, the practice of variolation slowly spread westwards. Via popular healers in Africa and the Near East, variolation evolved to involve the scratching of the skin with a sharp object and inserting "serum" material extracted from fresh smallpox scabs.

The efforts of the Greek James Pylarino further propagated the use of variolation, initially throughout the Ottoman Empire (Alivisatos, 1934). After completing his medical studies in 1679 in Padua and wandering through Europe as a court physician, he embarked on studying variolation in Constantinople by 1701. Shortly after his arrival in Constantinople Pylarino successfully variolated three children and thereby protected them from a local smallpox epidemic. The success of his approach was quickly recognized and spread accordingly as "the Greek method." Pylarino's accomplice Emanuel Timoni further propelled the method to popularity. He communicated a paper on effective variolation to the English Royal Society of Medicine in 1713. It was not until 1717 that variolation was introduced broadly to Europe, after Lady Mary Wortly Montagu undertook a trip to Turkey and Constantinople. Via her subsequent efforts variolation was introduced to the royalty of Europe and eventually to the common people.

Being a relatively common (although still risky and potentially mutilating) practice at the end of the 1700s, Reinders basically extrapolated variolation to his cows in an attempt to protect his cattle. In the process, he described the foundations of adaptive immunity. Jenner likely knew about the immunization practices of Geert Reinders, since Reinders published his discoveries 22 years before Jenner actually conducted his human experiments. Apparently citation principles could do with improvement even then. Jenner combined smallpox variolation with Reinders' cowpox inoculum since he knew that milkmaids working with cowpox-diseased cows rarely contracted smallpox. Thereby he made the first truly effective and highly safe human vaccine in history.

The use of vaccination was propagated further by the attenuated microbes of Pasteur and colleagues in the late 1800s (Pasteur *et al.*, 2002). Around this time also scientific interest in systematic immunity arose from the medical microbiology field of Pasteur and Koch. It was importantly propelled by the discoveries of Paul Ehrlich and Elie Metchnikoff who for the first time illustrated different mechanisms by which the host apparently fought back at invading pathogens. This was a revolutionary step forward from the traditional view of the host passively enduring microbial assault. Thereby, it is astounding that the fields of immunology and vaccination have never fully intermingled, which may be attributed to the practical approach of vaccinology and the conceptual state of immunological science in the late 1800s.

The knowledgeable decision of the Nobel committee to award the 1908 Nobel Prize for Medicine to both Elie Metchnikoff and Paul Ehrlich as "founders of immunology" could not unite the diverging sentiments of both founding fathers. While both scientists had common grounds in the study of cellular nutrient-uptake, the young scientific field of immunology split. On the one hand the "cellularist" discipline followed Metchnikoff's concept that it were the responses of migratory phagocytic cells that protected the host from infection. On the other side were Ehrlich's "humoralists" who were convinced that it rather were microbe neutralizing, molecular cell side chains coined "antibodies" that protected from infection (Kaufmann, 2008). While both would now likely be united in delight when observing the mosaic of complex immunological processes that deal with both systems, vaccinology in time got acquainted with the humoralist view and practically stuck with it. Hence, the aim has always been to induce protective titers of neutralizing antibodies in preventing pathogen infection. Certainly this approach has saved an innumerable number of lives by yielding very effective vaccines, like the outstanding yellow fever vaccine and the smallpox-eradicating vaccine, as well as bringing poliomyelitis a step closer to extinction. Still, effective vaccines do not exist against major diseases like tuberculosis, leprosy, human immunodeficiency virus (HIV), or parasitic infections like malaria and leishmaniasis. Current vaccination approaches are ineffective here, since neutralizing antibodies alone cannot control these pathogens. Instead, they require strong cellular cytotoxic responses to accompany the humoral response, leading us to re-aim vaccines toward a multilineage response.

2. THE IMMUNE SYSTEM AS SENSORY TISSUE

By variolation or vaccination one of the body's first lines of defense is breached: the physical barrier of the skin. Being the largest organ of the human body it has several essential functions. Its impermeability, mainly mediated by the outermost *stratum corneum*, protects the body from invading pathogens, noxious agents and dehydration. Furthermore, the resident pigment cells (melanocytes) aid in the shielding against harmful ultraviolet-radiation. Importantly, together with the internal mucosa, the skin employs an intricate network of immune cells, the skin immune system (SIS) and thereby mediates the initial response against many invading- or introduced agents (Bos, 2005).

2.1. Innate immune cell activation

The first immune cells to react to invading pathogens are those of the innate system. They employ a set of cross-species evolutionarily conserved receptors on their surface, in their endosomal vesciles or their cytosol, termed pattern-recognition receptors (PRRs). While the tissue distribution of PRR is outside the scope of this review, it is noteworthy that Toll-like receptors (TLRs) or C-type lectins are mainly expressed in immune cells, especially professional antigen presenting cells (APC) and macrophages (Barbalat *et al.*, 2011; Takeda *et al.*, 2003). Nonetheless, certain somatic cells can also express TLRs. For example, keratinocytes express functional TLR 3, 4, 5, and 9 (Lebre *et al.*, 2007). Activation of TLR in nonimmune cells can induce production of different cytokines or chemokines. Nevertheless, the TLR-triggered production of interferon-alpha is generally mediated by immune cells, in particular plasmacytoid dendritic cells (PDC). Other PRR have more broad tissue distributions, like the nod-like receptors and inflammasomes (Barbalat *et al.*, 2011; Martinon *et al.*, 2002; Sirard *et al.*, 2007), and some are basically expressed in all nucleated cells of the body, like the RIG-I-like helicases (Barbalat *et al.*, 2011; Schlee *et al.*, 2009). The latter should not be seen as an under appreciation of nonnucleated cells, like blood platelets. In contrast to their common exclusion from any immunological process, these small entities have distinct immune modulating properties which now start to be appreciated (Semple *et al.*, 2011).

By their PRR, innate immune cells recognize conserved structures widely expressed across families of microorganisms, termed pathogen-associated molecular patterns (PAMPs; Akira *et al.*, 2006; Barbalat *et al.*, 2011; Medzhitov, 2007). PRRs enable rapid recognition of pathogen classes by the innate immune cells, facilitating an evolutionary tailored response aimed at timely clearance. However, innate cells only display standardized response patterns and they lack the capability to form so-called "immunological memory." This memory is essential for the immune response to quickly respond upon persistent or repetitive infection with similar pathogen. It is the main feature exploited by vaccines, and is the hallmark of the adaptive immune system. The latter responds to very specific parts of the pathogen (antigens), which are not necessarily evolutionarily conserved. Adaptive immune cells are the CD4+ and CD8+ T cells, and B lymphocytes. Prior to carrying out their full function, these cells need precise activation by their innate counterparts.

2.2. Adaptive immune cell activation

The T cells from the adaptive immune system are activated by recognizing specific antigens on APC, typically the dendritic cells (DCs). Discovered initially in 1868 by Paul Langerhans, Ralph Steinman *et al.* in 1973 characterized DCs as stellar cells (Steinman and Cohn, 1973) with distinct immunostimulatory properties (Steinman *et al.*, 1983). Since then the understanding of DC function has advanced, and many functional subsets have been identified (Heath and Carbone, 2009; Kushwah and Hu, 2011). By their immune stimulatory properties, DCs have become central to an array of immunotherapeutic regimens (Melief, 2008; Steinman and Banchereau, 2007). Besides DCs, other innate immune cells are also able to act as effective APC, in particular macrophages (Hume, 2008; Paveley *et al.*, 2009) and basophils (Perrigoue *et al.*, 2009; Sokol *et al.*, 2009; Yoshimoto *et al.*, 2009). Important for this review, DCs are the essential APC initiating CD8+ T cell immunity against skin-derived and vaccinated antigen in general, as demonstrated by different DC antigen-targeting and *in vivo* depletion studies (Bonifaz *et al.*, 2004; Jung *et al.*, 2002).

Immature DCs reside in the peripheral tissues, preferentially at sites near the exterior. Upon antigen uptake and subsequent cellular activation by their PRR for example, the DC migrates to a nearby lymph node where it acquires a stimulatory phenotype. Here, it expresses T cell costimulatory molecules such as CD83 and CD86 together with high levels of surface MHC class-I and -II molecules loaded with processed antigenic peptides. Furthermore, it attracts naïve T cells by producing the chemokine CCL18 (Adema *et al.*, 1997). Principally, DCs present ingested lysosome-degraded antigenic material to CD4+ T cells in MHC class-II, while proteasomal degradation products are presented to CD8+ T cells in MHC class-I. Antigen for proteasomal breakdown can be acquired biosynthetically, for example by direct infections of DCs, or from ingested extracellular material via the so-called cross-presentation process (Jondal *et al.*, 1996). The latter is an important mechanism in the priming of CD8+ T cells against antigens from vaccines and virus-infected or malignant cells. Figure 1.1 schematically shows the initiation routes of adaptive immunity.

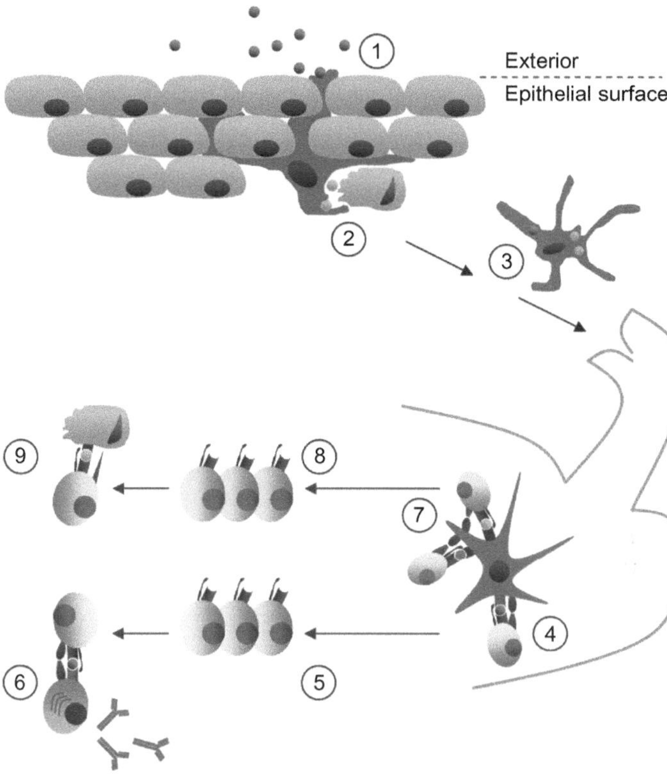

FIGURE 1.1 Initiation of the adaptive immune response. Antigen presenting cells such as dendritic cells (DCs) can reside near the exterior and engulf extracellular antigenic matter, like microbial constituents or vaccinated agents (1) or debris from stressed or dying cells (2). Upon activation, the DCs migrate to the local lymph node via afferent lymph vessels (3). In the lymph node, these DCs acquire a highly stimulatory phenotype and process the acquired antigens into peptides to be presented in their surface MHC class-I or -II. DCs can activate CD4+ T cells by presenting extracellular-derived antigen in their surface MHC-class-II molecules (4). The activated CD4+ T cells will subsequently proliferate (5) and are then able to mature local B cells displaying the CD4+ T cell's cognate antigen in their surface MHC class-II. These mature B cells can differentiate into antibody-producing plasma cells, secreting monoclonal antibodies directed against the antigen initially displayed to them (6). Alternatively, DCs can activate CD8+ T cells by presenting intracellular-derived antigen or extracellular-derived antigen via cross-presentation, in their surface MHC class-I (7). Following initial proliferation (8), activated CD8+ T cells will enter the circulation via efferent lymph vessels. In the peripheral tissues, these T cells can kill nucleated cells on which they recognize their specific antigenic peptide in the context of surface-expressed MHC class-I (9). (See Color Insert.)

3. WHY SOME VACCINES JUST DO NOT WORK

Most vaccines prime an adaptive immune response by the controlled delivery of live-attenuated or inactivated pathogen to the individual, generally by intramuscular injection. The basic readout hereafter has classically been the formation of protective antibody titers that are thought sufficient to protect from specific pathogen-mediated disease by neutralization and/or opsonization of the invading pathogen. In distinct cases, however, this response is fruitless.

3.1. Live attenuated vaccines

One of the most effective means of vaccination is the use of live attenuated pathogens. These encompass all pathogen-specific antigens and intrinsically carry numerous PRR-triggering determinants, all of which they spread locally in the host upon exercising their limited replicative potential following vaccination. A classic example of such a vaccine is yellow fever 17D. The vaccine strain briefly infects human DCs for 5–7 days upon vaccination without excessive multiplication (Querec *et al.*, 2006). This appears to deliver adequate antigen levels to the DC enabling it to initiate effective antigen processing and presentation to both CD4+ and CD8+ T cells (Barba-Spaeth *et al.*, 2005). The attenuated virus triggers multiple PRR simultaneously to activate the DC; it triggers TLR 2 and 8 on myeloid DC, TLR 7 and 9 in plasmacytoid DC, as well as the cytosolic immune sensors retinoic acid-inducible gene-1 (RIG-I), melanoma differentiation-associated gene 5 (MDA5), the NLRP3 inflammasome, and the DC-activating complement components C1qA and C1qB (Csomor *et al.*, 2007; Gaucher *et al.*, 2008; Querec *et al.*, 2006, 2009). The result is a robust multilineage innate- and adaptive response which, although being variable between individuals (Gaucher *et al.*, 2008), is able to induce a protective antibody response in 99% of vaccinees within 10 days (Monath *et al.*, 2002). After a single vaccination, the vaccine can protect for practically a lifetime against yellow fever disease (Barrett and Teuwen, 2009). The live attenuated 17D vaccine can thereby be regarded as an excellent example for further vaccine design. Albeit that much still needs to be deciphered about its true mode of action, a process which has been initiated recently (Barba-Spaeth *et al.*, 2005; Gaucher *et al.*, 2008).

By its limited proliferation, the associated innate immune activation induced by 17D can extend to up to 15 days (Gaucher *et al.*, 2008; Querec *et al.*, 2009). Also, a vigorous T cell response to numerous antigens in the yellow fever polyprotein is initiated by 17D vaccination (Miller *et al.*, 2008; Querec *et al.*, 2006), ensuring a broad adaptive mixed T_{h1}/T_{h2} response. Nevertheless, the 17D vaccine is also associated with serious adverse effects, like acute viscero- and neurotropic events closely resembling disseminated yellow fever disease (Lindsey *et al.*, 2008; Monath, 2010). These adverse effects have a high mortality rate of 64% on average, and preclude the use of the live attenuated 17D vaccine in high-risk individuals such as immunosuppressed or thymectomized persons, young children or pregnant women. Occurring at 0.4 and 0.8 cases per 100,000 vaccinees for viscero- and neurotropic events respectively, these are considerable adverse factors with near to 20 million vaccines administered yearly (Hayes, 2010). Hence, a safer yellow fever vaccine without replicative potential was required to enable vaccination of these high-risk groups.

3.2. Inactivated vaccines

An alternative inactivated vaccine has recently been developed from cellular cultivation of the 17D strain (Monath *et al.*, 2010, 2011). While it is less readily protective as its classic 17D counterpart, since it requires booster immunization, it is a breakthrough that an alternative now exists which can practically induce equal protection. A likewise situation is applicable to Leishmaniasis. For long, the only means of acquiring protection was vaccination with live attenuated parasites or undergoing natural infection, since vaccination with inactivated parasites or peptides did not readily induce protection from disease (Okwor *et al.*, 2009). Recently, however, it was established that repetitive inoculation with inactivated parasites could confer immune protection from Leishmaniasis in mice (Okwor *et al.*, 2010). These two examples illustrate that by rule of thumb inactivating a pathogen readily reduces its immunogenicity, while still the basic makeup of the pathogen remains equal. This relates less to the proliferative spread of the pathogen, but more to the actual sites where PAMPs encounter their PRR in local DCs. While live attenuated pathogens direct PAMPs to sites where evolutionary conserved PRR reside to recognize them briskly, inactivated vaccine pathogens must rely on active uptake and antigen processing by DCs, a process during which multiple PAMPs could be directed to divergent cellular compartments leading to incomplete triggering of the available reactive PRR repertoire. For example, the use of inactivated pathogens omits the presence of pathogen-derived nucleic acids in the cytosol of host cells.

3.3. *Mycobacterium tuberculosis*: Differentially expressed antigens

Apart from differences between live attenuated and inactivated vaccines concerning their capacity to trigger innate immunity, the specific antigens present in the pathogen's vaccine strain may also interfere with priming protective immunity. For example, *M. tuberculosis* expresses distinct antigen sets during acute or latent infection (Commandeur *et al.*, 2011a; Lin *et al.*, 2007). The live attenuated vaccine strain *Mycobacterium bovis* Bacillus Calmette-Guérin (BCG) predominantly expresses antigens related to acute infection (Lin *et al.*, 2007). While BCG is a poor vaccine by its temporary protection of young children and incapability to protect adults from pulmonary *M. tuberculosis* infection, it hereby is also incapable to counteract reactivation of latent *M. tuberculosis* infections. The latter is of grave concern, since one-third of the world population is latently infected with pulmonary *M. tuberculosis*, of which 10% will likely experience reactivated tuberculosis during their lifetime. Moreover, this percentage is expected to rise along with increasing numbers of HIV-infected immune compromised individuals (Corbett *et al.*, 2003; Lin and Ottenhoff, 2008). The situation around tuberculosis thus calls for incorporating its chronic infection-related dormancy-regulon (DosR) antigens into the vaccine strain. Since it is these antigens that actually relate to immune control of latent *M. tuberculosis* infection (Black *et al.*, 2009; Commandeur *et al.*, 2011b; Leyten *et al.*, 2006; Schuck *et al.*, 2009). Adaptation of the BCG vaccine strain, which actually is capable of expressing the DosR antigens (Lin *et al.*, 2007), can prove a fruitful strategy.

3.4. Dengue virus: Antibody-dependent enhancement of infection

Besides differentially expressed antigen sets, antigenic similarity between distinct pathogen strains can also hamper protective immunity. The mosquito-transmitted dengue flavivirus family comprises four different strains that can infect humans (DENV-1 to -4). While natural infection can protect from reinfection by the same strain, and shortly to infection by the other three strains, it can eventually enhance the infection of another dengue strain. Moreover, it augments the chances for developing deadly dengue haemorrhagic fever upon secondary infection (Rothman, 2011). Dengue shows tropism for monocytes, macrophages, and DCs (Jessie *et al.*, 2004), which all express Fc-receptors. Neutralizing antibodies induced by the primary infection that appear of insufficient titer, low avidity or insufficient specificity can enhance viral uptake through these Fc-receptors, a process named antibody-dependent enhancement of infection (Rothman, 2011). Empirical vaccination approaches have thereby been counter-effective, since they increase the risk of a severe morbidity and additionally do not protect against all four subtypes (Rothman, 2011). Still, natural dengue infection induces a predominantly Th_1-oriented T cell response focusing around the NS3 and NS4b proteins within the polyprotein (Mangada and Rothman, 2005), which are highly conserved and shared between the four DENV serotypes (Mongkolsapaya *et al.*, 2003; Rothman, 2011). Hence, development of a protein (subunit) vaccine that strictly elicits specific CD8+ T cell responses to these shared T_{h1} antigens could provide us with an effective dengue vaccine, in analogy to the development of influenza vaccines targeting the shared surface glycoprotein hemagglutinins in pursuit of a broadly protective vaccine to overcome the need for seasonal vaccinations (Chen *et al.*, 2011).

3.5. HIV: High antigenic drift

Posing an even greater challenge to vaccine development and practically impossible to target via empirical vaccination, are pathogens with high antigenic drift. One such pathogen for which a vaccine is highly desirable is the HIV. The agility by which HIV escapes immunity is twofold: Firstly, by nature, the HIV retrovirus has a highly error-prone reverse transcriptase that lacks proofreading capability. During the generation of the DNA copy of its viral genome that is inserted into the host cell genome, it introduces about one translational mutation per replication cycle. Combined with template-switching and recombination, this ensures that HIV continuously generates unique viral subtypes during infection (Gaschen *et al.*, 2002; Malim and Emerman, 2001). In the most common "M" group of HIV strains, subtypes can differ up to 40% in their genetic makeup. This can result in sequence variations in envelope-proteins to as high as 20%. While a variation of only 2% in influenza protein composition is sufficient to render the seasonal vaccine ineffective and require the selection of a new strain (Gaschen *et al.*, 2002). Secondly, via its pliable character HIV has adapted to human humoral immunity at the population level. A recent study shows how the virus from the 1980s up to the 2000s has evaded antibody neutralization with increasing efficiency by increasing the length of the variable loops and the number of possible *N*-linked glycosylation sites on its gp120 envelope subunit proteins (Bunnik *et al.*, 2010). Combined with its mutational potency this makes HIV constantly outrun the adaptive immune system, which will eventually succumb to clonal exhaustion (Nikolich-Zugich *et al.*, 2004).

However, also for HIV there is an intriguing new T cell part to the story that suggests new opportunities in the direction of a CD8+ T cell-activating vaccine. For long, it has been recognized that effective CD8+ T cell immunity is essential in controlling HIV infection (McMichael and Rowland-Jones, 2001). This is underlined by the association of certain human leukocyte antigen (HLA) class-I subtypes with delayed progression from HIV infection to acquired immunodeficiency syndrome (AIDS) development (Kaslow *et al.*, 1996). In particular, the expression of the autoimmunity-associated HLA-B*27 and HLA-B*57 alleles appears to be highly beneficial. While in the majority of HIV-infected individuals the CD8+ T cell response collapses in time, many HIV-infected long-term nonprogressors appear to have populations of HLA-B*27 and HLA-B*57 restricted CD8+ T cells which retain their proliferative and killing potential. These virus-specific T cells have been directly related to a significantly improved AIDS-free survival (Dinges *et al.*, 2010). Moreover, they actively evade T_{reg}-mediated immune-suppressive mechanisms by actively killing T_{reg} cells in a granzyme-B-dependent manner and by expressing significantly diminished levels of the T cell inhibitory receptor Tim-3 (T cell immunoglobulin domain and mucin domain 3). Tim-3 negatively regulates T_{h1} responses upon interaction with its ligand gallectin-9, which is expressed on different lymphocyte populations and constitutively on T_{reg} (Elahi *et al.*, 2011). The deeper understanding of these HLA-B*27 and HLA-B*57-restricted killer T cells is a key advance in understanding the immune control of HIV infection and resulting long-term nonprogression. Moreover, it suggests a path to designing a vaccine-based approach against HIV, targeting CD8+ T cells against one of the few conserved HIV proteins, p24 (Gaschen *et al.*, 2002), and ideally would provide them with low Tim-3 levels and an effector profile alike the HLA-B*27 and HLA-B*57-restricted T cells.

Hence, in many neutralizing antibody insensitive diseases there still appears to exist a possibility for intervention using targeted CD8+ T cells. The degree of specific antigen cross-presentation by DCs is crucial to induce cytotoxic T cell responses and can be greatly influenced by the adjuvants employed in the vaccine, skewing the outcome of vaccination.

4. SYNERGIZING INNATE IMMUNE STIMULI

While the multilineage responses to live attenuated vaccines often induce protective immunity after one dose, inactivated or protein (subunit) vaccines are often not readily immunogenic. The latter therefore need addition of adjuvants to boost their immunogenicity, which provide additional PRR triggers. Especially when strong antigen cross-presentation is needed, the choice of adjuvant is crucial since the select few approved for clinical use have distinct effects. Here, the recently uncovered functions of the cytosolic nucleic acid sensors could be essential.

With the discovery of PRR came the realization that a potent and timely activation of such innate immune receptors was a major reason why live inactivated vaccines are able to induce protective and lasting immunity. Many of the PRR-triggering PAMPs have been used as potent adjuvants in experimental vaccinations in mice (Coffman *et al.*, 2010; Higgins and Mills, 2010). However, as an apparent paradox, mice lacking individual innate immune receptors, or the signaling adapters MyD88, TRIF, IPS-1, NLRP3/ASC, Syk/CARD9 that mediate the signaling of groups of innate receptors often display only modest impairments in humoral and cellular adaptive immune responses (Gavin *et al.*, 2006;

Ishii *et al.*, 2008; Koyama *et al.*, 2007). This indicates a robust redundancy in the innate immune pathways that are activated by microbes. Furthermore, there apparently exists a strong synergistic potential between the signaling pathways of PRR like nucleic acid receptors, illustrated by the before mentioned yellow fever vaccine.

Indeed, bacteria and viruses have been shown to activate multiple innate immune pathways simultaneously (Delaloye *et al.*, 2009; Gaucher *et al.*, 2008; Ichinohe *et al.*, 2009; Rhee *et al.*, 2010; Saiga *et al.*, 2011). Moreover, contemporaneous activation of innate immune signaling pathways has been shown to synergistically enhance adaptive responses (Napolitani *et al.*, 2005), as well as a potentiated adjuvant effect (Kasturi *et al.*, 2011). Activation profiles of innate immune pathways that are typical for classes of pathogens also instruct the adaptive immune system on how to optimally respond (Iwasaki and Medzhitov, 2010). While opsonizing high affinity antibodies should be appropriate against extracellularly replicating bacteria, cytotoxic $CD8^+$ T cells excel at detecting and eliminating virus-infected cells. In the following, we discuss approaches that focus on employing agonists of nucleic acid receptors of the innate immune system, that is, on the receptors that predominantly mediate the recognition of viruses.

4.1. TLR9 activation by CpG ODN

Oligonucleotides containing CpG dinucleotides (CpG ODN) were among the first molecular structures explicitly designed to model a PAMP (Krieg *et al.*, 1995). The innate immune receptor responsive to DNA that reaches the endosome, including CpG ODN was later defined to be TLR9 (Bauer *et al.*, 2001). Since then the potential of CpG ODN to act as vaccine adjuvant has been extensively evaluated in over 600 preclinical studies including rodents and nonhuman primates (Bode *et al.*, 2011). For the induction of Ab responses, potent adjuvancy by the addition of CpG ODN has been observed for example with anthrax (Klinman *et al.*, 2006) and hepatitis B antigen (Davis *et al.*, 1998)(Zhang *et al.*, 2011), Toxoplasma lysate (El-Malky *et al.*, 2005), or vaccinia virus (Moldoveanu *et al.*, 1998).

Most of these studies have been performed using CpG-B ODN that efficiently stimulate B-cells but elicit little or no type I IFN from plasmacytoid DC. In contrast, CpG-A ODN form higher order structures and strongly induce type I IFN in PDC (Krug *et al.*, 2001). A recent paper concluded that CpG-A ODN were a superior vaccine adjuvant for the generation of cytotoxic T cells (Katsuda *et al.*, 2011). One hypothesis for this finding is that CpG-A ODN remain better associated with the antigen, and via type I IFN promote cross-presentation and prolongs $CD8^+$ T cell proliferation (Le Bon *et al.*, 2003, 2006). In fact, physically linking or coencapsulating CpG ODN with the soluble antigen, or also with apoptotic tumor cells was shown to potently enhance $CD8^+$ T cell responses (Heit *et al.*, 2005, 2007; Shirota and Klinman, 2011).

Boosted Ab titers using CpG ODN as vaccine adjuvant have been achieved also in clinical trials in humans, for example when combined with Engerix B (Cooper *et al.*, 2004) or Malaria antigen (Ellis *et al.*, 2009). In contrast, CpG ODN adjuvanted induction of $CD8^+$ T cells in humans was less successful compared to mice, which may be due to the fact that TLR9 expression in humans is restricted to PDC and B-cells (Hornung *et al.*, 2002), while in mice TLR9 is active also in conventional DCs that are essential for the cross-priming of $CD8^+$ T cells (Heit *et al.*, 2003).

4.2. Small molecule and single stranded RNA (ssRNA) agonists of TLR7/8

Endosomal detection of ssRNA is mediated by TLRs 7 and 8 (Diebold *et al.*, 2004; Heil *et al.*, 2004). As with TLR9 there are notable differences between the human and mouse expression patterns. In humans, TLR7 is expressed in PDC and neutrophils, and is inducible in B-cells, while macrophages and conventional DC express TLR8. In contrast, murine TLR7 is active in macrophages and DC subsets, with the notable exception of $CD8\alpha^+$ DC, whereas TLR8 appears nonfunctional for RNA detection (Barchet *et al.*, 2008). Besides ssRNA, TLR7 and 8 are activated also by small molecule agonists, including imidazoquinolines and guanosine analogs (Hemmi *et al.*, 2002). Some imidazoquinoline derivates exclusively activate TLR7 or TLR8, which is pharmacologically relevant to limit toxicity by restricting the cell types activated. The TLR7 selective agonist imiquimod is now widely used to treat dermatological disorders including genital warts, keratosis, and basal cell carcinoma (A Gaspari *et al.*, 2009). Immobilized, antigen-linked, or coencapsulated imidazoquinolines show promise as enhancers of vaccine immunogenicity (Oh *et al.*, 2011; Russo *et al.*, 2011; Shukla *et al.*, 2011; Smirnov *et al.*, 2011; Wille-Reece *et al.*, 2005). Also, imiquimod has been used successfully in humans as a vaccination adjuvant when applied topically at the vaccination site (Adams *et al.*, 2008).

It is not yet clear whether adjuvants inducing predominantly type I IFN via TLR7, or the T_{h1} polarizing cytokine IL-12 via TLR8 or both will prove superior for adjuvancy with respect to efficacy and safety in humans. In rhesus macaques immunized with Influenza H1N1 together with synergizing adjuvants, a TLR7/8 agonist led to slightly higher neutralizing antibody titers compared to a TLR7 selective imidazoquinoline (Kasturi *et al.*, 2011). Alternatively, also synthetic ssRNAs protected from RNAse degradation by chemical modification or encapsulation have successfully been used as vaccine adjuvants for soluble and cell-associated antigens (Bourquin *et al.*, 2010; Hamm *et al.*, 2007; Westwood *et al.*, 2006).

4.3. Poly I:C and derivatives activate TLR3 in the endosome and MDA-5 in the cytosol

The enzymatically generated polynucleotide Poly I:C is considered a mimic of viral double stranded RNA, and has for decades been known as a potent inducer of type I IFN (Field *et al.*, 1967). Poly I:C has been shown to engage both TLR3 (Alexopoulou *et al.*, 2001) as well as the cytosolic helicase MDA-5 (Gitlin *et al.*, 2006; Kato *et al.*, 2006). Although originally deemed too toxic for human use, recently the potent adjuvant activity of poly I:C has been newly appreciated in vaccine formulations targeted to DCs (Longhi *et al.*, 2009; Tewari *et al.*, 2010; Trumpfheller *et al.*, 2008). Wang and colleagues discovered that the superior qualities of poly I:C as a vaccine adjuvant are due to the synergy between TLR3 and MDA-5 activation. While TLR3 was required for $CD8^+$ T cell activation by cross-priming, survival of CD8 memory T cells depended on functional MDA-5 in stromal cells (Wang *et al.*, 2010). A poly I:C variant stabilized by lysine and carboxymethylcellulose with improved pharmacokinetic and pharmacodynamic parameters (poly ICLC or Hiltonol) is currently evaluated in clinical trials and has successfully been employed as stimulant in cancer immunotherapy (Okada *et al.*, 2011).

However, also RNA forms that selectively trigger TLR3, but not MDA-5, are able to increase vaccine immunogenicity. The modified dsRNA poly $I{:}C_{12}U$ (Ampligen) has been shown to exclusively activate TLR3, while still exhibiting potent adjuvant function (Jasani *et al.*, 2009). Similarly, oligonucleotide dsRNAs that were designed to selectively interact with the TLR3 extracellular domain were shown to be potent adjuvants promoting cross-priming of $CD8^+$ T cells, leading to protection from lethal doses of influenza (Jelinek *et al.*, 2011).

4.4. 5′-Triphosphate RNA detection by RIG-I

The cytosolic helicase RIG-I is structurally related to MDA-5. In contrast to MDA-5, the viral RNA structure recognized by RIG-I has been identified as 5′-triphosphate (Hornung *et al.*, 2006; Pichlmair *et al.*, 2006). This allowed the design of defined synthetic RIG-I agonists, and thereby revealed that blunt ended dsRNA at the triphosphate end was essential for activity (Schlee *et al.*, 2009). So far, synthetic RIG-I agonists have not been evaluated as vaccine adjuvants. However, an initial step was recently undertaken, when RIG-I agonistic RNA transcribed from an influenza virus DNA vaccine vector promoted the subsequent humoral response (Luke *et al.*, 2011). This does, however, not reserve RIG-I triggering for the T_{h2} side of immunity. While the CD8+ T cell response-skewing potential of 5′-triphosphate RNA ligands for RIG-I remains as yet unexplored, this is likely to be present by the ligand's natural viral origin.

Interestingly, RIG-I triggering was recently shown to mediate apoptosis in melanoma cells via the proapoptotic BH3-only proteins Puma and Noxa. While melanoma cells showed high sensitivity to RIG-I induced apoptosis, both *in vitro* and *in vivo*, normal Bcl-x_L expression rescued nonmalignant cells from RIG-I induced apoptosis (Besch *et al.*, 2009). Thereby 5′-triphosphate RNA has the unique property of exhibiting tumoricidal activity besides being a potent PRR trigger. Moreover, this tumoricidal effect liberates additional antigens for the immune response to react upon, and could modulate the tumor microenvironment from immunosuppressive toward inflammatory. RIG-I triggering could thus very well be employed in a therapeutic vaccination setting against cancer, in an as yet to be uncovered spectrum of therapeutic combinations.

4.5. Recognition of cytosolic DNA by STING-dependent pathways and the AIM2 inflammasome

Recent reports strongly suggest that activation of the STING/MITA and/or AIM2 pathways contributes to the immunogenicity of DNA vaccines (Ishii *et al.*, 2008), DNA viruses, bacteria (Rathinam *et al.*, 2010) and malaria parasites (Sharma *et al.*, 2011). However, so far no adjuvants designed to explicitly target these pathways have been described. While not DNA molecules, the bacterial PAMPs cyclic-di-AMP and cyclic-di-GMP could be contenders for such an adjuvant as they are able to induce potent humoral and cellular immune responses (Ebensen *et al.*, 2011), and have recently been found to activate the STING pathway (Sauer *et al.*, 2011). The importance of cytosolic DNA recognition for vaccine adjuvancy has recently been highlighted by the surprising discovery that genomic DNA released upon alum induced cell death was a critical contributor to its immune function (Marichal *et al.*, 2011).

5. THERAPEUTIC VACCINATION: JUST A SHOT AWAY?

Prophylactic vaccines have caused the disappearance of many childhood diseases and provided control of many infectious illnesses. In certain cases, notably cancer and chronic infections, a therapeutic vaccine is rather required. Thus far, therapeutic vaccination has been largely unsuccessful. This is because most experimental vaccines failed to induce both CD4+ and CD8+ T cell responses of sufficient size and avidity against a broad antigen pool. This relates to the before mentioned predominant use of adjuvants that skew toward T_{h2} oriented immunity and humoral responses, once more emphasizing the need for T_{h1}-skewing adjuvants like the viral origin nucleic acids.

A recent study emphasizes that a therapeutic vaccine can manage to achieve durable and complete remissions of cancer, when it uses a setup aiming for a powerful mixed T cell response. Herein, grade 3 vulvar intraepithelial neoplasias in 47% of the vaccinees regressed completely. The vaccine contained synthetic long overlapping peptides of human papilloma virus type 16 E6- and E7-protein, formulated in the T_{h1} immunity-associated adjuvant Montanide ISA-51 adjuvant (HPV16 SLP vaccine). Clinical outcome highly correlated with the magnitude of the interferon-gamma (IFN-gamma)-associated CD4+ and CD8+ T cell proliferative responses following vaccination (Kenter *et al.*, 2009). The vaccine illustrates, alike the yellow fever 17D vaccine, that a potent and broadly antigen-specific response of both CD4+ and CD8+ T cells is an essential goal in achieving effective immune control of malignancies or chronic infections by vaccination. Importantly, it shows that the recent dimming of interest in immunotherapy by therapeutic vaccination is unjustified.

5.1. Therapeutic cancer immunization

William Coley already demonstrated the potential of therapeutic immunization against cancer in 1891. Inspired by the effective cancer treatments using bacterial preparations that Friedrich Fehleisen published a decade earlier (Fehleisen, 1883), he injected the tumors of patients with inoperable cancer with a specific streptococcal preparation (known as *Coley's toxins*) and observed the tumors regress alongside a florid infection (Coley, 1891). Since then, immunological knowledge has advanced to develop more specific forms of therapeutic antitumor vaccination, which unfortunately are still not superior in efficacy to Coley's toxins. The added difficulty with anticancer vaccination in contrast to antipathogen vaccination, which targets foreign antigens, is to restrain the specificity of the immune activation toward the malignant tissue without allowing uncontrollable immunity toward broadly expressed autoantigens. Also, while in both cancer and chronic infection the vaccine must boost an otherwise ineffective immune response, in the case of tumors there is often additional active suppression of the (local) immune system involved. By these characteristics therapeutic vaccination against cancer is the most challenging.

5.2. Immunosurveillance and immunomodulation

Alike chronic infection, tumorigenesis does not go unnoticed by the immune system. In 1957, Frank Burnet proposed the principle of immune surveillance (Burnet, 1957), which suggests that frequently the immune system clears microscopic subclinical tumors before they grow unimpeded. This is likely for virus-induced tumors (Melief, 2008) since these cancers regularly express viral antigens able to initiate protective immunity, and also for some nonviral tumors displaying native immunogenicity such as melanoma and renal cell cancer. Besides this direct clearance, tumors can also become dormant and kept in an equilibrium state between growth and attack by the adaptive immune system (Koebel *et al.*, 2007; Melief, 2007). This situation may last for decades and seems to be applicable to nonviral chemically induced tumors. It is supported by the finding that immunosuppressed individuals show a significantly higher cancer incidence (MacKie *et al.*, 2003; Vajdic and van Leeuwen, 2009). By this immune control, tumors have developed many ways of evading the immune response, like down regulating antigen processing pathways (Lankat-Buttgereit and Tampé, 2002) or surface MHC expression (Pandha *et al.*, 2007) to minimize the chances for T cell recognition. Additionally, myeloid-derived suppressor cells (Gabrilovich and Nagaraj, 2009) or regulatory T cells (Ménétrier-Caux *et al.*, 2009) can be recruited to actively suppress local antitumor immunity. The efficiency by which a tumor can suppress T cell reactivity is strikingly illustrated by the observation that in vitiligo patients melanocyte antigen-specific T cells progressively destroy melanocytes, while T cells with identical specificities found in melanomas display a deteriorated functional phenotype (Palermo *et al.*, 2005).

Nonetheless, successes booked with passive immunization strategies like adoptive T cell transfer (Dudley *et al.*, 2008) or active immunizations like the HPV-16 SLP vaccine (Kenter *et al.*, 2009), illustrate that a T cell response of sufficient magnitude and broad specificity is able to effectively battle tumors. Moreover, yellow fever 17D and Coley's toxins illustrate that broad stimulation of PRR pathways is highly important for the induction of protective adaptive immunity, prophylactic as well as therapeutic. In pursuit of a potent multilineage-activating vaccine, engaging CD8+ T cell reactivity, vaccinated antigens need to be correctly presented and cross-presented to ensure a strong response able to overrule the ineffective existing one. Recently discovered mechanisms could bring such a vaccine closer to application.

6. TOWARD THE INTEGRATED RESPONSE: CROSS-PRIMING OF CYTOTOXIC T CELL IMMUNITY

Like vaccinating with live attenuated pathogens, the design of CD8+ T cell-targeting vaccines should learn from the natural routes employed to prime cytotoxic T cell responses. This sounds obvious, still our understanding of exploitable cross-priming mechanisms is in its early days.

In practice, the priming of CD8+ T cell immunity toward a tumor or virally infected cell, raises a population of cytotoxic T cells that will undertake the task of selectively destroying the host's own tissues. It is not surprising that a mechanism like this is under tight natural control.

The wish to unleash cross-priming to the benefit of protection requires a twofold strategy: targeting the antigen to the right processing route and correctly activating the right type of DC.

6.1. Negative regulation of cross-presentation by NK cells via DR5

Effective cross-priming of CD8+ T cells results from an intimate interplay between immune cells, involving CD4+ T cells, NK and NKT cells, DCs, and ultimately CD8+ T cells. Recent evidence shows that NK cells can negatively regulate cross-priming in a TRAIL-DR5 receptor-dependent manner (Iyori *et al.*, 2011). Crosslinking of DR5 receptors on DC resulted in a significantly decreased expression of MHC class-I-antigen complexes loaded with exogenous antigen, while presentation of endogenous antigen was largely uninfluenced. Illustrating the maintenance of reactive homeostasis between NK cells and CD8+ T cells in the response against virally infected or malignant cells, this study by Iyori *et al.* showed that blocking the DR5-dependent interaction between NK cells and DCs augmented DC cross-priming capabilities *in vivo*. Systemic blocking of DR5 using monoclonal antibodies during vaccination is, however, undesirable. Particularly in a therapeutic setting, since it deteriorates NK cell-mediated killing of target cells via the TRAIL/FADD pathway (Schneider *et al.*, 1997). Nonetheless it may be fruitful to incorporate anti-DR5 antibodies to enhance DC antigen cross-presentation in the local vaccination context.

6.2. Augmentation of cross-presentation by NKT cells

In contrast to NK cells, NKT cells can augment cross-presentation by DCs. Alternatively to the classical CD40-CD40L based "cognate license" of cross-presentation provided to the DC by CD4+ T cells recognizing their cognate antigen on their surface (Schoenberger *et al.*, 1998), NKT cells can provide the same contact-dependent license following their recognition of bacterial components or synthetic glycolipid antigens in DC surface-expressed CD1d (Semmling *et al.*, 2010). Moreover, in their recent study Semmling *et al.* showed that the cognate licensing of DC by CD4+ T cells and NKT cells can show functional synergism. Hence, to boost cross-presentation of antigens to CD8+ T cells it can be profitable to include CD1d-dependent NKT cell antigens such as α-glycuronosylceramide as adjuvant to the vaccine next to classic PRR ligands, to exploit this synergism. Indeed, Semmling *et al.* showed that subcutaneous vaccination of OVA together with α-glycuronosylceramide and CpG as adjuvants, yielded far superior numbers of activated CD8+ T cells in the vaccine-draining lymph node, as was to be expected from the two adjuvants alone.

6.3. Cross-presentation depends on the DC subset

While CD4+ or CD4− CD8− DC most readily activate CD4+ T cells, the DCs that most potently cross-present are those that express the antigens CD24, CD207 (Langerin), CD103 (alphaE integrin) and in particular CD8alpha. With the latter being the most potent cross-presenting DC. While these subtypes may dominate the cross-presentation market, it is known that under certain tissue or antigen conditions other DC types can also cross-present antigen. For example, T cell responses to antigen encapsulated in poly(D,L-lactate-co-glycolate) acid (PLGA) microvesicles have been shown to depend on cross-presentation by both CD8− DC and macrophages *in vivo* (Schliehe *et al.*, 2011). Interestingly for the cross-presentation of PLGA-encapsulated antigens, CD8alpha+ DCs were actually dispensable. Nonetheless, the latter does not hold true for all encapsulated antigens, since immuno stimulating complex (ISCOM) vaccines, consisting of multimeric viral membrane proteins encaging the antigen of choice (Morein *et al.*, 1984), rather depend on CD8alpha+ instead of CD8alpha− and CD207+ DCs (Duewell *et al.*, 2011). This discrepancy between cross-presentation of particulate antigen by CD8alpha DC likely reflects the differential precursor origin of this DC subset as well as the demands of the local tissue microenvironment. For example, in the thymus these DCs have cross-priming capabilities more readily omitting cognate licensing procedures, than do CD8alpha+ DC found in the spleen (Dresch *et al.*, 2011).

For vaccination purposes, a population of activated vaccine antigen cross-presenting DCs in the local lymph node is crucial to the proper activation of CD8+ T cell immunity. A recent study using an antigen-TLR7-agonist complex vaccine shows that it could potently activate both CD8alpha+ and CD207+ DCs to cross-present the antigen to T cells in the local lymph node. The coordinated recruitment and activation of these cell types depended on both type I interferons and interleukin-12 (Oh *et al.*, 2011), which may further clarify the role of these cytokines in the generation of effective CD8+ T cell immunity.

6.4. Antigen targeting to specific DC subsets

A complexed antigen like the TLR7-agonist coupled vaccine used above can enhance the magnitude of the CD8+ T cell response. Still, a complexed antigen like this depends on active uptake by the DC, and processing through the endosomal route where it will ultimately meet its TLR7 PRR. Active targeting of antigen complexes to specialized uptake receptors can further enhance cross-presentation by DC. CD8alpha+ DCs can potently present antigens derived from necrotic cells, like dying tumor- or virally infected cells, by their expression of the C-type lectin domain family 9A (CLEC9a or DNGR1), a receptor for necrotic debris (Sancho *et al.*, 2009). While predominantly CD8alpha+ DC express CLEC9a at high levels (plasmacytoid DC do so at low levels) targeting of antigen to this receptor does not readily induce cross-presentation. Rather, it yields potent activation of CD4+ T cells even when the antigen is coadministered with an adjuvant like CpG (Lahoud *et al.*, 2011). While this suggests rigidity in CLEC9a function, the receptor actually allows careful manipulation of the resulting T cell response, depending on the adjuvant context. Administration of low levels of antigen bound to CLEC9a-specific monoclonal antibodies without added adjuvants, can induce antigen-specific Foxp3+ CD4+ regulatory T cells (T_{reg}) (Joffre *et al.*, 2010). In the same study, addition of polyIC adjuvant rather resulted in cross-presentation of the antigen and induction of potent T_{h1} immunity, while the use of curdlan adjuvant instead primed T_{h17} cells. A powerful tool in the precise design of vaccines, it also shows the need for educated vaccine-design since antigen/adjuvant context can induce such divergent states of immunity.

Besides targeting CLEC9a, other uptake receptors are also rewarding targets for enhancing antigen endocytosis, like CLEC7a (Dectin-1), DC-SIGN (CD209), DEC205 (CD205) and the mannose receptor-1 (CD206). All these receptors are expressed on CD8alpha DCs, embodying probably one reason why these DCs excel at cross-presentation. A recent study has illustrated the potency of targeting these receptors during vaccination against the before mentioned HIV p24 protein. Complexes of this protein with anti-CD207, -CD205, and -CLEC9a monoclonal antibodies, together with anti-CD40 stimulation, yielded specific T_{h1} and cytotoxic CD8+ T cell immunity against this conserved HIV protein (Idoyaga *et al.*, 2011). Further illustrating the potency of targeting the right DC subtype in the right context, are other studies that have effectively skewed specific immunity toward T_{h1} and CD8+ T cell responses by targeting antigen to the mannose-1 receptor (Singh *et al.*, 2011) or the novel neck-region of DC-SIGN (Tacken *et al.*, 2011).

7. CONCLUSION

By the current knowledge the design of a vaccine that maximally induces T_{h1} and CD8+ T cell immunity to a broad antigen array comes within experimental reach. Apart from empirically injecting live attenuated, inactivated or protein (subunit) vaccines in basic adjuvant, an array of fine-skewing options is now emerging. Broad antigen panels in the form of synthetic long overlapping peptides could be combined with DR5 inhibition and CD1d-restricted NKT antigens to specifically improve cross-priming. Also, antigen targeting to specific uptake receptors like CLEC9a ensures delivery to cross-presenting DC. In addition, a specific adjuvant context can skew the immune outcome during vaccination. Depending on the aim, induction of CD4+ T cell and humoral immunity or a focused CD8+ T cell activation can be "programmed" into the vaccine. Moreover, the design of therapeutic vaccines will greatly benefit from a number of novel nucleic acid adjuvants. Specifically innate immunoreceptors responsible for nucleic acid recognition in the cytoplasm (RIG-I-like helicases) provide the immunological signals required to trigger a cytotoxic T cell response capable to eliminate infected cells or tumor cells. RIG-I like helicases are employed by nature to induce strong CD8+ T cell based immunity against viruses. We should learn from this example, the same way we learned to master smallpox vaccination by mimicking natural infection. Synthetic oligonucleotides are being developed carrying a 5′-triphosphate moiety and stabilizing modifications show high potency and selectivity for RIG-I. Similarly to previous developments of TLR9 stimulating CpG oligonucleotides that have become the strongest humoral vaccine adjuvant, we now have the molecular tools in our hands that may allow us to replace attenuated vaccines with completely synthetic vaccines without cutting back on immunogenicity. Such vaccines hold great promise for improved treatment of chronic viral infections and cancer. Finally, vaccinology may indeed benefit from the molecular principles of immunology that have been uncovered over the last few years.

ACKNOWLEDGMENTS

This work was supported by KFO177, SFB670 and SFB704 of the German Research Council (DFG), and a Biofuture and a Go-Bio grant of the Bundesministerium für Bildung und Forschung (BMBF) to G.H., a DFG Emmy Noether Grant (BA3544 1-1) to W.B., and a Junior Research Group Grant (2011-1-3) from the BONFOR-Forschungskommision to J.G.v.d.B.

REFERENCES

Adams, S., O'Neill, D. W., Nonaka, D., Hardin, E., Chiriboga, L., Siu, K., Cruz, C. M., Angiulli, A., Angiulli, F., Ritter, E., Holman, R. M., Shapiro, R. L., *et al.* (2008). Immunization of malignant melanoma patients with full-length NY-ESO-1 protein using TLR7 agonist imiquimod as vaccine adjuvant. *J. Immunol.* **181,** 776–784.

Adema, G. J., Hartgers, F., Verstraten, R., de Vries, E., Marland, G., Menon, S., Foster, J., Xu, Y., Nooyen, P., McClanahan, T., Bacon, K. B., and Figdor, C. G. (1997). A dendritic-cell-derived C-C chemokine that preferentially attracts naive T cells. *Nature* **387,** 713–717.

Akira, S., Uematsu, S., and Takeuchi, O. (2006). Pathogen recognition and innate immunity. *Cell* **124,** 783–801.

Alexopoulou, L., Holt, A. C., Medzhitov, R., and Flavell, R. A. (2001). Recognition of double-stranded RNA and activation of NF-kappaB by Toll-like receptor 3. *Nature* **413,** 732–738.

Alivisatos, C. N. (1934). The first immunologist, James Pylarino (1659–1718), and the introduction of variolation: (Section of the history of medicine). *Proc. R. Soc. Med.* **27,** 1099.

Barbalat, R., Ewald, S. E., Mouchess, M. L., and Barton, G. M. (2011). Nucleic acid recognition by the innate immune system. *Annu. Rev. Immunol.* **29,** 185–214.

Barba-Spaeth, G., Longman, R. S., Albert, M. L., and Rice, C. M. (2005). Live attenuated yellow fever 17D infects human DCs and allows for presentation of endogenous and recombinant T cell epitopes. *J. Exp. Med.* **202,** 1179–1184.

Barchet, W., Wimmenauer, V., Schlee, M., and Hartmann, G. (2008). Accessing the therapeutic potential of immunostimulatory nucleic acids. *Curr. Opin. Immunol.* **20,** 389–395.

Barrett, A. D. T., and Teuwen, D. E. (2009). Yellow fever vaccine—How does it work and why do rare cases of serious adverse events take place? *Curr. Opin. Immunol.* **21,** 308–313.

Bauer, S., Kirschning, C. J., Häcker, H., Redecke, V., Hausmann, S., Akira, S., Wagner, H., and Lipford, G. B. (2001). Human TLR9 confers responsiveness to bacterial DNA via species-specific CpG motif recognition. *Proc. Natl. Acad. Sci. USA* **98,** 9237–9242.

Besch, R., Poeck, H., Hohenauer, T., Senft, D., Häcker, G., Berking, C., Hornung, V., Endres, S., Ruzicka, T., Rothenfusser, S., and Hartmann, G. (2009). Proapoptotic signaling induced by RIG-I and MDA-5 results in type I interferon–independent apoptosis in human melanoma cells. *J. Clin. Invest.* **119,** 2399–2411.

Black, G. F., Thiel, B. A., Ota, M. O., Parida, S. K., Adegbola, R., Boom, W. H., Dockrell, H. M., Franken, K. L. M. C., Friggen, A. H., Hill, P. C., Klein, M. R., Lalor, M. K., *et al.* (2009). Immunogenicity of novel DosR regulon-encoded candidate antigens of *Mycobacterium tuberculosis* in three high-burden populations in Africa. *Clin. Vaccine Immunol.* **16,** 1203–1212.

Bode, C., Zhao, G., Steinhagen, F., Kinjo, T., and Klinman, D. M. (2011). CpG DNA as a vaccine adjuvant. *Expert Rev. Vaccines* **10,** 499–511.

Bonifaz, L. C., Bonnyay, D. P., Charalambous, A., Darguste, D. I., Fujii, S.-I., Soares, H., Brimnes, M. K., Moltedo, B., Moran, T. M., and Steinman, R. M. (2004). In vivo targeting of antigens to maturing dendritic cells via the DEC-205 receptor improves T cell vaccination. *J. Exp. Med.* **199,** 815–824.

Bos, J. (2005). Cutaneous Immunology and Clinical Immunodermatology. Skin Immune System (SIS) CRC Press, Boca Raton, FL.

Bourquin, C., Wurzenberger, C., Heidegger, S., Fuchs, S., Anz, D., Weigel, S., Sandholzer, N., Winter, G., Coester, C., and Endres, S. (2010). Delivery of immunostimulatory RNA oligonucleotides by gelatin nanoparticles triggers an efficient antitumoral response. *J. Immunother.* **33,** 935–944.

Bunnik, E. M., Euler, Z., Welkers, M. R. A., Boeser-Nunnink, B. D. M., Grijsen, M. L., Prins, J. M., and Schuitemaker, H. (2010). Adaptation of HIV-1 envelope gp120 to humoral immunity at a population level. *Nat. Med.* **16,** 995–997.

Burnet, M. (1957). Cancer: A biological approach. III. Viruses associated with neoplastic conditions. IV. Practical applications. *Br. Med. J.* **1,** 841–847.

Chen, J.-R., Ma, C., and Wong, C.-H. (2011). Vaccine design of hemagglutinin glycoprotein against influenza. *Trends Biotechnol.* **29,** 426–434.

Coffman, R., Sher, A., and Seder, R. (2010). Vaccine adjuvants: Putting innate immunity to work. *Immunity* **33,** 12.

Coley, W. B. (1891). II. Contribution to the Knowledge of Sarcoma. *Ann. Surg.* **14,** 199.

Commandeur, S., Lin, M. Y., van Meijgaarden, K. E., Friggen, A. H., Franken, K. L. M. C., Drijfhout, J. W., Korsvold, G. E., Oftung, F., Geluk, A., and Ottenhoff, T. H. M. (2011a). Double- and monofunctional CD4(+) and CD8(+) T-cell responses to *Mycobacterium tuberculosis* DosR antigens and peptides in long-term latently infected individuals. *Eur. J. Immunol.* **41,** 2925–2936.

Commandeur, S., van Meijgaarden, K. E., Lin, M. Y., Franken, K. L. M. C., Friggen, A. H., Drijfhout, J. W., Oftung, F., Korsvold, G. E., Geluk, A., and Ottenhoff, T. H. M. (2011b). Identification of human T-cell responses to *Mycobacterium tuberculosis* resuscitation-promoting factors in long-term latently infected individuals. *Clin. Vaccine Immunol.* **18,** 676–683.

Cooper, C. L., Davis, H. L., Morris, M. L., Efler, S. M., Adhami, M. A., Krieg, A. M., Cameron, D. W., and Heathcote, J. (2004). CPG 7909, an immunostimulatory TLR9 agonist oligodeoxynucleotide, as adjuvant to Engerix-B HBV vaccine in healthy adults: A double-blind phase I/II study. *J. Clin. Immunol.* **24,** 693–701.

Corbett, E. L., Watt, C. J., Walker, N., Maher, D., Williams, B. G., Raviglione, M. C., and Dye, C. (2003). The growing burden of tuberculosis: Global trends and interactions with the HIV epidemic. *Arch. Intern. Med.* **163,** 1009–1021.

Csomor, E., Bajtay, Z., Sándor, N., Kristóf, K., Arlaud, G. J., Thiel, S., and Erdei, A. (2007). Complement protein C1q induces maturation of human dendritic cells. *Mol. Immunol.* **44,** 3389–3397.

Davis, H., Davis, H., Davis, H., Weeranta, R., Weeranta, R., Weeranta, R., Waldschmidt, T., Waldschmidt, T., Waldschmidt, T., Tygrett, L., Tygrett, L., Tygrett, L., *et al.* (1998). CpG DNA is a potent enhancer of specific immunity in mice immunized with recombinant hepatitis B surface antigen. *J. Immunol.* **160,** 870–876.

Delaloye, J., Roger, T., Steiner-Tardivel, Q.-G., Le Roy, D., Knaup Reymond, M., Akira, S., Pétrilli, V., Gomez, C. E., Perdiguero, B., Tschopp, J., Pantaleo, G., Esteban, M., *et al.* (2009). Innate immune sensing of modified vaccinia virus Ankara (MVA) is mediated by TLR2-TLR6, MDA-5 and the NALP3 inflammasome. *PLoS Pathog.* **5,** e1000480.

Diebold, S. S., Kaisho, T., Hemmi, H., Akira, S., and Reis e Sousa, C. (2004). Innate antiviral responses by means of TLR7-mediated recognition of single-stranded RNA. *Science* **303,** 1529–1531.

Dinges, W. L., Richardt, J., Friedrich, D., Jalbert, E., Liu, Y., Stevens, C. E., Maenza, J., Collier, A. C., Geraghty, D. E., Smith, J., Moodie, Z., Mullins, J. I., *et al.* (2010). Virus-specific CD8+ T-cell responses better define HIV disease progression than HLA genotype. *J. Virol.* **84,** 4461–4468.

Dresch, C., Ackermann, M., Vogt, B., de Andrade Pereira, B., Shortman, K., and Fraefel, C. (2011). Thymic but not splenic CD8(+) DCs can efficiently cross-prime T cells in the absence of licensing factors. *Eur. J. Immunol.* **41,** 2544–2555.

Dudley, M. E., Yang, J. C., Sherry, R., Hughes, M. S., Royal, R., Kammula, U., Robbins, P. F., Huang, J., Citrin, D. E., Leitman, S. F., Wunderlich, J., Restifo, N. P., *et al.* (2008). Adoptive cell therapy for patients with metastatic melanoma: Evaluation of intensive myeloablative chemoradiation preparative regimens. *J. Clin. Oncol.* **26,** 5233–5239.

Duewell, P., Kisser, U., Heckelsmiller, K., Hoves, S., Stoitzner, P., Koernig, S., Morelli, A., Clausen, B., Dauer, M., Eigler, A., Anz, D., Bourquin, C., *et al.* (2011). ISCOMATRIX adjuvant combines immune activation with antigen delivery to dendritic cells in vivo leading to effective cross-priming of CD8+ T cells. *J. Immunol.* **187,** 10.

Ebensen, T., Libanova, R., Schulze, K., Yevsa, T., Morr, M., and Guzmán, C. A. (2011). Bis-(3″,5″)-cyclic dimeric adenosine monophosphate: Strong Th1/Th2/Th17 promoting mucosal adjuvant. *Vaccine* **29,** 5210–5220.

Elahi, S., Dinges, W. L., Lejarcegui, N., Laing, K. J., Collier, A. C., Koelle, D. M., McElrath, M. J., and Horton, H. (2011). Protective HIV-specific CD8+ T cells evade Treg cell suppression. *Nat Med.* **17,** 989–995.

Ellis, R. D., Mullen, G. E. D., Pierce, M., Martin, L. B., Miura, K., Fay, M. P., Long, C. A., Shaffer, D., Saul, A., Miller, L. H., and Durbin, A. P. (2009). A Phase 1 study of the blood-stage malaria vaccine candidate AMA1-C1/Alhydrogel with CPG 7909, using two different formulations and dosing intervals. *Vaccine* **27,** 4104–4109.

El-Malky, M., Shaohong, L., Kumagai, T., Yabu, Y., Noureldin, M. S., Saudy, N., Maruyama, H., and Ohta, N. (2005). Protective effect of vaccination with Toxoplasma lysate antigen and CpG as an adjuvant against Toxoplasma gondii in susceptible C57BL/6 mice. *Microbiol. Immunol.* **49,** 639–646.

Fehleisen, F. (1883). Die Aetiologie des Erysipels. Verlag T. Fischer. Berlin.

Field, A. K., Tytell, A. A., Lampson, G. P., and Hilleman, M. R. (1967). Inducers of interferon and host resistance. II. Multistranded synthetic polynucleotide complexes. *Proc. Natl. Acad. Sci. USA* **58,** 1004–1010.

Gabrilovich, D. I., and Nagaraj, S. (2009). Myeloid-derived suppressor cells as regulators of the immune system. *Nat. Rev. Immunol.* **9,** 162–174.

Gaschen, B., Taylor, J., Yusim, K., Foley, B., Gao, F., Lang, D., Novitsky, V., Haynes, B., Hahn, B. H., Bhattacharya, T., and Korber, B. (2002). Diversity considerations in HIV-1 vaccine selection. *Science* **296,** 2354–2360.

A Gaspari, A., Tyring, S. K., and Rosen, T. (2009). Beyond a decade of 5% imiquimod topical therapy. *J. Drugs Dermatol.* **8,** 467–474.

Gaucher, D., Therrien, R., Kettaf, N., Angermann, B. R., Boucher, G., Filali-Mouhim, A., Moser, J. M., Mehta, R. S., Drake, D. R., Castro, E., Akondy, R., Rinfret, A., *et al.* (2008). Yellow fever vaccine induces integrated multilineage and polyfunctional immune responses. *J. Exp. Med.* **205,** 3119–3131.

Gavin, A. L., Hoebe, K., Duong, B., Ota, T., Martin, C., Beutler, B., and Nemazee, D. (2006). Adjuvant-enhanced antibody responses in the absence of toll-like receptor signaling. *Science* **314,** 1936–1938.

Gitlin, L., Barchet, W., Gilfillan, S., Cella, M., Beutler, B., Flavell, R. A., Diamond, M. S., and Colonna, M. (2006). Essential role of mda-5 in type I IFN responses to polyriboinosinic: polyribocytidylic acid and encephalomyocarditis picornavirus. *Proc. Natl. Acad. Sci. USA* **103,** 8459–8464.

Hamm, S., Heit, A., Koffler, M., Huster, K. M., Akira, S., Busch, D. H., Wagner, H., and Bauer, S. (2007). Immunostimulatory RNA is a potent inducer of antigen-specific cytotoxic and humoral immune response in vivo. *Int. Immunol.* **19,** 297–304.

Hayes, E. B. (2010). Is it time for a new yellow fever vaccine? *Vaccine* **28,** 8073–8076.

Heath, W. R., and Carbone, F. R. (2009). Dendritic cell subsets in primary and secondary T cell responses at body surfaces. *Nat. Immunol.* **10,** 1237–1244.

Heil, F., Hemmi, H., Hochrein, H., Ampenberger, F., Kirschning, C., Akira, S., Lipford, G., Wagner, H., and Bauer, S. (2004). Species-specific recognition of single-stranded RNA via toll-like receptor 7 and 8. *Science* **303,** 1526–1529.

Heit, A., Maurer, T., Hochrein, H., Bauer, S., Huster, K. M., Busch, D. H., and Wagner, H. (2003). Cutting edge: Toll-like receptor 9 expression is not required for CpG DNA-aided cross-presentation of DNA-conjugated antigens but essential for cross-priming of CD8 T cells. *J. Immunol.* **170,** 2802–2805.

Heit, A., Schmitz, F., O'Keeffe, M., Staib, C., Busch, D. H., Wagner, H., and Huster, K. M. (2005). Protective CD8 T cell immunity triggered by CpG-protein conjugates competes with the efficacy of live vaccines. *J. Immunol.* **174,** 4373–4380.

Heit, A., Schmitz, F., Haas, T., Busch, D. H., and Wagner, H. (2007). Antigen co-encapsulated with adjuvants efficiently drive protective T cell immunity. *Eur. J. Immunol.* **37,** 2063–2074.

Hemmi, H., Kaisho, T., Takeuchi, O., Sato, S., Sanjo, H., Hoshino, K., Horiuchi, T., Tomizawa, H., Takeda, K., and Akira, S. (2002). Small anti-viral compounds activate immune cells via the TLR7 MyD88-dependent signaling pathway. *Nat. Immunol.* **3,** 196–200.

Higgins, S. C., and Mills, K. H. G. (2010). TLR, NLR agonists, and other immune modulators as infectious disease vaccine adjuvants. *Curr. Infect. Dis. Rep.* **12,** 4–12.

Hornung, V., Rothenfusser, S., Britsch, S., Krug, A., Jahrsdörfer, B., Giese, T., Endres, S., and Hartmann, G. (2002). Quantitative expression of toll-like receptor 1-10 mRNA in cellular

subsets of human peripheral blood mononuclear cells and sensitivity to CpG oligodeoxynucleotides. *J. Immunol.* **168,** 4531–4537.
Hornung, V., Ellegast, J., Kim, S., Brzózka, K., Jung, A., Kato, H., Poeck, H., Akira, S., Conzelmann, K.-K., Schlee, M., Endres, S., and Hartmann, G. (2006). 5′-Triphosphate RNA is the ligand for RIG-I. *Science* **314,** 994–997.
Hume, D. A. (2008). Macrophages as APC and the dendritic cell myth. *J. Immunol.* **181,** 5829–5835.
Ichinohe, T., Lee, H. K., Ogura, Y., Flavell, R., and Iwasaki, A. (2009). Inflammasome recognition of influenza virus is essential for adaptive immune responses. *J. Exp. Med.* **206,** 79–87.
Idoyaga, J., Lubkin, A., Fiorese, C., Lahoud, M. H., Caminschi, I., Huang, Y., Rodriguez, A., Clausen, B. E., Park, C. G., Trumpfheller, C., and Steinman, R. M. (2011). Comparable T helper 1 (Th1) and CD8 T-cell immunity by targeting HIV gag p24 to CD8 dendritic cells within antibodies to Langerin, DEC205, and Clec9A. *Proc. Natl. Acad. Sci. USA* **108,** 2384–2389.
Ishii, K., Kawagoe, T., Koyama, S., Matsui, K., Kumar, H., Kawai, T., Uematsu, S., Takeuchi, O., Takeshita, F., Coban, C., and Akira, S. (2008). TANK-binding kinase-1 delineates innate and adaptive immune responses to DNA vaccines. *Nature* **451,** 6.
Iwasaki, A., and Medzhitov, R. (2010). Regulation of adaptive immunity by the innate immune system. *Science* **327,** 291–295.
Iyori, M., Zhang, T., Pantel, H., Gagne, B. A., and Sentman, C. L. (2011). TRAIL/DR5 plays a critical role in NK cell-mediated negative regulation of dendritic cell cross-priming of T cells. *J. Immunol.* **187**(6), 3087–3095.
Jasani, B., Navabi, H., and Adams, M. (2009). Ampligen: A potential toll-like 3 receptor adjuvant for immunotherapy of cancer. *Vaccine* **27,** 3401–3404.
Jelinek, I., Leonard, J. N., Price, G. E., Brown, K. N., Meyer-Manlapat, A., Goldsmith, P. K., Wang, Y., Venzon, D., Epstein, S. L., and Segal, D. M. (2011). TLR3-specific double-stranded RNA oligonucleotide adjuvants induce dendritic cell cross-presentation, CTL responses, and antiviral protection. *J. Immunol.* **186,** 2422–2429.
Jenner, E. (1798). An Inquiry Into the Causes and Effects of the Variolae Vacciniae, a Disease Discovered in Some of the Western Counties of England, Particularly Gloucestershire, and Known by the Name of the Cow Pox (London).
Jessie, K., Fong, M. Y., Devi, S., Lam, S. K., and Wong, K. T. (2004). Localization of dengue virus in naturally infected human tissues, by immunohistochemistry and in situ hybridization. *J. Infect. Dis.* **189,** 1411–1418.
Joffre, O. P., Sancho, D., Zelenay, S., Keller, A. M., and Reis e Sousa, C. (2010). Efficient and versatile manipulation of the peripheral CD4+ T-cell compartment by antigen targeting to DNGR-1/CLEC9A. *Eur. J. Immunol.* **40,** 1255–1265.
Jondal, M., Schirmbeck, R., and Reimann, J. (1996). MHC class I-restricted CTL responses to exogenous antigens. *Immunity* **5,** 295–302.
Jung, S., Unutmaz, D., Wong, P., Sano, G.-I., De los Santos, K., Sparwasser, T., Wu, S., Vuthoori, S., Ko, K., Zavala, F., Pamer, E. G., Littman, D. R., *et al.* (2002). In vivo depletion of CD11c+ dendritic cells abrogates priming of CD8+ T cells by exogenous cell-associated antigens. *Immunity* **17,** 211–220.
Kaslow, R. A., Carrington, M., Apple, R., Park, L., Muñoz, A., Saah, A. J., Goedert, J. J., Winkler, C., O'Brien, S. J., Rinaldo, C., Detels, R., Blattner, W., *et al.* (1996). Influence of combinations of human major histocompatibility complex genes on the course of HIV-1 infection. *Nat. Med.* **2,** 405–411.
Kasturi, S. P., Skountzou, I., Albrecht, R. A., Koutsonanos, D., Hua, T., Nakaya, H. I., Ravindran, R., Stewart, S., Alam, M., Kwissa, M., Villinger, F., Murthy, N., *et al.* (2011). Programming the magnitude and persistence of antibody responses with innate immunity. *Nature* **470,** 543–547.

Kato, H., Takeuchi, O., Sato, S., Yoneyama, M., Yamamoto, M., Matsui, K., Uematsu, S., Jung, A., Kawai, T., Ishii, K. J., Yamaguchi, O., Otsu, K., *et al.* (2006). Differential roles of MDA5 and RIG-I helicases in the recognition of RNA viruses. *Nature* **441,** 101–105.

Katsuda, M., Iwahashi, M., Matsuda, K., Miyazawa, M., Nakamori, M., Nakamura, M., Ojima, T., Iida, T., Hayata, K., and Yamaue, H. (2011). Comparison of different classes of CpG-ODN in augmenting the generation of human epitope peptide-specific CTLs. *Int. J. Oncol.* **39,** 1295–1302.

Kaufmann, S. (2008). Elie Metchnikoff's and Paul Ehrlich's impact on infection biology. *Microbes Infect.* **10,** 1417–1419.

Kenter, G. G., Welters, M. J. P., Valentijn, A. R. P. M., Lowik, M. J. G., Berends-van der Meer, D. M. A., Vloon, A. P. G., Essahsah, F., Fathers, L. M., Offringa, R., Drijfhout, J. W., Wafelman, A. R., Oostendorp, J., *et al.* (2009). Vaccination against HPV-16 oncoproteins for vulvar intraepithelial neoplasia. *N. Engl. J. Med.* **361,** 1838–1847.

Klinman, D. M., Xie, H., and Ivins, B. E. (2006). CpG oligonucleotides improve the protective immune response induced by the licensed anthrax vaccine. *Ann. N. Y. Acad. Sci.* **1082,** 137–150.

Koebel, C. M., Vermi, W., Swann, J. B., Zerafa, N., Rodig, S. J., Old, L. J., Smyth, M. J., and Schreiber, R. D. (2007). Adaptive immunity maintains occult cancer in an equilibrium state. *Nature* **450,** 903–907.

Koyama, S., Ishii, K. J., Kumar, H., Tanimoto, T., Coban, C., Uematsu, S., Kawai, T., and Akira, S. (2007). Differential role of TLR- and RLR-signaling in the immune responses to influenza A virus infection and vaccination. *J. Immunol.* **179,** 4711–4720.

Krieg, A. M., Yi, A. K., Matson, S., Waldschmidt, T. J., Bishop, G. A., Teasdale, R., Koretzky, G. A., and Klinman, D. M. (1995). CpG motifs in bacterial DNA trigger direct B-cell activation. *Nature* **374,** 546–549.

Krug, A., Rothenfusser, S., Hornung, V., Jahrsdörfer, B., Blackwell, S., Ballas, Z. K., Endres, S., Krieg, A. M., and Hartmann, G. (2001). Identification of CpG oligonucleotide sequences with high induction of IFN-alpha/beta in plasmacytoid dendritic cells. *Eur. J. Immunol.* **31,** 2154–2163.

Kushwah, R., and Hu, J. (2011). Complexity of dendritic cell subsets and their function in the host immune system. *Immunology* **133,** 409–419, (DC subsets and classification.)

Lahoud, M. H., Ahmet, F., Kitsoulis, S., Wan, S. S., Vremec, D., Lee, C. N., Phipson, B., Shi, W., Smyth, G. K., Lew, A. M., Kato, Y., Mueller, S. N., *et al.* (2011). Targeting antigen to mouse dendritic cells via Clec9A induces potent CD4 T cell responses biased toward a follicular helper phenotype. *J. Immunol.* **187,** 842–850.

Lankat-Buttgereit, B., and Tampé, R. (2002). The transporter associated with antigen processing: Function and implications in human diseases. *Physiol. Rev.* **82,** 187–204.

Le Bon, A., Etchart, N., Rossmann, C., Ashton, M., Hou, S., Gewert, D., Borrow, P., and Tough, D. F. (2003). Cross-priming of CD8+ T cells stimulated by virus-induced type I interferon. *Nat. Immunol.* **4,** 1009–1015.

Le Bon, A., Durand, V., Kamphuis, E., Thompson, C., Bulfone-Paus, S., Rossmann, C., Kalinke, U., and Tough, D. F. (2006). Direct stimulation of T cells by type I IFN enhances the CD8+ T cell response during cross-priming. *J. Immunol.* **176,** 4682–4689.

Lebre, M. C., van der Aar, A. M. G., van Baarsen, L., van Capel, T. M. M., Schuitemaker, J. H. N., Kapsenberg, M. L., and de Jong, E. C. (2007). Human keratinocytes express functional toll-like receptor 3, 4, 5, and 9. *J. Invest. Dermatol.* **127,** 331–341.

Leyten, E. M. S., Lin, M. Y., Franken, K. L. M. C., Friggen, A. H., Prins, C., van Meijgaarden, K. E., Voskuil, M. I., Weldingh, K., Andersen, P., Schoolnik, G. K., Arend, S. M., Ottenhoff, T. H. M., *et al.* (2006). Human T-cell responses to 25 novel antigens encoded by genes of the dormancy regulon of *Mycobacterium tuberculosis*. *Microbes Infect.* **8,** 2052–2060.

Lin, M. Y., and Ottenhoff, T. H. M. (2008). Not to wake a sleeping giant: new insights into host-pathogen interactions identify new targets for vaccination against latent *Mycobacterium tuberculosis* infection. *Biol. Chem.* **389,** 497–511.

Lin, M. Y., Geluk, A., Smith, S. G., Stewart, A. L., Friggen, A. H., Franken, K. L. M. C., Verduyn, M. J. C., van Meijgaarden, K. E., Voskuil, M. I., Dockrell, H. M., Huygen, K., Ottenhoff, T. H. M., *et al.* (2007). Lack of immune responses to *Mycobacterium tuberculosis* DosR regulon proteins following Mycobacterium bovis BCG vaccination. *Infect. Immun.* **75,** 3523–3530.

Lindsey, N. P., Schroeder, B. A., Miller, E. R., Braun, M. M., Hinckley, A. F., Marano, N., Slade, B. A., Barnett, E. D., Brunette, G. W., Horan, K., Staples, J. E., Kozarsky, P. E., *et al.* (2008). Adverse event reports following yellow fever vaccination. *Vaccine* **26,** 6077–6082.

Longhi, M. P., Trumpfheller, C., Idoyaga, J., Caskey, M., Matos, I., Kluger, C., Salazar, A. M., Colonna, M., and Steinman, R. M. (2009). Dendritic cells require a systemic type I interferon response to mature and induce CD4+ Th1 immunity with poly IC as adjuvant. *J. Exp. Med.* **206,** 1589–1602.

Luke, J., Simon, G., Soderholm, J., Errett, J., August, J., Gale, M., Hodgson, C., and Williams, J. (2011). Coexpressed RIG-I agonist enhances humoral immune response to influenza virus DNA vaccine. *J. Virol.* **85,** 14.

MacKie, R. M., Reid, R., and Junor, B. (2003). Fatal melanoma transferred in a donated kidney 16 years after melanoma surgery. *N. Engl. J. Med.* **348,** 567–568.

Malim, M. H., and Emerman, M. (2001). HIV-1 sequence variation: Drift, shift, and attenuation. *Cell* **104,** 469–472.

Mangada, M. M., and Rothman, A. L. (2005). Altered cytokine responses of dengue-specific CD4+ T cells to heterologous serotypes. *J. Immunol.* **175,** 2676–2683.

Marichal, T., Ohata, K., Bedoret, D., Mesnil, C., Sabatel, C., Kobiyama, K., Lekeux, P., Coban, C., Akira, S., Ishii, K., Bureau, F., and Desmet, C. (2011). DNA released from dying host cells mediates aluminum adjuvant activity. *Nat. Med.* **17**(8), 996–1002.

Martinon, F., Burns, K., and Tschopp, J. (2002). The inflammasome: A molecular platform triggering activation of inflammatory caspases and processing of proIL-beta. *Mol. Cell* **10,** 417–426.

McMichael, A. J., and Rowland-Jones, S. L. (2001). Cellular immune responses to HIV. *Nature* **410,** 980–987.

Medzhitov, R. (2007). Recognition of microorganisms and activation of the immune response. *Nature* **449,** 819–826.

Melief, C. J. M. (2007). Cancer: Immune pact with the enemy. *Nature* **450,** 803–804.

Melief, C. J. M. (2008). Cancer immunotherapy by dendritic cells. *Immunity* **29,** 372–383.

Ménétrier-Caux, C., Gobert, M., and Caux, C. (2009). Differences in tumor regulatory T-cell localization and activation status impact patient outcome. *Cancer Res.* **69,** 7895–7898.

Miller, J. D., van der Most, R. G., Akondy, R. S., Glidewell, J. T., Albott, S., Masopust, D., Murali-Krishna, K., Mahar, P. L., Edupuganti, S., Lalor, S., Germon, S., Del Rio, C., *et al.* (2008). Human effector and memory CD8+ T cell responses to smallpox and yellow fever vaccines. *Immunity* **28,** 710–722.

Moldoveanu, Z., Love-Homan, L., Huang, W. Q., and Krieg, A. M. (1998). CpG DNA, a novel immune enhancer for systemic and mucosal immunization with influenza virus. *Vaccine* **16,** 1216–1224.

Monath, T. P. (2010). Suspected yellow fever vaccine-associated viscerotropic adverse events (1973 and 1978), United States. *Am. J. Trop. Med. Hyg.* **82,** 919–921.

Monath, T. P., Nichols, R., Archambault, W. T., Moore, L., Marchesani, R., Tian, J., Shope, R. E., Thomas, N., Schrader, R., Furby, D., and Bedford, P. (2002). Comparative safety and immunogenicity of two yellow fever 17D vaccines (ARILVAX and YF-VAX) in a phase III multicenter, double-blind clinical trial. *Am. J. Trop. Med. Hyg.* **66,** 533–541.

Monath, T. P., Lee, C. K., Julander, J. G., Brown, A., Beasley, D. W., Watts, D. M., Hayman, E., Guertin, P., Makowiecki, J., Crowell, J., Levesque, P., Bowick, G. C., *et al.* (2010). Inactivated yellow fever 17D vaccine: Development and nonclinical safety, immunogenicity and protective activity. *Vaccine* **28,** 3827–3840.

Monath, T. P., Fowler, E., Johnson, C. T., Balser, J., Morin, M. J., Sisti, M., and Trent, D. W. (2011). An inactivated cell-culture vaccine against yellow fever. *N. Engl. J. Med.* **364,** 1326–1333.

Mongkolsapaya, J., Dejnirattisai, W., Xu, X.-N., Vasanawathana, S., Tangthawornchaikul, N., Chairunsri, A., Sawasdivorn, S., Duangchinda, T., Dong, T., Rowland-Jones, S., Yenchitsomanus, P.-T., McMichael, A., *et al.* (2003). Original antigenic sin and apoptosis in the pathogenesis of dengue hemorrhagic fever. *Nat. Med.* **9,** 921–927.

Morein, B., Sundquist, B., Höglund, S., Dalsgaard, K., and Osterhaus, A. (1984). Iscom, a novel structure for antigenic presentation of membrane proteins from enveloped viruses. *Nature* **308,** 457–460.

Napolitani, G., Rinaldi, A., Bertoni, F., Sallusto, F., and Lanzavecchia, A. (2005). Selected toll-like receptor agonist combinations synergistically trigger a T helper type 1-polarizing program in dendritic cells. *Nat. Immunol.* **6,** 769–776.

Nikolich-Zugich, J., Slifka, M. K., and Messaoudi, I. (2004). The many important facets of T-cell repertoire diversity. *Nat. Rev. Immunol.* **4,** 123–132.

Oh, J. Z., Kurche, J. S., Burchill, M. A., and Kedl, R. M. (2011). TLR7 enables cross-presentation by multiple dendritic cell subsets through a type I IFN-dependent pathway. *Blood* **118,** 3028–3038.

Okada, H., Kalinski, P., Ueda, R., Hoji, A., Kohanbash, G., Donegan, T. E., Mintz, A. H., Engh, J. A., Bartlett, D. L., Brown, C. K., Zeh, H., Holtzman, M. P., *et al.* (2011). Induction of CD8+ T-cell responses against novel glioma-associated antigen peptides and clinical activity by vaccinations with type 1 polarized dendritic cells and polyinosinic-polycytidylic acid stabilized by lysine and carboxymethylcellulose in patients with recurrent malignant glioma. *J. Clin. Oncol.* **29,** 330–336.

Okwor, I., Liu, D., and Uzonna, J. (2009). Qualitative differences in the early immune response to live and killed Leishmania major: Implications for vaccination strategies against Leishmaniasis. *Vaccine* **27,** 2554–2562.

Okwor, I., Kuriakose, S., and Uzonna, J. (2010). Repeated inoculation of killed Leishmania major induces durable immune response that protects mice against virulent challenge. *Vaccine* **28,** 5451–5457.

Palermo, B., Garbelli, S., Mantovani, S., Scoccia, E., Da Prada, G. A., Bernabei, P., Avanzini, M. A., Brazzelli, V., Borroni, G., and Giachino, C. (2005). Qualitative difference between the cytotoxic T lymphocyte responses to melanocyte antigens in melanoma and vitiligo. *Eur. J. Immunol.* **35,** 3153–3162.

Pandha, H., Rigg, A., John, J., and Lemoine, N. (2007). Loss of expression of antigen-presenting molecules in human pancreatic cancer and pancreatic cancer cell lines. *Clin. Exp. Immunol.* **148,** 127–135.

Pasteur, L., Chamberland, L., and Roux, L. (2002). Summary report of the experiments conducted at Pouilly-le-Fort, near Melun, on the anthrax vaccination, 1881. *Yale J. Biol. Med.* **75,** 59–62.

Paveley, R. A., Aynsley, S. A., Cook, P. C., Turner, J. D., and Mountford, A. P. (2009). Fluorescent imaging of antigen released by a skin-invading helminth reveals differential uptake and activation profiles by antigen presenting cells. *PLoS Negl. Trop. Dis.* **3,** e528.

Perrigoue, J. G., Saenz, S. A., Siracusa, M. C., Allenspach, E. J., Taylor, B. C., Giacomin, P. R., Nair, M. G., Du, Y., Zaph, C., van Rooijen, N., Comeau, M. R., Pearce, E. J., *et al.* (2009). MHC class II-dependent basophil-CD4+ T cell interactions promote T(H)2 cytokine-dependent immunity. *Nat. Immunol.* **10,** 697–705.

Pichlmair, A., Schulz, O., Tan, C. P., Näslund, T. I., Liljeström, P., Weber, F., and Reis e Sousa, C. (2006). RIG-I-mediated antiviral responses to single-stranded RNA bearing 5′-phosphates. *Science* **314,** 997–1001.

Plotkin, S. L., and Plotkin, S. A. (2008). A short history of vaccination. *In* "Vaccines", (S. Plotkin, , W. A. Orenstein, and P. A. Offit, eds.), pp. 1–16. Elsevier-Saunders, Philadelphia, PA.

Querec, T., Bennouna, S., Alkan, S., Laouar, Y., Gorden, K., Flavell, R., Akira, S., Ahmed, R., and Pulendran, B. (2006). Yellow fever vaccine YF-17D activates multiple dendritic cell subsets via TLR2, 7, 8, and 9 to stimulate polyvalent immunity. *J. Exp. Med.* **203,** 413–424.

Querec, T. D., Akondy, R. S., Lee, E. K., Cao, W., Nakaya, H. I., Teuwen, D., Pirani, A., Gernert, K., Deng, J., Marzolf, B., Kennedy, K., Wu, H., *et al.* (2009). Systems biology approach predicts immunogenicity of the yellow fever vaccine in humans. *Nat. Immunol.* **10,** 116–125.

Rathinam, V. A. K., Jiang, Z., Waggoner, S. N., Sharma, S., Cole, L. E., Waggoner, L., Vanaja, S. K., Monks, B. G., Ganesan, S., Latz, E., Hornung, V., Vogel, S. N., *et al.* (2010). The AIM2 inflammasome is essential for host defense against cytosolic bacteria and DNA viruses. *Nat. Immunol.* **11,** 395–402.

Rhee, E. G., Blattman, J. N., Kasturi, S. P., Kelley, R. P., Kaufman, D. R., Lynch, D. M., La Porte, A., Simmons, N. L., Clark, S. L., Pulendran, B., Greenberg, P. D., and Barouch, D. H. (2010). Multiple innate immune pathways contribute to the immunogenicity of recombinant adenovirus vaccine vectors. *J. Virol.* **85,** 315–323.

Rothman, A. L. (2011). Immunity to dengue virus: A tale of original antigenic sin and tropical cytokine storms. *Nat. Rev. Immunol.* **11,** 532–543.

Russo, C., Cornella-Taracido, I., Galli-Stampino, L., Jain, R., Harrington, E., Isome, Y., Tavarini, S., Sammicheli, C., Nuti, S., Mbow, M. L., Valiante, N. M., Tallarico, J., *et al.* (2011). Small molecule Toll-like receptor 7 agonists localize to the MHC class II loading compartment of human plasmacytoid dendritic cells. *Blood* **117,** 5683–5691.

Saiga, H., Shimada, Y., and Takeda, K. (2011). Innate immune effectors in mycobacterial infection. *Clin. Dev. Immunol.* **2011,** 347594.

Sancho, D., Joffre, O. P., Keller, A. M., Rogers, N. C., Martínez, D., Hernanz-Falcón, P., Rosewell, I., and Sousa, C. R. E. (2009). Identification of a dendritic cell receptor that couples sensing of necrosis to immunity. *Nature* **458,** 899–903.

Sauer, J.-D., Sotelo-Troha, K., Moltke von, J., Monroe, K. M., Rae, C. S., Brubaker, S. W., Hyodo, M., Hayakawa, Y., Woodward, J. J., Portnoy, D. A., and Vance, R. E. (2011). The *N*-ethyl-*N*-nitrosourea-induced Goldenticket mouse mutant reveals an essential function of Sting in the in vivo interferon response to Listeria monocytogenes and cyclic dinucleotides. *Infect. Immun.* **79,** 688–694.

Schlee, M., Roth, A., Hornung, V., Hagmann, C. A., Wimmenauer, V., Barchet, W., Coch, C., Janke, M., Mihailovic, A., Wardle, G., Juranek, S., Kato, H., *et al.* (2009). Recognition of 5′ triphosphate by RIG-I helicase requires short blunt double-stranded RNA as contained in panhandle of negative-strand virus. *Immunity* **31,** 25–34.

Schliehe, C., Redaelli, C., Engelhardt, S., Fehlings, M., Mueller, M., van Rooijen, N., Thiry, M., Hildner, K., Weller, H., and Groettrup, M. (2011). CD8-dendritic cells and macrophages cross-present poly(D,L-lactate-co-glycolate) acid microsphere-encapsulated antigen in vivo. *J. Immunol.* **187,** 2112–2121.

Schneider, P., Thome, M., Burns, K., Bodmer, J.-L., Hofmann, K., Kataoka, T., Holler, N., and Tschopp, J. (1997). TRAIL receptors 1 (DR4) and 2 (DR5) signal FADD-dependent apoptosis and activate NF-κB. *Immunity* **7,** 831–836.

Schoenberger, S. P., Toes, R. E., van der Voort, E. I., Offringa, R., and Melief, C. J. (1998). T-cell help for cytotoxic T lymphocytes is mediated by CD40-CD40L interactions. *Nature* **393,** 480–483.

Schuck, S. D., Mueller, H., Kunitz, F., Neher, A., Hoffmann, H., Franken, K. L. C. M., Repsilber, D., Ottenhoff, T. H. M., Kaufmann, S. H. E., and Jacobsen, M. (2009). Identification of T-cell antigens specific for latent *Mycobacterium tuberculosis* infection. *PLoS One* **4,** e5590.
Semmling, V., Lukacs-Kornek, V., Thaiss, C. A., Quast, T., Hochheiser, K., Panzer, U., Rossjohn, J., Perlmutter, P., Cao, J., Godfrey, D. I., Savage, P. B., Knolle, P. A., *et al.* (2010). Alternative cross-priming through CCL17-CCR4-mediated attraction of CTLs toward NKT cell-licensed DCs. *Nat. Immunol.* **11,** 313–320U57.
Semple, J. W., Italiano, J. E., and Freedman, J. (2011). Platelets and the immune continuum. *Nat. Rev. Immunol.* **11,** 264–274.
Sharma, S., Deoliveira, R. B., Kalantari, P., Parroche, P., Goutagny, N., Jiang, Z., Chan, J., Bartholomeu, D. C., Lauw, F., Hall, J. P., Barber, G. N., Gazzinelli, R. T., *et al.* (2011). Innate immune recognition of an AT-rich stem-loop DNA motif in the plasmodium falciparum genome. *Immunity* **35,** 194–207.
Shirota, H., and Klinman, D. M. (2011). CpG-conjugated apoptotic tumor cells elicit potent tumor-specific immunity. *Cancer Immunol. Immunother.* **60,** 659–669.
Shukla, N., Lewis, T., Day, T., Mutz, C., Ukani, R., Hamilton, C., Balakrishna, R., and David, S. (2011). Toward self-adjuvanting subunit vaccines: Model peptide and protein antigens incorporating covalently bound toll-like receptor-7 agonistic imidazoquinolines. *Bioorg. Med. Chem. Lett.* **5,** 3232–3236.
Singh, S. K., Streng-Ouwehand, I., Litjens, M., Kalay, H., Burgdorf, S., Saeland, E., Kurts, C., Unger, W. W., and van Kooyk, Y. (2011). Design of neo-glycoconjugates that target the mannose receptor and enhance TLR-independent cross-presentation and Th1 polarization. *Eur. J. Immunol.* **41,** 916–925.
Sirard, J.-C., Vignal, C., Dessein, R., and Chamaillard, M. (2007). Nod-like receptors: Cytosolic watchdogs for immunity against pathogens. *PLoS Pathog.* **3,** e152.
Smirnov, D., Schmidt, J. J., Capecchi, J. T., and Wightman, P. D. (2011). Vaccine adjuvant activity of 3M-052: An imidazoquinoline designed for local activity without systemic cytokine induction. *Vaccine* **29,** 5434–5442.
Sokol, C. L., Chu, N.-Q., Yu, S., Nish, S. A., Laufer, T. M., and Medzhitov, R. (2009). Basophils function as antigen-presenting cells for an allergen-induced T helper type 2 response. *Nat. Immunol.* **10,** 713–720.
Steinman, R. M., and Banchereau, J. (2007). Taking dendritic cells into medicine. *Nature* **449,** 419–426.
Steinman, R. M., and Cohn, Z. A. (1973). Identification of a novel cell type in peripheral lymphoid organs of mice. I. Morphology, quantitation, tissue distribution. *J. Exp. Med.* **137,** 1142–1162.
Steinman, R. M., Gutchinov, B., Witmer, M. D., and Nussenzweig, M. C. (1983). Dendritic cells are the principal stimulators of the primary mixed leukocyte reaction in mice. *J. Exp. Med.* **157,** 613–627.
Tacken, P. J., Ginter, W., Berod, L., Cruz, L. J., Joosten, B., Sparwasser, T., Figdor, C. G., and Cambi, A. (2011). Targeting DC-SIGN via its neck region leads to prolonged antigen residence in early endosomes, delayed lysosomal degradation and cross-presentation. *Blood* **118,** 4111–4119.
Takeda, K., Kaisho, T., and Akira, S. (2003). Toll-like receptors. *Annu. Rev. Immunol.* **21,** 335–376.
Tewari, K., Flynn, B. J., Boscardin, S. B., Kastenmueller, K., Salazar, A. M., Anderson, C. A., Soundarapandian, V., Ahumada, A., Keler, T., Hoffman, S. L., Nussenzweig, M. C., Steinman, R. M., *et al.* (2010). Poly(I:C) is an effective adjuvant for antibody and multi-functional CD4+ T cell responses to Plasmodium falciparum circumsporozoite protein (CSP) and αDEC-CSP in non human primates. *Vaccine* **28,** 7256–7266.
Trumpfheller, C., Caskey, M., Nchinda, G., Longhi, M. P., Mizenina, O., Huang, Y., Schlesinger, S., Colonna, M., and Steinman, R. M. (2008). The microbial mimic poly IC

induces durable and protective CD4+ T cell immunity together with a dendritic cell targeted vaccine. *Proc. Natl. Acad. Sci. USA* **105,** 6.

Vajdic, C. M., and van Leeuwen, M. T. (2009). Cancer incidence and risk factors after solid organ transplantation. *Int. J. Cancer* **125,** 1747–1754.

Wang, Y., Cella, M., Gilfillan, S., and Colonna, M. (2010). Cutting edge: Polyinosinic:polycytidylic acid boosts the generation of memory CD8 T cells through melanoma differentiation-associated protein 5 expressed in stromal cells. *J. Immunol.* **184,** 2751–2755.

Westwood, A., Elvin, S. J., Healey, G. D., Williamson, E. D., and Eyles, J. E. (2006). Immunological responses after immunisation of mice with microparticles containing antigen and single stranded RNA (polyuridylic acid). *Vaccine* **24,** 1736–1743.

Wille-Reece, U., Wu, C.-Y., Flynn, B. J., Kedl, R. M., and Seder, R. A. (2005). Immunization with HIV-1 Gag protein conjugated to a TLR7/8 agonist results in the generation of HIV-1 Gag-specific Th1 and CD8+ T cell responses. *J. Immunol.* **174,** 7676–7683.

Yoshimoto, T., Yasuda, K., Tanaka, H., Nakahira, M., Imai, Y., Fujimori, Y., and Nakanishi, K. (2009). Basophils contribute to T(H)2-IgE responses in vivo via IL-4 production and presentation of peptide-MHC class II complexes to CD4+ T cells. *Nat. Immunol.* **10,** 706–712.

Zhang, X., He, P., Hu, Z., Wang, X., and Liang, Z. (2011). Enhanced specific immune responses by CpG DNA in mice immunized with recombinant hepatitis B surface antigen and HB vaccine. *Virol. J.* **8,** 78.

CHAPTER 2

Structure-Based Design for High-Hanging Vaccine Fruits

Jaap W. Back* and **Johannes P.M. Langedijk**[†,1]

Contents

Abstract

Although vaccines have proven life saving against a myriad of infectious diseases, various pathogens have remained refractory to prophylaxis of their host by active immunization. New insights in the three dimensional (3D) structure, domain organization and dynamics of viral and bacterial surface proteins can guide the design of effective vaccines in several ways. In this review we highlight recent developments in structure-based vaccine design that are aimed at stabilization of native conformations and focusing immune response to conserved epitopes. Detailed 3D structures of pathogen surface proteins provide knowledge on how to minimize complex antigens or how to redesign the surface of an immunogen in order to induce only relevant neutralizing antibodies against a broad range of serotypes. Structure – based vaccines with reduced complexity and broad efficacy could greatly enhance the number of people that might benefit from the therapies that are developed.

* Pepscan Therapeutics, Lelystad, The Netherlands
† Crucell, Innovation and Discovery Laboratory, Leiden, The Netherlands
1 Corresponding author. E-mail address: hans.langedijk@crucell.com

Advances in Immunology, Volume 114
ISSN 0065-2776, DOI: 10.1016/B978-0-12-396548-6.00002-0

Vaccines are by far the most successful life-saving medical developments in modern times. Very successful vaccines have been developed with little knowledge of either the pathogen or the human immune system. Due to better understanding of the complex biology of viruses, bacteria, and the immune system and because of technological advances in biotechnology, vaccines are now available against a large assortment of microorganisms. Yet despite our advanced knowledge, no vaccine is available to protect against notorious infectious life-threatening diseases like AIDS, TBC, and malaria. Decades of research have not delivered a vaccine against respiratory syncytial virus (RSV), which is a major cause of pneumonia and bronchiolitis in infants and the elderly. The low-hanging fruit of the easy targets has been picked and this early success strengthened the hope and belief that infectious diseases would be held in check and could be eradicated given enough effort. Eradication has only been achieved for smallpox and is being pursued for other viruses like polio. However, this early optimism has disappeared. Even infectious diseases that are kept in check with effective vaccines still pose a threat because continuous evolution of microbial reservoirs can cause a return of the disease because of mismatch with the vaccine. Such recurrent update of the vaccine strain is common practice for influenza virus which is continuously sampled around the globe in order to select the matching vaccine for next year's epidemic.

The problem of considerable antigenic variation of viruses that are controlled by efficacious vaccines is costly, but manageable. For other viruses, like HIV and HCV, the antigenic diversity is so high that it will be a major challenge to develop a vaccine that can protect in a heterologous challenge and will be effective against all circulating variants. Novel approaches are needed to combat these resilient pathogens and reach the high-hanging fruit.

To tackle these problems, a thorough understanding of the host defense is needed, and new tools such as structural biology, system biology, development of vectors, novel adjuvants, and prime–boost vaccination strategies will be needed.

The growing insights into the structural details of viral surface proteins have opened the way to use this knowledge for structure-based design of antigens that can be used for a highly directed immune response against hitherto intractable targets.

1. TARGETS FOR STRUCTURAL VACCINOLOGY

Most examples of structural vaccinology in this review will deal with HIV-1 because it is one of the best-studied pathogens. Although the antigenic variability problem is huge, structural details of HIV envelope proteins are emerging, and many different approaches including cutting edge rational design approaches have been used. Although this has not yet yielded an effective vaccine, capable of containing the HIV epidemic, impressive progress has been booked and the spin-off of this research has spurred other vaccine discovery efforts.

The spike on the HIV surface is composed of a trimer of heterodimers of glycoproteins gp120 and gp41. The precursor gp160 is cleaved into a gp120 region that is the head of the spike and contains the CD4 receptor binding site and the large hypervariable loops, and a gp41 region that is the membrane-anchored stem of the spike and like other class I fusogenic proteins contains an N-terminal fusion peptide (FP) and a C-terminal transmembrane helical membrane anchor. Like other class I fusion proteins, fusion occurs in a multistep process. In the case of HIV-1, binding of gp120 to the receptor induces a conformational change that exposes the coreceptor binding site. After coreceptor binding, a subsequent conformational change results in detachment of the gp120 head region from the gp41 stem which subsequently goes through a dramatic conformational change which results in the liberation of the occluded FP that swings out and inserts in the target membrane. After the viral membrane and target membrane are bridged in this way, the three C-terminal heptad repeat 2 (HR2) regions of gp41 coil through antiparallel packing onto the N-terminal HR1 helical trimer forming a six-helix bundle (6HB). 6HB formation is the final stable conformation of gp41, and at that stage, fusion has occurred because in the 6HB the transmembrane region, originally anchored in the viral membrane, is next to the FP anchored in the fused target membrane (Chan *et al.*, 1997; Wyatt and Sodroski, 1998).

To understand this difficult target, impressive advances have been made to resolve the unique three-dimensional (3D) structure of the surface proteins which are different from any known structure (Kwong *et al.*, 1998, 2002). The gp120 structure consists of a highly glycosylated, double β-barrel outer domain, an inner domain, and a four-strand "bridging sheet" composed of two strands from the inner domain and two strands from the outer domain (Kwong *et al.*, 1998). These studies show that the tips of the first three variable loops (V1–V3) and the conserved, highly discontinuous CD4 binding site (CD4bs) are the only significantly exposed protein surfaces on the native trimer (Fig. 2.1). CD4 binds in a depression between the inner and outer domain and the bridging sheet, which is thought to be stabilized after binding of CD4 (Kwong *et al.*, 1998; Wyatt and Sodroski, 1998; Wyatt *et al.*, 1995). The structural studies showed that apart from the variation and glycosylation problem, also the relatively labile and dynamic structures poses problem for antigen stability and may preclude presentation of a genuine mimic to the immune system in order to induce antibodies that will cross-react with the native trimer (Kwong *et al.*, 2002; Wei *et al.*, 2003).

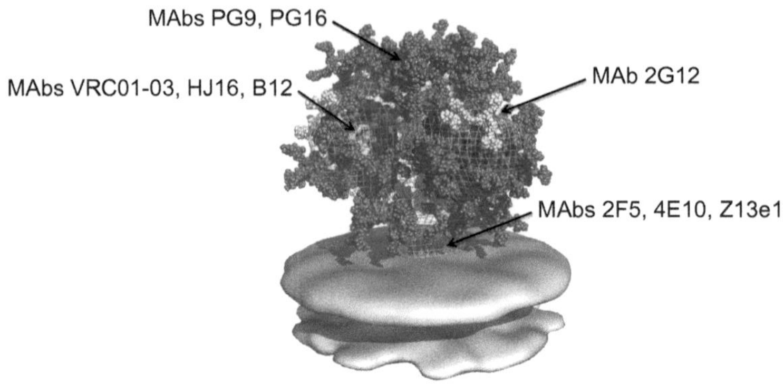

FIGURE 2.1 Fully glycosylated model of HIV trimeric spike from Schief *et al.* (2009). HIV gp160 trimer shown as a transparent mesh representing the density based on cryo-electron tomography (Liu *et al.*, 2008). The mesh is filled with the available higher resolution structure of gp120 (Zhou *et al.*, 2007). Modeled carbohydrates are shown as blue spheres, and the glycans implicated in Mab 2G12 binding are highlighted in white. Binding site for broadly neutralizing antibodies against the CD4 binding site (yellow), against the gp41 MPER, and against the complex quaternary epitopes are indicated. (See Color Insert.)

Many HIV vaccine studies have been described, but very low titers of neutralizing antibodies were induced against the homologous virus and no neutralization was observed against heterologous viruses (Barouch, 2008; Karlsson Hedestam *et al.*, 2008; Wei *et al.*, 2003). In contrast, some individuals who are chronically infected with HIV can mount a broadly neutralizing immune response. Several monoclonal antibodies obtained from such individuals can neutralize a diverse set of HIV-1 strains and some even neutralize across clades. Research on the binding sites of these broadly neutralizing antibodies has shown several interesting conserved epitopes that should ideally be the basic target for efficacious vaccines that can induce broad neutralization. Several regions on the spike have been indicated as the binding site of broadly neutralizing antibodies (Fig. 2.1). An important neutralization site is located at the base of the gp41 stem of the viral spike in the membrane proximal extracellular region (MPER).

This structurally dynamic region becomes exposed during the fusion process and is the target site for several broadly neutralizing antibodies that inhibit the fusion process (Brunel *et al.*, 2006; Frey *et al.*, 2008; Muster *et al.*, 1993; Ofek *et al.*, 2004; Pejchal *et al.*, 2009; Stiegler *et al.*, 2001). Another class of neutralizing antibodies binds conserved sites that are not present on the native prefusion spike but are exposed transiently on an intermediate conformation of the viral spike during the fusion process.

These epitopes are exposed after gp120 binding to CD4 and are therefore called "CD4-induced," and another neutralization site is exposed on the HR1 trimer of gp41 after the FP has been released and before refolding into the final 6HB (Corti *et al.*, 2010; Luftig *et al.*, 2006). Another important target for neutralizing antibodies that block virus attachment is the highly discontinuous and conserved CD4 binding site in gp120. Interestingly, this region is targeted not only by both relatively weak and narrow neutralizing antibodies but also by several very potent and broad antibodies like VRC01 (Wu *et al.*, 2010; Zhou *et al.*, 2010). Also, the exposed hypervariable regions are targets for neutralizing antibodies, and some unique antibodies have been described against the third variable region (V3) that neutralize many different strains with high potency despite the variable nature of the loop (Conley *et al.*, 1994; Corti *et al.*, 2010; Gorny *et al.*, 2002). However, an additional problem for the V3 regions is that on top of the variability, epitopes on its tip can also be masked in such a way that even a pan-V3 binding antibody can no longer bind.

Recently, the term of broad neutralization needed redefinition because a set of much broader neutralizing antibodies were discovered that bind to epitopes that have not yet been fully characterized. Several of these antibodies bind discontinuous epitopes that depend on the correct quaternary assembly of the membrane-bound native trimeric spike (Walker *et al.*, 2009). Binding of these antibodies shows a strong carbohydrate dependency. The interaction of some of these antibodies can be competed by the neutralizing high-mannose-specific 2G12 antibody (Scanlan *et al.*, 2002) and with antibodies either directed against V3 or the CD4 binding site (Walker *et al.*, 2011). It has not yet been clarified whether the carbohydrate contributes to binding or whether it is responsible for maintaining the correct structure of the epitope.

2. STABILIZING ANTIGENS

The detailed structural knowledge on many neutralization sites, the location of some conserved exposed surfaces on the native viral spike, and the general architecture and dynamics of the labile structure reveals some clues of how to stabilize the spike in order to induce such broadly neutralizing antibodies.

One way of using the structural knowledge for a recombinant protein-based vaccine is to engineer, modify, or stabilize the labile spike in such a way that the recombinant soluble protein mimics the prefusion native trimer that can cross-react with all the broadly neutralizing antibodies and remains stable in a vaccine adjuvant. Several approaches have been applied successfully to stabilize the spike.

In case the immunogen is based on the soluble envelope protein, the deletion of the membrane anchor destabilizes the trimer which can be compensated by inclusion of heterologous trimerization domains (Yang *et al.*, 2000). Additionally, the prefusion conformation can be stabilized by preventing the FP from swinging out and the gp120 head to detach. A straightforward solution to fix the FP in its prefusion position and obstruct the refolding of gp41 into the stable postfusion conformation is to prevent the cleavage of the precursor gp160 into mature gp120–gp41 heterodimer (Yang *et al.*, 2000). Alternatively, to increase the chance of maintaining the FP in its native, probably buried, position, gp120 and gp41 can be covalently linked by the introduction of an intermolecular disulfide bridge (Binley *et al.*, 2000; Yang *et al.*, 2000). Although it has been possible to engineer a disulfide with trial and error, high-resolution detail of the structure would permit rational introduction of stabilizing disulfide bonds that connect the heterodimer. Disulfide bridges have also been used for the intramolecular stabilization of the flexible regions within the subunits (Dey *et al.*, 2009; Zhou *et al.*, 2007). Constructing a heat-stable foot-and-mouth disease vaccine by disulfide engineering came within reach when the crystal structure of the viral capsid was solved (Mateo *et al.*, 2008) and also the atomic-level resolution of the complete prefusion spike of HIV will undoubtedly contribute to structure-based design of inter- and intramolecular disulfides without going through the arduous path of trial and error.

3. ENGINEERING IMMUNOGENICITY AND IMMUNODOMINANCE

Because many viral surface proteins are heavily glycosylated, epitopes are masked by relatively immunosilent and variable sugars. Deglycosylation can therefore be a strategy to expose the viral surface and increase access of antibodies to otherwise buried sites that are difficult to reach (Li *et al.*, 2008). In contrast, in order to focus the immune response to the Achilles heel of the protein surface, for example, the conserved CD4 binding site, it is has also been tried to introduce extra glycosylation sites in a structure-guided way to cover sites that attract nonbroadly neutralizing antibodies that may dominate the immune response (Pantophlet *et al.*, 2003). However, the recent discovery of very potent and broad antibodies that depend on glycosylation for binding renders this approach questionable and implies that the protein surface and glycosylation sites should preferably be kept as native as possible (Walker *et al.*, 2009, 2011). Alternatively, the immune response may be focused on the conserved CD4 binding site and diverted from the immunodominant variable regions by resurfacing of gp120. In a resurfaced gp120, all variable residues were mutated that were not part of the CD4 binding region and not masked by carbohydrates. These residues were mutated to SIV homologues or other non-HIV-1 residues and the resulting recombinant protein that also lacked the large variable loops was used to isolate potent broadly neutralizing antibodies against the CD4 binding site (Wu *et al.*, 2010). Using a prime–boost strategy with several different resurfaced gp120 that only share the conserved CD4 binding site could perhaps elicit broadly neutralizing antibodies.

Instead of concealing antigenic regions, resurfacing of protein can also be used to increase the amount of essential antigenic information. Scarselli *et al.* (2011) have merged the antigenic determinants that convey protective immunity against group B *meningococci* into one fusion protein. The authors used a clever divide-and-conquer strategy to reduce the high sequence variance of the highly variable complement factor H binding protein (fHBP), that protects this bacterium against host complement-mediated elimination, into a single variant immunogen that elicits broadly protective antibodies. First, the variants were binned into three classes covering most sequence variation. Prototypes of these variants yielded antibodies binding to a large region (type1) or an overlapping region (type 2 and 3) on the protein surface. The surface was then divided into 11 discrete regions into which series of mutants that are common in groups 2 and 3 were applied, totaling 54 chimeras. Two copies of the best resurfaced protein were fused with a meningococcal antigen to enhance stability and immunogenicity. Immunization with this protein induced broad protection against 10 different strains of all three serogroups and is predicted to be protective against all 300 natural variants of *meningococcus B*.

4. FOCUS ON DOMAINS

To focus the immune response to conserved neutralization sites, it would be helpful if the immunogen could be minimized in order to induce primarily broadly neutralizing antibodies. The success of this approach depends on a suitable architecture of the immunogen. If the immunogen is composed of multiple independently folding domains, it may be minimized based on the domain boundaries. A perfect example of such a conveniently organized protein is the extracellular region of attachment protein G of RSV which is composed of a small independently folding globular domain bounded by two extended mucin-like regions (Langedijk *et al.*, 1996). Vaccination with this minimal domain reduced pulmonary inflammation and virus replication in mice after challenge (Zhang *et al.*, 2010).

A combination of reverse vaccinology and structure-based design was used for the construction of an artificial protein consisting of six variants of the major immunogenic domain of a group B *Streptococcus* pilus protein. After dissection of the immune response and epitope mapping of the most prominent protective antibodies, it was found that most of these mapped to a single domain of a heterotetrameric shaft-forming subunit of pili, which was variable between bacterial strains, and therefore precluded broad protection. Immunization with a chimeric recombinant protein with a string of variant protective domains, spaced with a serine glycine motif, induced full protection in mice against challenge with the respective pilus-carrying strains (Nuccitelli *et al.*, 2011). It is planned to include more variants of this pilus protein in a next generation immunogen.

Although the influenza spike is not composed of such clear discrete domains, its architecture does hold some possibilities for minimization. The influenza spike is composed of a highly variable head domain comprising a large part of hemagglutinin 1 (HA1) and a more conserved stem domain comprising both HA1 and HA2 that is the target of several very broadly neutralizing Mabs. A structure-based vaccine based on headless HA was able to provide full protection from lethal challenge suggesting that this vaccine may be able to induce broadly neutralizing antibodies directed against the conserved stem that could lead to a universal influenza vaccine (Bommakanti *et al.*, 2010; Steel *et al.*, 2010).

Clear boundaries between independently folding protein domains are lacking in the HIV spike and because there is no structure of the native spike, designs of a discrete head or stem are not within reach. However, there is knowledge on the intermediary, so-called prehairpin conformation of gp41, a transitional state between the prefusion stem and the postfusion 6HB that is a target of broadly neutralizing antibodies (Corti *et al.*, 2010; Luftig *et al.*, 2006). In this conformational state, gp120 is detached and gp41 is stretched out, exposing regions of gp41 with clear, albeit transient, domain boundaries. Therefore, the gp41 N-terminal HR1 trimer that comprises the conserved neutralization site (Corti *et al.*, 2010; Luftig *et al.*, 2006) is a potential target for vaccine development, amenable to immunogen minimization and rational design. A trimeric, helical coiled coil is a typical example of an independently folding structural domain that can be easily generated as a miniprotein. Because the prehairpin structure of gp41 is transient, stable, soluble trimeric mimetics have been designed by optimization of the leucine zipper motif, addition of Cys-Cys-Gly motifs for interhelical disulfide bridges and extension with short charged helical trimerization motifs (Eckert and Kim, 2001; Eckert *et al.*, 1999; Langedijk *et al.*, 2011). Vaccination of guinea pigs with stable, soluble mimetics of the gp41 HR1 helical trimer could induce a cross-neutralizing antibody response against a number of tier-1 viral isolates of HIV-1 (Bianchi *et al.*, 2010).

5. FOCUS ON MINIMAL ANTIGENIC SITE

The ultimate way to focus the immune response to the antigenic site of interest is the use of epitope-based vaccines. A peptide or miniprotein that holds just the epitope information, the footprint of a broadly neutralizing antibody, should in theory suffice to re-elicit a neutralizing humoral immune response that can cross-react with and neutralize the virus. In the case of simple linear sites, immunization with a single epitope has proven very successful for inducing a protective response against parvovirus and foot-and-mouth disease (Dalsgaard *et al.*, 1997; DiMarchi *et al.*, 1986; Langeveld *et al.*, 1994). However, with structurally more complex or constrained antigenic sites, this has proven to be difficult. Also, linear peptides that mimic complex discontinuous sites and bind the broadly neutralizing Mab with high affinity were not able to elicit antibodies that cross-react with the viral surface (Saphire *et al.*, 2007). Even for less complex linear epitopes like the extended epitope of Mab 2F5 (Ofek *et al.*, 2004), immunization with peptides or peptide inserts induced no or only poorly neutralizing antibodies (Arnold *et al.*, 2009; Chakrabarti *et al.*, 2005; Coeffier *et al.*, 2000; Eckhart *et al.*, 1996; Ho *et al.*, 2005; Joyce *et al.*, 2002; Law *et al.*, 2007; Liang *et al.*, 1999; McGaughey *et al.*, 2003; Muster *et al.*, 1994; Zhang *et al.*, 2004). Because the correct mimicry of the antigenic region is crucial for an epitope-based vaccine, the exposed V3 region is actually the best target for structure-based design because it is an unglycosylated, independently folding, protruding loop (Huang *et al.*, 2005b) and is highly immunogenic, constituting the binding site of strongly neutralizing antibodies (Carrow *et al.*, 1991; Goudsmit *et al.*, 1988; Vogel *et al.*, 1994). The problem is that the amino acid sequence is highly variable, and therefore, the antibodies that bind the V3 region have limited breadth of neutralization (Davis *et al.*, 2009). However, in recent years, several very broadly neutralizing antibodies have been isolated (Binley *et al.*, 2004; Corti *et al.*, 2010; Gorny *et al.*, 2006; Hioe *et al.*, 2010) that are directed against some conserved features at the tip of the V3 loop and also recognize the side of the loop in a relatively sequence-independent manner (Bell *et al.*, 2008; Burke *et al.*, 2009; Stanfield *et al.*, 2006). Therefore, the hope is raised that minimal immunogens can be designed based on the variable loop that would be presented in such a way that only the conserved elements would elicit antibodies that show broad neutralization. This design problem is complicated because a variable immunogen will most likely induce a strain-specific antibody response. There is no clear structural improvement that can be applied to optimize mimicry because the 35-residue loop folds as a relatively featureless independent domain that is only constrained by a disulfide bridge at the termini. There is no reason to scaffold a structure that needs no further support, and introduction of any kind of scaffolding or linkers can divert the immune response to a cryptic epitope that hampers cross-reaction with the native protein. The variability problem can be limited slightly by truncation of the V3-based immunogen, causing focusing of the immune response to the V3 sequence that is recognized by most anti-V3 and all broadly neutralizing anti-V3 antibodies. Further, the truncated V3 sequence should be cyclized at positions that allow the geometries observed in most of the X-ray structures of the V3 regions (Bell *et al.*, 2008; Burke *et al.*, 2009; Stanfield *et al.*, 2006). It has been shown that the difference between the broad and the narrow neutralizing anti-V3 Mabs can be explained by the presence of very selective binding pockets for charged residues in the paratopes of the Mabs with narrow specificity (Burke *et al.*, 2009). Therefore, perhaps the variability problem at the tip of the loop may be circumvented to some extent by selecting or designing a V3 sequence with a minimal amount of charges that will not elicit antibodies with the typical selective pocket for a complementary charge in the paratope. Several of these criteria were met in a recent study using stabilized matched synthetic peptides (Rachel P. J. Lai, submitted for publication) and by using full-length V3 designs that were inserted in acceptor proteins (Zolla-Pazner *et al.*, 2011), that were able to induce cross-clade neutralizing antibodies in a prime–boost regimen.

To avoid variability problems, most efforts have been concentrated on the mimicry of the epitopes in the MPER because of its high conservation, low complexity, and continuous nature. In addition to 2F5 that binds residues $_{662}$ELDKWASL$_{669}$, MAbs Z13e1 and 4E10 also bind epitopes within the gp41 MPER. Z13e1 binds residues $_{670}$WNWFDITN$_{677}$ and the more potent MAb 4E10 binds residues $_{672}$WFDITNWLW$_{680}$ (Brunel *et al.*, 2006; Muster *et al.*, 1993; Stiegler *et al.*, 2001).

In contrast to the extended 2F5 epitope, 4E10 recognizes a fully helical epitope conformation. Such a single secondary structure is relatively easy to mimic and stabilize with helical templates or cross-linkers (Cardoso *et al.*, 2007; Langedijk *et al.*, 2011). The templates promote alpha helix formation, and cross-linkers limit peptide flexibility without affecting the interaction with 4E10 (Cardoso *et al.*, 2007). These minimal stabilized helical epitopes show increased affinity for MAb 4E10, and in the crystal structure, the side chains are similarly oriented as the side chains of the unconstrained gp41 peptide in the original crystal structure. Despite the mimicry and high affinity for the neutralizing antibody, it has not yet been possible to induce cross-reactive neutralizing antibodies with helical mimics.

6. NATURAL SCAFFOLDS

An elegant approach to mimic the surface of a protein or epitope of interest is to use a small miniprotein scaffold with identical 3D structure as the target that can be used as a template to mimic the surface of interest. A scaffold is suitable if residues can be mutated and transplanted by the side chains of the target surface that needs to be mimicked. Short helical homodimeric peptides based on leucine zippers are amenable examples because the stable helical dimers tolerate side-chain transplants in principle on all positions of the heptads in the dimer except for the position of the leucine zipper at the interface of the helical dimer. Apart from these simple model secondary structural scaffolds, more complicated scaffolds based on natural proteins have also been used successfully. Because protein evolution has selected for a large collection of successful stable folds, it is possible to exploit this natural diversity of shapes and assess/evaluate which fold can be used for side-chain transplantation. For this goal, the function of the protein is no longer important and the only feature that counts is whether the template has a stable fold and allows manipulation and mutation of surface-exposed residues that do not influence folding. In this way, all components of the epitope can be transferred into regions of the template that are structurally compatible and are permissive for sequence mutations.

Various protein–scaffold platforms have been described in which structural elements of scaffold proteins act as acceptors of functional or antigenic regions from other proteins. Versatile examples of such stable folds with promiscuous sequences are the cysteine-rich small toxins. Part of the backbone of the small scyllatoxin shows local structural similarity with the gp120-binding site on CD4. By transplanting the side chains of CD4 important for gp120 binding on the scyllatoxin scaffold, the small toxin was resurfaced and the CD4 mimicry was such that the scyllatoxin miniprotein hybrid exceeded the affinity of sCD4 for gp120 (Huang *et al.*, 2005a; Martin and Vita, 2000; Vita *et al.*, 1995; Stricher *et al.*, 2006).

Also for vaccine design, this approach can expand the possibilities of presenting epitopes on scaffolds for induction of a focused immune response. In order to tap into the full potential of all possible natural scaffolds, new algorithms have been developed to search the complete protein database for a protein that has the best structural similarity with segments of the query epitope that can be used as acceptor for the epitope transplantation. In addition, computational redesign allows the correct exposure of the epitope to the original prototype antibody and correct folding of the scaffold protein in the region in close proximity to the transplanted epitope. Rotamer and sequence optimization protocols are developed to identify amino acids that form good electrostatic interactions, packing interactions, and hydrogen bonds at target interfaces (Correia *et al.*, 2010; Das and Baker, 2008; Kuhlman *et al.*, 2003; Ofek *et al.*, 2010; Ortiz *et al.*, 2002).

In general, after expression of the redesigned candidate hybrid proteins, affinity can be measured with the prototype broadly neutralizing antibody, and if possible, the structure of the recombinant protein scaffolds in complex with the antibody or the single scaffold should be solved to validate the similarity with the target.

For such epitope-based vaccine approaches, detailed high-resolution 3D knowledge is vital for the correct reconstruction of the epitope. These are available for the 2F5 epitope, and it was possible to reconstruct the extended loop structure in several different acceptor proteins (Ofek *et al.*, 2004, 2010). These 2F5-epitope scaffolds with the right structure and high affinity for MAb 2F5 were used to immunize guinea pigs and were able to elicit an antibody response that matched the prototype 2F5 very closely. Interestingly, these studies showed that epitope flexibility enhances immunogenicity, and conversely, that graft rigidity reduces immunogenicity. Therefore, a prime–boost immunization vaccination regimen was applied in which a primary response with a relatively flexible, grafted scaffold could be boosted with a more rigid grafted scaffold (Guenaga *et al.*, 2011; Ofek *et al.*, 2010). Although no neutralization could be detected, the antibody specificity was very similar as the specificity of prototype 2F5 and the crystal structure of a monoclonal antibody (11f10) that was elicited with the 2F5 scaffolds that was solved in complex with a gp41 peptide adopted a conformation and side-chain orientations that were remarkably similar to that induced by 2F5 (Fig. 2.2A and B).

Although the electrostatic potentials on the 11f10 and 2F5 antibody surfaces show a high degree of similarity, there are some apparent differences which are also exemplified in the minor differences in the fine specificity of binding with a library of MPER peptide variants. When binding of both Mabs was tested in a peptide library in which each position of the epitope was mutated (Figure 2.2D and E), a preference for arginine residues at position 663, 668, and 669 was observed for Mab 11f10 that would fit into the extra acidic patch on the surface of Mab 11f10 (Fig. 2.2C).

The antibodies induced by the described MPER mimics are actually not expected to have the same biological effect as the prototype antibodies because it is believed that an essential part of the epitope is still missing. The hydrophobic tip of the long protruding CDR3 of the heavy chain is probably responsible for binding lipids in the viral membrane and contributes to HIV neutralization. This essential membrane-binding component of 2F5 and 4E10 binding was not addressed, and incorporation could improve future vaccine studies. Therefore, it is not known whether the

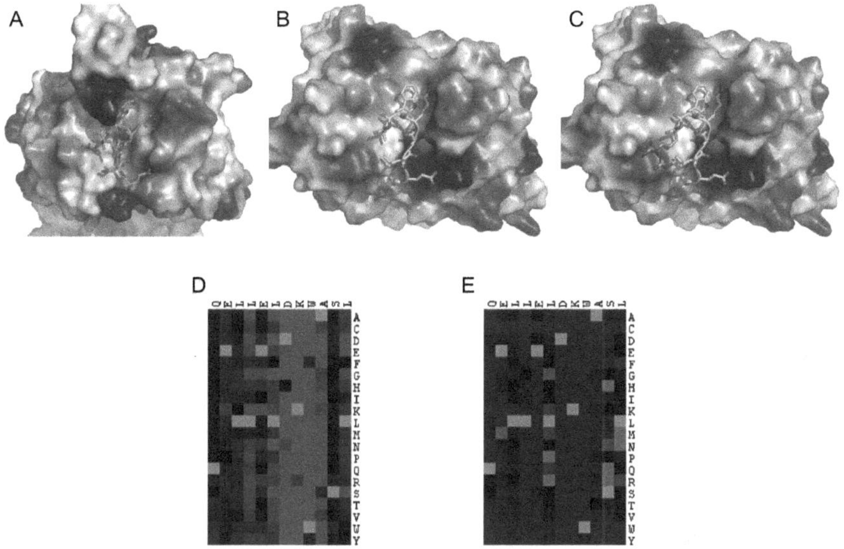

FIGURE 2.2 The MPER peptide cocrystallized with Fabs 2F5 and 11f10. (A) gp41 peptide bound in the 2F5 paratope. (B) The same peptide in the similar 11f10 paratope. (C) As B with arginine substitutions at positions 663 and 668 responsible for higher binding according to pepscan analysis of (E). Either of these substitutions would allow guanidyl side chain packing onto the negatively charged surface of 11f10, explaining its enhanced affinity for these substituted MPER peptides. The average binding activity of FAb 2F5 at 12.5 ng/ml (D) and Mab 11f10 (E) at 1 μg/ml with the seed peptide (sequence QELLELDKWASL) is taken as the zero point for the heat map of the replacements. Signal decrease is shown in shades of red and signal increase in shades of green. (See Color Insert.)

mimicry of the gp41 surface in the epitope scaffolds is sufficient. The dissimilar negatively charged patch on the surface of Mab 11f10 suggests that the positive charge of the opposing region of the scaffold that elicited the antibody should perhaps be reduced. Fine-tuning the surface of the scaffold and incorporation of a lipid component hold promise for rational vaccine design as well as might prove a hard nut to crack.

Similar results have been achieved with epitope scaffolds based on a neutralizing Mab against the fusion protein (F) of RSV. In this case, the total resolved surface of the epitope, a peptide in complex with the neutralizing antibody, was both larger and discontinuous. Epitope scaffolds were produced that were very similar to the structure of the original antibody complexed with the RSV-F peptide (McLellan *et al.*, 2010, 2011). These epitope scaffolds were able to elicit antibodies that were able to cross-react with the native RSV-F protein but no neutralization could be detected (McLellan *et al.*, 2011). Although the RSV epitope was larger and more complex, like the HIV-1 epitope scaffolds, the target epitope was based on a crystal structure of an antibody:peptide complex and not on the complete footprint of the antibody on the surface of the native viral protein. Therefore, more knowledge on the structure of native surface proteins and other developments in vaccinology like adjuvants and prime–boost regimens will certainly foster this new and exciting field of atomic-level rational vaccine design.

7. CONCLUDING REMARKS

Although very effective vaccines are available that did not rely on extensive knowledge of pathogen structure or of the complexity of immunological networks, new developments in these fields will certainly improve the efficacy of available vaccines and, more importantly, facilitate the development of vaccines directed against targets that are now still intractable. Structural knowledge will provide the necessary insights that are needed for stabilizing the native conformation and also for modifying surface proteins by the introduction of new protective epitopes, reconstruction of an epitope mosaic that match several serotypes, and removal or masking of protein domains that do not contribute to broad protection. Although several of these approaches have already paid off, the ultimate minimization of a highly focused immune response to a single protective epitope has not yet resulted in a straightforward vaccine solution. However, impressive breakthroughs have been reached with epitope transplants on natural scaffolds, and this encouraging development will stimulate future research. Perhaps not as an ultimate minimization of an epitope-based vaccine but merged with other structure-based approaches as an add-on of larger subunit vaccines, virus-like particles, live attenuated, or vector-based vaccines.

ACKNOWLEDGMENTS

We like to thank Gilad Ofek, Bill Schief Joris Benschop, Mariet Zekveld for their contributions. This work was supported by the International AIDS Vaccine Initiative.

REFERENCES

Arnold, G. F., Velasco, P. K., Holmes, A. K., Wrin, T., Geisler, S. C., Phung, P., Tian, Y., Resnick, D. A., Ma, X., Mariano, T. M., Petropoulos, C. J., Taylor, J. W., *et al.* (2009). Broad neutralization of human immunodeficiency virus type 1 (HIV-1) elicited from human rhinoviruses that display the HIV-1 gp41 ELDKWA epitope. *J. Virol.* **83,** 5087–5100.

Barouch, D. H. (2008). Challenges in the development of an HIV-1 vaccine. *Nature* **455,** 613–619.

Bell, C. H., Pantophlet, R., Schiefner, A., Cavacini, L. A., Stanfield, R. L., Burton, D. R., and Wilson, I. A. (2008). Structure of antibody F425-B4e8 in complex with a V3 peptide reveals a new binding mode for HIV-1 neutralization. *J. Mol. Biol.* **375,** 969–978.

Bianchi, E., Joyce, J. G., Miller, M. D., Finnefrock, A. C., Liang, X., Finotto, M., Ingallinella, P., McKenna, P., Citron, M., Ottinger, E., Hepler, R. W., Hrin, R., *et al.* (2010). Vaccination with peptide mimetics of the gp41 prehairpin fusion intermediate yields neutralizing antisera against HIV-1 isolates. *Proc. Natl. Acad. Sci. USA* **107,** 10655–10660.

Binley, J. M., Sanders, R. W., Clas, B., Schuelke, N., Master, A., Guo, Y., Kajumo, F., Anselma, D. J., Maddon, P. J., Olson, W. C., and Moore, J. P. (2000). A recombinant human immunodeficiency virus type 1 envelope glycoprotein complex stabilized by an intermolecular disulfide bond between the gp120 and gp41 subunits is an antigenic mimic of the trimeric virion-associated structure. *J. Virol.* **74,** 627–643.

Binley, J. M., Wrin, T., Korber, B., Zwick, M. B., Wang, M., Chappey, C., Stiegler, G., Kunert, R., Zolla-Pazner, S., Katinger, H., Petropoulos, C. J., and Burton, D. R. (2004). Comprehensive cross-clade neutralization analysis of a panel of anti-human immunodeficiency virus type 1 monoclonal antibodies. *J. Virol.* **78,** 13232–13252.

Bommakanti, G., Citron, M. P., Hepler, R. W., Callahan, C., Heidecker, G. J., Najar, T. A., Lu, X., Joyce, J. G., Shiver, J. W., Casimiro, D. R., ter Meulen, J., Liang, X., *et al.* (2010). Design of an HA2-based Escherichia coli expressed influenza immunogen that protects mice from pathogenic challenge. *Proc. Natl. Acad. Sci. USA* **107,** 13701–13706.

Brunel, F. M., Zwick, M. B., Cardoso, R. M., Nelson, J. D., Wilson, I. A., Burton, D. R., and Dawson, P. E. (2006). Structure-function analysis of the epitope for 4E10, a broadly neutralizing human immunodeficiency virus type 1 antibody. *J. Virol.* **80,** 1680–1687.

Burke, V., Williams, C., Sukumaran, M., Kim, S. S., Li, H., Wang, X. H., Gorny, M. K., Zolla-Pazner, S., and Kong, X. P. (2009). Structural basis of the cross-reactivity of genetically related human anti-HIV-1 mAbs: implications for design of V3-based immunogens. *Structure* **17,** 1538–1546.

Cardoso, R. M., Brunel, F. M., Ferguson, S., Zwick, M., Burton, D. R., Dawson, P. E., and Wilson, I. A. (2007). Structural basis of enhanced binding of extended and helically constrained peptide epitopes of the broadly neutralizing HIV-1 antibody 4E10. *J. Mol. Biol.* **365,** 1533–1544.

Carrow, E. W., Vujcic, L. K., Glass, W. L., Seamon, K. B., Rastogi, S. C., Hendry, R. M., Boulos, R., Nzila, N., and Quinnan, G. V., Jr. (1991). High prevalence of antibodies to the gp120 V3 region principal neutralizing determinant of HIV-1MN in sera from Africa and the Americas. *AIDS Res. Hum. Retroviruses* **7,** 831–838.

Chakrabarti, B. K., Ling, X., Yang, Z. Y., Montefiori, D. C., Panet, A., Kong, W. P., Welcher, B., Louder, M. K., Mascola, J. R., and Nabel, G. J. (2005). Expanded breadth of virus neutralization after immunization with a multiclade envelope HIV vaccine candidate. *Vaccine* **23,** 3434–3445.

Chan, D. C., Fass, D., Berger, J. M., and Kim, P. S. (1997). Core structure of gp41 from the HIV envelope glycoprotein. *Cell* **89,** 263–273.

Coeffier, E., Clement, J. M., Cussac, V., Khodaei-Boorane, N., Jehanno, M., Rojas, M., Dridi, A., Latour, M., El Habib, R., Barre-Sinoussi, F., Hofnung, M., and Leclerc, C. (2000). Antigenicity and immunogenicity of the HIV-1 gp41 epitope ELDKWA inserted into permissive sites of the MalE protein. *Vaccine* **19,** 684–693.

Conley, A. J., Gorny, M. K., Kessler, J. A., 2nd, Boots, L. J., Ossorio-Castro, M., Koenig, S., Lineberger, D. W., Emini, E. A., Williams, C., and Zolla-Pazner, S. (1994). Neutralization of primary human immunodeficiency virus type 1 isolates by the broadly reactive anti-V3 monoclonal antibody. *J. Virol.* **68,** 6994–7000.

Correia, B. E., Ban, Y. E., Holmes, M. A., Xu, H., Ellingson, K., Kraft, Z., Carrico, C., Boni, E., Sather, D. N., Zenobia, C., Burke, K. Y., Bradley-Hewitt, T., *et al.* (2010). Computational

design of epitope-scaffolds allows induction of antibodies specific for a poorly immunogenic HIV vaccine epitope. *Structure* **18,** 1116–1126.
Corti, D., Langedijk, J. P., Hinz, A., Seaman, M. S., Vanzetta, F., Fernandez-Rodriguez, B. M., Silacci, C., Pinna, D., Jarrossay, D., Balla-Jhagjhoorsingh, S., Willems, B., Zekveld, M. J., *et al.* (2010). *PLoS One* **5,** e8805.
Dalsgaard, K., Uttenthal, A., Jones, T. D., Xu, F., Merryweather, A., Hamilton, W. D., Langeveld, J. P., Boshuizen, R. S., Kamstrup, S., Lomonossoff, G. P., Porta, C., Vela, C., *et al.* (1997). *Nat. Biotechnol.* **15,** 248.
Das, R., and Baker, D. (2008). *Annu. Rev. Biochem.* **77,** 363.
Davis, K. L., Gray, E. S., Moore, P. L., Decker, J. M., Salomon, A., Montefiori, D. C., Graham, B. S., Keefer, M. C., Pinter, A., Morris, L., Hahn, B. H., and Shaw, G. M. (2009). *Virology* **387,** 414.
Dey, B., Svehla, K., Xu, L., Wycuff, D., Zhou, T., Voss, G., Phogat, A., Chakrabarti, B. K., Li, Y., Shaw, G., Kwong, P. D., Nabel, G. J., *et al.* (2009). *PLoS Pathog.* **5,** e1000445.
DiMarchi, R., Brooke, G., Gale, C., Cracknell, V., Doel, T., and Mowat, N. (1986). *Science* **232,** 639.
Eckert, D. M., and Kim, P. S. (2001). *Proc. Natl. Acad. Sci. USA* **98,** 11187.
Eckert, D. M., Malashkevich, V. N., Hong, L. H., Carr, P. A., and Kim, P. S. (1999). *Cell* **99,** 103.
Eckhart, L., Raffelsberger, W., Ferko, B., Klima, A., Purtscher, M., Katinger, H., and Ruker, F. (1996). *J. Gen. Virol.* **77** (Pt 9), 2001.
Frey, G., Peng, H., Rits-Volloch, S., Morelli, M., Cheng, Y., and Chen, B. (2008). *Proc. Natl. Acad. Sci. USA* **105,** 3739.
Gorny, M. K., Williams, C., Volsky, B., Revesz, K., Cohen, S., Polonis, V. R., Honnen, W. J., Kayman, S. C., Krachmarov, C., Pinter, A., and Zolla-Pazner, S. (2002). *J. Virol.* **76,** 9035.
Gorny, M. K., Williams, C., Volsky, B., Revesz, K., Wang, X. H., Burda, S., Kimura, T., Konings, F. A., Nadas, A., Anyangwe, C. A., Nyambi, P., Krachmarov, C., *et al.* (2006). *J. Virol.* **80,** 6865.
Goudsmit, J., Debouck, C., Meloen, R. H., Smit, L., Bakker, M., Asher, D. M., Wolff, A. V., Gibbs, C. J., Jr., and Gajdusek, D. C. (1988). *Proc. Natl. Acad. Sci. USA* **85,** 4478.
Guenaga, J., Dosenovic, P., Ofek, G., Baker, D., Schief, W. R., Kwong, P. D., Karlsson Hedestam, G. B., and Wyatt, R. T. (2011). *PLoS One* **6,** e16074.
Hioe, C. E., Wrin, T., Seaman, M. S., Yu, X., Wood, B., Self, S., Williams, C., Gorny, M. K., and Zolla-Pazner, S. (2010). *PLoS One* **5,** e10254.
Ho, J., Uger, R. A., Zwick, M. B., Luscher, M. A., Barber, B. H., and MacDonald, K. S. (2005). *Vaccine* **23,** 1559.
Huang, C. C., Stricher, F., Martin, L., Decker, J. M., Majeed, S., Barthe, P., Hendrickson, W. A., Robinson, J., Roumestand, C., Sodroski, J., Wyatt, R., Shaw, G. M., *et al.* (2005a). *Structure* **13,** 755.
Huang, C. C., Tang, M., Zhang, M. Y., Majeed, S., Montabana, E., Stanfield, R. L., Dimitrov, D. S., Korber, B., Sodroski, J., Wilson, I. A., Wyatt, R., and Kwong, P. D. (2005b). *Science* **310,** 1025.
Joyce, J. G., Hurni, W. M., Bogusky, M. J., Garsky, V. M., Liang, X., Citron, M. P., Danzeisen, R. C., Miller, M. D., Shiver, J. W., and Keller, P. M. (2002). *J. Biol. Chem.* **277,** 45811.
Karlsson Hedestam, G. B., Fouchier, R. A., Phogat, S., Burton, D. R., Sodroski, J., and Wyatt, R. T. (2008). *Nat. Rev. Microbiol.* **6,** 143.
Kuhlman, B., Dantas, G., Ireton, G. C., Varani, G., Stoddard, B. L., and Baker, D. (2003). *Science* **302,** 1364.
Kwong, P. D., Doyle, M. L., Casper, D. J., Cicala, C., Leavitt, S. A., Majeed, S., Steenbeke, T. D., Venturi, M., Chaiken, I., Fung, M., Katinger, H., Parren, P. W., *et al.* (2002). *Nature* **420,** 678.
Kwong, P. D., Wyatt, R., Robinson, J., Sweet, R. W., Sodroski, J., and Hendrickson, W. A. (1998). *Nature* **393,** 648.

Langedijk, J. P., Schaaper, W. M., Meloen, R. H., and van Oirschot, J. T. (1996). *J. Gen. Virol.* **77** (Pt 6), 1249.
Langedijk, J. P., Zekveld, M. J., Ruiter, M., Corti, D., and Back, J. W. (2011). *Anal. Biochem.* **417,** 149.
Langeveld, J. P., Casal, J. I., Osterhaus, A. D., Cortes, E., de Swart, R., Vela, C., Dalsgaard, K., Puijk, W. C., Schaaper, W. M., and Meloen, R. H. (1994). *J. Virol.* **68,** 4506.
Law, M., Cardoso, R. M., Wilson, I. A., and Burton, D. R. (2007). *J. Virol.* **81,** 4272.
Li, Y., Cleveland, B., Klots, I., Travis, B., Richardson, B. A., Anderson, D., Montefiori, D., Polacino, P., and Hu, S. L. (2008). *J. Virol.* **82,** 638.
Liang, X., Munshi, S., Shendure, J., Mark, G., 3rd, Davies, M. E., Freed, D. C., Montefiori, D. C., and Shiver, J. W. (1999). *Vaccine* **17,** 2862.
Liu, J., Bartesaghi, A., Borgnia, M. J., Sapiro, G., and Subramaniam, S. (2008). Molecular architecture of native HIV-1 gp120 trimers. *Nature* **455,** 109–113.
Luftig, M. A., Mattu, M., Di Giovine, P., Geleziunas, R., Hrin, R., Barbato, G., Bianchi, E., Miller, M. D., Pessi, A., and Carfi, A. (2006). *Nat. Struct. Mol. Biol.* **13,** 740.
Martin, L., and Vita, C. (2000). Engineering novel bioactive mini-proteins from small size natural and de novo designed scaffolds. *Curr. Protein Pept. Sci.* **1,** 403–430.
Mateo, R., Luna, E., Rincon, V., and Mateu, M. G. (2008). *J. Virol.* **82,** 12232.
McGaughey, G. B., Citron, M., Danzeisen, R. C., Freidinger, R. M., Garsky, V. M., Hurni, W. M., Joyce, J. G., Liang, X., Miller, M., Shiver, J., and Bogusky, M. J. (2003). *Biochemistry* **42,** 3214.
McLellan, J. S., Chen, M., Kim, A., Yang, Y., Graham, B. S., and Kwong, P. D. (2010). *Nat. Struct. Mol. Biol.* **17,** 248.
McLellan, J. S., Correia, B. E., Chen, M., Yang, Y., Graham, B. S., Schief, W. R., and Kwong, P. D. (2011). *J. Mol. Biol.* **409,** 853.
Muster, T., Guinea, R., Trkola, A., Purtscher, M., Klima, A., Steindl, F., Palese, P., and Katinger, H. (1994). *J. Virol.* **68,** 4031.
Muster, T., Steindl, F., Purtscher, M., Trkola, A., Klima, A., Himmler, G., Ruker, F., and Katinger, H. (1993). *J. Virol.* **67,** 6642.
Nuccitelli, A., Cozzi, R., Gourlay, L. J., Donnarumma, D., Necchi, F., Norais, N., Telford, J. L., Rappuoli, R., Bolognesi, M., Maione, D., Grandi, G., and Rinaudo, C. D. (2011). *Proc. Natl. Acad. Sci. USA* **108,** 10278.
Ofek, G., Guenaga, F. J., Schief, W. R., Skinner, J., Baker, D., Wyatt, R., and Kwong, P. D. (2010). *Proc. Natl. Acad. Sci. USA* **107,** 17880.
Ofek, G., Tang, M., Sambor, A., Katinger, H., Mascola, J. R., Wyatt, R., and Kwong, P. D. (2004). *J. Virol.* **78,** 10724.
Ortiz, A. R., Strauss, C. E., and Olmea, O. (2002). *Protein Sci.* **11,** 2606.
Pantophlet, R., Wilson, I. A., and Burton, D. R. (2003). *J. Virol.* **77,** 5889.
Pejchal, R., Gach, J. S., Brunel, F. M., Cardoso, R. M., Stanfield, R. L., Dawson, P. E., Burton, D. R., Zwick, M. B., and Wilson, I. A. (2009). *J. Virol.* **83,** 8451.
Saphire, E. O., Montero, M., Menendez, A., van Houten, N. E., Irving, M. B., Pantophlet, R., Zwick, M. B., Parren, P. W., Burton, D. R., Scott, J. K., and Wilson, I. A. (2007). *J. Mol. Biol.* **369,** 696.
Scanlan, C. N., Pantophlet, R., Wormald, M. R., Ollmann Saphire, E., Stanfield, R., Wilson, I. A., Katinger, H., Dwek, R. A., Rudd, P. M., and Burton, D. R. (2002). *J. Virol.* **76,** 7306.
Scarselli, M., Arico, B., Brunelli, B., Savino, S., Di Marcello, F., Palumbo, E., Veggi, D., Ciucchi, L., Cartocci, E., Bottomley, M. J., Malito, E., Lo Surdo, P., *et al.* (2011). *Sci. Transl. Med.* **3,** 91ra62.
Schief, W. R., Ban, Y. E., and Stamatatos, L. (2009). Challenges for structure-based HIV vaccine design. *Curr. Opin. HIV AIDS* **4,** 431–440.
Stanfield, R. L., Gorny, M. K., Zolla-Pazner, S., and Wilson, I. A. (2006). *J. Virol.* **80,** 6093.

Steel, J., Lowen, A. C., Wang, T. T., Yondola, M., Gao, Q., Haye, K., Garcia-Sastre, A., and Palese, P. (2010). *MBio* **1,** e00018.

Stiegler, G., Kunert, R., Purtscher, M., Wolbank, S., Voglauer, R., Steindl, F., and Katinger, H. (2001). *AIDS Res. Hum. Retroviruses* **17,** 1757.

Stricher, F., Martin, L., and Vita, C. (2006). *Methods Mol. Biol.* **340,** 113.

Vita, C., Roumestand, C., Toma, F., and Menez, A. (1995). *Proc. Natl. Acad. Sci. USA* **92,** 6404.

Vogel, T., Kurth, R., and Norley, S. (1994). *J. Immunol.* **153,** 1895.

Walker, L. M., Huber, M., Doores, K. J., Falkowska, E., Pejchal, R., Julien, J. P., Wang, S. K., Ramos, A., Chan-Hui, P. Y., Moyle, M., Mitcham, J. L., Hammond, P. W., *et al.* (2011). *Nature* **477,** 466.

Walker, L. M., Phogat, S. K., Chan-Hui, P. Y., Wagner, D., Phung, P., Goss, J. L., Wrin, T., Simek, M. D., Fling, S., Mitcham, J. L., Lehrman, J. K., Priddy, F. H., *et al.* (2009). *Science* **326,** 285.

Wei, X., Decker, J. M., Wang, S., Hui, H., Kappes, J. C., Wu, X., Salazar-Gonzalez, J. F., Salazar, M. G., Kilby, J. M., Saag, M. S., Komarova, N. L., Nowak, M. A., *et al.* (2003). *Nature* **422,** 307.

Wu, X., Yang, Z. Y., Li, Y., Hogerkorp, C. M., Schief, W. R., Seaman, M. S., Zhou, T., Schmidt, S. D., Wu, L., Xu, L., Longo, N. S., McKee, K., *et al.* (2010). *Science* **329,** 856.

Wyatt, R., Moore, J., Accola, M., Desjardin, E., Robinson, J., and Sodroski, J. (1995). *J. Virol.* **69,** 5723.

Wyatt, R., and Sodroski, J. (1998). *Science* **280,** 1884.

Yang, X., Florin, L., Farzan, M., Kolchinsky, P., Kwong, P. D., Sodroski, J., and Wyatt, R. (2000). *J. Virol.* **74,** 4746.

Zhang, H., Huang, Y., Fayad, R., Spear, G. T., and Qiao, L. (2004). *J. Virol.* **78,** 8342.

Zhang, W., Choi, Y., Haynes, L. M., Harcourt, J. L., Anderson, L. J., Jones, L. P., and Tripp, R. A. (2010). *J. Virol.* **84,** 1148.

Zhou, T., Georgiev, I., Wu, X., Yang, Z. Y., Dai, K., Finzi, A., Kwon, Y. D., Scheid, J. F., Shi, W., Xu, L., Yang, Y., Zhu, J., *et al.* (2010). *Science* **329,** 811.

Zhou, T., Xu, L., Dey, B., Hessell, A. J., Van Ryk, D., Xiang, S. H., Yang, X., Zhang, M. Y., Zwick, M. B., Arthos, J., Burton, D. R., Dimitrov, D. S., *et al.* (2007). *Nature* **445,** 732.

Zolla-Pazner, S., Kong, X. P., Jiang, X., Cardozo, T., Nadas, A., Cohen, S., Totrov, M., Seaman, M. S., Wang, S., and Lu, S. (2011). *J. Virol.* **85,** 9887.

CHAPTER 3

Mechanisms of Peptide Vaccination in Mouse Models: Tolerance, Immunity, and Hyperreactivity

Thorbald van Hall and Sjoerd H. van der Burg

Contents

Department of Clinical Oncology, Experimental Cancer Immunology and Therapy, Leiden University Medical Center, Albinusdreef 2, Leiden, Netherlands

Advances in Immunology, Volume 114
ISSN 0065-2776, DOI: 10.1016/B978-0-12-396548-6.00003-2

Abstract

The development of synthetic peptide vaccines capable of inducing strong and protective T-cell immunity has taken more than 20 years. Peptide vaccines come in many flavors and although their design is simple, their use is more complicated as the success of a particular peptide vaccine is influenced by many parameters. In fact, peptide vaccination may lead to tolerance, immunity or even hyper-reactivity causing death of the animals. Here we systematically dissect the parameters that influence the final outcome of peptide vaccines as examined in mouse models and this will guide the rational design of new vaccines in the future.

1. INTRODUCTION

Vaccination is a powerful method to induce humoral and cellular adaptive immune responses aiming to control bacterial and viral infections as well as tumor growth. After the great success of antibody-inducing prophylactic vaccines, starting with cowpox and extending now to an ever expanding list of infectious pathogens, therapeutic vaccines enter the stage of medicine. Whereas the prevention of infections relies on neutralizing antibodies, the treatment of chronic intracellular infections and cancers strongly depends on the activation of antigen-specific CD4 and CD8 T cells, and this requires different types of vaccines. Therefore, the aim of immunotherapeutic vaccines for cancer is to mount a robust and effective antitumor response in the patient, with the ultimate aim to destroy the tumor by T-cell effector mechanisms of the immune system. The success and the progress in this field is illustrated by the recent FDA approval of a vaccine for the treatment of prostate cancer (Provenge/Sipuleucel-T®) as well as a T-cell stimulating therapeutic antibody for the treatment of melanoma (Ipilimumab/Yervoy®). In addition, we recently reported that vaccination with long synthetic peptides (25–35 amino acids) resulted in complete and durable regressions of human papilloma virus-induced premalignant lesions by induction of a strong and broad multifunctional CD4 and CD8 T-cell reaction (Kenter *et al.*, 2008, 2009; Welters *et al.*, 2008). The development of peptide vaccines started in the late 1980s, indicating that it took more than 20 years to show their clinical efficacy. At first sight, the design and use of peptide vaccines seem very simple. However, mechanistic studies with peptide vaccines in different mouse models revealed that the success of a particular peptide vaccine is influenced by many parameters. In fact, peptide vaccination may lead to tolerance, immunity, or even hyperreactivity causing death of the animals. In this review, we dissect how a number of parameters, including presence of helper T-cell epitopes, necessity of uptake by professional antigen-presenting cells (APCs), biodistribution, influence of adjuvants, peptide length, peptide affinity, and mode of administration, can affect the final outcome of such a vaccine. A good understanding of the underlying mechanisms will guide the rational design of new vaccines in the future.

2. ONCE UPON A TIME

2.1. The molecular definition of T-cell recognition

Cytotoxic $CD8^{+}$ T lymphocytes recognize short peptides of 8–11 amino acids folded in MHC class I molecules (MHC-I) (Bjorkman *et al.*, 1987a,b; Rotzschke *et al.*, 1990a,b; Zinkernagel and Doherty, 1974). The T-cell receptor heterodimer docks unto the surface of this peptide/MHC-I complex and makes molecular interactions with the upstanding alpha-helixes of the MHC-I and single amino acid residues of the stretched and bound peptide-antigen (Bjorkman *et al.*, 1987a,b). This molecular interface ultimately determines the clinical outcome of immune responses to not only invading viruses and growing tumors but also tissue-destructive autoimmune diseases, like type I diabetes. The recognition of these peptide-antigens by CD8 T cells is both selective and extremely sensitive. One amino acid change can turn an agonistic epitope into a nonstimulating peptide.

Virtually, all cells of the body express a wide array of different peptide-filled MHC-I molecules at their cell surface, and by sensing these structures, CD8 T cells detect if unknown (e.g., pathogen-derived) protein sequences are present within that cell. Before peptide/MHC-I complexes arrive at the cell surface, they experienced a long journey of intracellular processing. This processing route starts with intermediate degradation products of nuclear and cytosolic proteins destined for breakdown by the proteasome. Peptide products of around 20 amino acids are further degraded by other proteolytic enzymes and eventually saved from total disintegration by transport into the endoplasmic reticulum. A loading machinery with editing and quality control features in the ER certifies that stably binding peptides end up in the binding grooves of MHC-I molecules. Then peptide-MHC-I complexes are shuttled into the secretory route for display at the cell surface. In contrast, MHC-II molecules present exogenous antigens and depend on active uptake pathways and other processing mechanisms, which predominantly operate in APCs, to load peptides. These peptide-antigens are longer than those of MHC-I and vary in length, as both ends of the MHC-II binding groove are open.

2.2. Molecularly defined peptide vaccines induce protective T-cell immunity

The first peptide vaccination experiments were performed in the late 1980s and built on the landmark achievement that short peptides confer T-cell recognition (Townsend *et al.*, 1986). Small synthetically produced peptides mimicking known virus-derived CD8 T-cell epitopes were administered to mice, and apparently, these peptides found their way to MHC-I molecules *in vivo* and were able to effectively stimulate a response of T cells expressing the cognate T-cell receptor allowing the mice to resist a subsequent challenge with the relevant virus type (Aichele *et al.*, 1990; Gao *et al.*, 1991; Kast *et al.*, 1991; Schulz *et al.*, 1991). Single synthetic peptides from antigens of LCMV, influenza, or Sendai virus were tested in different labs, and in all cases, an otherwise lethal virus challenge prevented death of the mice. Although these vaccinations were performed in a prophylactic setting, immune control was clearly T-cell mediated and did not depend on neutralizing antibodies, suggesting that their use may be extended into therapeutic applications. A few years later, the first reports appeared showing that administration of synthetic peptides was also successful to control tumor outgrowth in mouse models (Feltkamp *et al.*, 1993, 1995; Mandelboim *et al.*, 1995; Noguchi *et al.*, 1994; Reinholdsson-Ljunggren *et al.*, 1992). Interestingly, in most of the early studies, synthetic peptides were used that were often longer than the 9–11 amino acids of the minimal peptide-sequence recognized by CD8 T cells. Such longer peptides are not likely to directly bind to MHC-I grooves at the cell's surface, as the length of the peptide that can be accommodated is restricted by the closed ends at both sides of the groove (Bjorkman *et al.*, 1987a,b). Injected elongated peptides, therefore, may need trimming, and this can occur in the extracellular matrix by serum proteases or by endo- and exopeptidases present at the cell surface of dendritic cell (DC) (Amoscato *et al.*, 1998; Falo *et al.*, 1992; Larsen *et al.*, 1996). Alternatively, longer peptides can be ingested by professional APC and there trimmed to minimal MHC-I-binding ligands inside cells by antigen processing enzymes. In later studies, the exact minimal CTL peptide-epitopes were successfully applied showing that the length of a peptide was not critical for the induction of protective CD8 T-cell responses (Feltkamp *et al.*, 1993, 1995; Kast *et al.*, 1993; Mandelboim *et al.*, 1995). Importantly, all studies made use of peptides mimicking the dominant CTL epitope of viruses or an epitope within a mutated self-protein that displayed strong binding affinity for MHC-I. Thus the recruited T-cell repertoires were not hampered by tolerance mechanisms of "self"-specificity. Together, these pioneering studies evoked enthusiasm and ignited clinical vaccination trials in small cohorts of patients with cancer. Overall, results of these vaccination trials were disappointing. The vaccines failed to install a convincing T-cell response, let alone clinical benefit for the patients, arguing that T-cell-based immunotherapy rather should focus on the adoptive transfer of effector cells (Mocellin *et al.*, 2004; Rosenberg *et al.*, 2004).

2.3. The dark side of peptide vaccines

Meanwhile, several groups reported that vaccination with the minimal MHC-I-binding peptide-epitopes (synthetic short peptides, SSPs) could have a detrimental effect on CD8 T-cell responses (Aichele *et al.*, 1995; Kyburz *et al.*, 1993; Toes *et al.*, 1996a,b). SSP vaccination in those models resulted in functional deletion of the antigen-specific T cells, leading to enhanced virus and tumor outgrowth. The finding that tumors following SSP vaccination grew faster than in untreated animals convincingly demonstrated that the antigen-specific immunity was actively destroyed by peptide vaccination. Indeed, CD8 T-cell reactivity was silenced by peripheral deletion and tolerance after an initial expansion phase. Antigen-unrelated responses were unaffected, confirming that the injected short peptides specifically targeted the cognate peptide-recognizing CD8 T lymphocytes. Comparison of these "failure" data with the successful peptide vaccination data did not immediately provide a likely explanation: both categories made use of peptides representing a dominant nonself epitopes that were emulsified in mineral oil (incomplete Freund's adjuvant, IFA), applied at comparable peptide doses of SSP, and all studies were done in the same mouse strain. The finding that elongation of the minimal CTL peptide-epitope, by adding a number of its natural flanking amino acids, prevented tolerance induction and led to priming of antigen-specific CD8 T cells instead, was a conceptual breakthrough. The strongest example of this was provided by the model antigen Ad5E1 from the adenovirus oncogene E1. Injecting the 10-mer SSP of this model antigen in a subcutaneous depot of IFA effectively destroys the cognate T-cell response, even in doses as low as 10μg (Toes *et al.*, 1996a,b). A 30-mer synthetic long peptide (SLP) comprising this minimal peptide in the middle region, flanked with the natural sequences, generates a large pool of activated peptide-specific cytotoxic T cells (Bijker *et al.*, 2007a) while the same IFA emulsion, equal molar doses of peptide, same mode of administration and mouse strain were used. Years of basic research were required to explain the outcomes between the different SSPs and between SSPs and SLPs. Some of the answers were not so surprising and pointed at common vaccination principles, whereas other results were more startling.

3. RULES OF ENGAGEMENT

3.1. The need for danger

Tolerance and immunity are opposing sides of the same coin. Where immunity is wanted for infections and cancer, tolerance is the preferred status in cases of autoimmunity. Since the late 1950s, immunologists reasoned along the lines of self/nonself distinction to predict immune responsiveness. The overall idea was that the immune system would function correctly when it responds to nonself, such as foreign pathogens, and that it should remain inactive when encountering self-proteins, like organ-specific structures. The T-cell repertoire is shaped during thymus education roughly along these lines and is curtailed to prevent emergence of T cells recognizing self-peptide/MHC-I complexes (Anderson and Su, 2011; Klein *et al.*, 2009). While about 20% of all tumors are induced by viruses and may present viral epitopes, the majority of tumors will express tumor antigens that represent aberrantly expressed self-proteins. The direct consequence of the thymic negative selection process is the absence or impaired quality of T cells directed at the latter type of tumor antigens. This T-cell pool is usually equipped with low-affinity T-cell receptors. Although the self/nonself model of the immune system was valuable, it is now overtaken by a modified version that includes the importance of APCs (Anderson *et al.*, 2001; Janeway and Medzhitov, 2002; Matzinger, 1994, 2002). APCs not only ingest proteins in their environment but also detect products from foreign pathogens and from tissue damage in this environment, respectively, named "pathogen-associated molecular patterns" (PAMPs) and "damage-associated molecular patterns" (DAMPs) (Piccinini and Midwood, 2010). These products are recognized by pattern-recognition receptors resulting in the activation and full maturation of APC allowing them to ignite a full-blown adaptive immune response. The principles of this "danger" model fully apply to the field of vaccination. When high doses of foreign antigens are administered, the immune system responds with tolerance, but when low doses of foreign antigens are combined with noxious substances (adjuvants), the immune system is activated and generates effector cells and memory. The central function of adjuvants is alarming the innate immune system, especially DCs, which are the most suited population of APC driving effective T-cell responses as shown in mouse models where depletion of DC strongly affected the priming T-cell responses (Jung *et al.*, 2002). Thus, vaccination should be considered as "mimicking an infection" (van der Burg *et al.*, 2006). Consequently, vaccines should mediate PAMP or DAMP type of exposure to the antigen-containing APC to prevent APC from taking a default course that results in the tolerization of the antigen-specific T-cell compartment (Bennett *et al.*, 1998; Carbone *et al.*, 1998; Heath and Carbone, 2001; Luckashenak *et al.*, 2008), not only via T-cell deletion or anergy but also via the induction of antigen-specific regulatory T cells (Bennett *et al.*, 1998; Carbone *et al.*, 1998; Daniel *et al.*, 2011; Heath and Carbone, 2001; Luckashenak *et al.*, 2008; Wells *et al.*, 2009). A number of approaches have been taken to provide the necessary "danger" signals to DC *in vivo*. Activation of DC can be accomplished by various synthetic adjuvant compounds that trigger Toll like receptors

(TLR) and other pattern-recognition receptors, for example, oligonucleotides, ssRNA, flagellin, and the lipid PAM3CSK (Duthie *et al.*, 2011). Alternatively, CD4 T cell-mediated activation of DC can be mimicked by targeting receptors of the TNF family by antibodies. For instance, the addition of an agonistic CD40 antibody may convert a SSP vaccine strategy associated with tolerance induction into an immunostimulatory treatment (Diehl *et al.*, 1999). Interestingly, targeting the T-cell expressed TNF-family members 4-1BB and OX40 results in a similar outcome (Diehl *et al.*, 2002; Salek-Ardakani *et al.*, 2011a). These artificial antibody adjuvants point at the natural role for TNF-family members in the priming of protective T-cell responses (Diehl *et al.*, 2000; Salek-Ardakani *et al.*, 2011b; Toes *et al.*, 1998a) and suggest that the costimulatory context in which peptide vaccines are delivered is decisive for their efficacy. Under appropriate conditions, this is delivered by fully activated DC but, alternatively, can be delivered by less optimal APC provided that the T cells are directly stimulated via 4-1BB or OX40 at their cell surface. For instance, in the above mentioned studies, vaccination with SSPs in IFA combined with either TLR agonists or agonistic antibodies to TNF-family members induced up to 70% peptide-specific CD8 T cells from the normal endogenous repertoire (Bilsborough *et al.*, 2002; Liu *et al.*, 2006; Salek-Ardakani *et al.*, 2011a) so that high numbers of T cells within the CD8 T-cell pool displayed a vaccine-induced monovalent specificity. Notably, this also holds true for nonviral epitopes, as comparable high frequencies were observed for the tumor-associated "self"-antigen TRP2 (tyrosinase-related protein 2). Here, APC stimulation was accomplished by combined application of agonistic anti-CD40 antibodies and multiple TLR ligands (Cho and Celis, 2009).

In conclusion, these findings emphasize that induction of tolerance or immunity is not an intrinsic factor of peptide vaccines but strongly depends on the context of antigen presentation in which the antigenic signal is delivered to the T cells.

3.2. Size matters

The first pioneering studies on peptide vaccination actually used peptides that varied in length between 14 and 16 amino acids (Aichele *et al.*, 1990; Gao *et al.*, 1991; Kast *et al.*, 1991; Schulz *et al.*, 1991), which is longer than the size of the corresponding MHC-I-binding epitopes (Rotzschke *et al.*, 1990a,b). Subsequent studies in mouse models commonly used the exact minimal peptide-epitope recognized by CD8 T cells, under the assumption that these peptides are optimal for immediate binding to MHC-I molecules and as such would form the best vaccines. A direct comparison between the efficacy of SSPs and SLPs was not performed until 2002. In this first study, the immunogenicity of a 35-mer SLP comprising the HPV16 E7 CTL epitope was compared to that of the same CTL epitope formulated as a 9-mer SSP. Frequencies of peptide-induced CTL and their tumor controlling capacity were significantly better in the mice receiving the SLP vaccine (Zwaveling *et al.*, 2002). Even when the strong adjuvants GM-CSF, MPL, or CpG were included, the SLPs performed better. Subsequent studies revealed comparable differences for other antigens, including ovalbumine (OVA) and Ad5E1 (Bijker *et al.*, 2007a, 2008). Although the OVA-derived CTL epitope (SIINFEKL) is a very strong T-cell antigen and certainly able to induce a good CTL responses when injected as SSPs in IFA, the 30-mer long peptides outperformed this small peptide in the long-term memory response. Thirty days after vaccination, the OVA-specific CD8 T cells in the mice receiving the SSPs in IFA were barely detectable and failed to kill peptide-loaded target cells *in vivo* (Bijker *et al.*, 2007a).

In contrast, vaccination with long peptides resulted in somewhat delayed but sustained CTL responses (Bijker *et al.*, 2007a). The SLPs-induced CTL displayed good cytolytic function as long as day 90. The delayed onset of immunity might relate to the requirement of antigen processing, a process that includes uptake of antigens, digestion by intracellular proteolytic enzymes, and routing of peptide/MHC-I complexes to the cell surface. As the OVA-derived SIINFEKL peptide is one of the best MHC-I binders known, we repeated these studies with a variant peptide for which the binding affinity and stability were decreased by exchanging the C-terminal position with an isoleucine, representing common tumor-associated antigens. This decreased binding affinity led to a much weakened CTL response when given in SSP formulation. Again, a longer version of this lower-affinity CTL epitope was highly immunogenic (Bijker *et al.*, 2008). Moreover, we recently found that comparable differences in immunogenicity between short and long peptides can also be observed for the melanoma-associated antigen gp100 (L. Ly and T. van Hall, unpublished observations), indicating that the better performance of long peptides is not restricted to "foreign" antigens OVA, HPV, and Ad5E1 but reflects a general feature in peptide vaccination. The fact that elongation of the peptides (1) converts a tolerizing peptide into an effective vaccine (2) improves the immunogenicity of low-affinity CTL epitopes, and (3) enhances the strength of vaccine-induced immunity even in the presence of good DC-activating agonists clearly illustrates that long peptides display properties which are fundamental to the design of peptide vaccines in general. So far, at least three responsible parameters have been identified and will be discussed in the succeeding sections: the inclusion of helper T-cell epitopes, which sustain the CD8 T-cell responses; the differences in biodistribution (pharmacokinetics), which might uncouple antigen from danger signals; and the type of APC that picks up and presents the antigen, as not all APC behave professional.

3.3. Help!

Helper T cells are pivotal for the development of protective immune responses, and these CD4 T cells orchestrate the direction of immune attack in the effector phase. Based on the instructions that CD4 helper T cells receive from their activating APC, immunity will develop into tissue-destructive responses needed, for instance, to kill intracellular pathogens by antigen-specific cytotoxic CD8 T cells, or into antibody responses in order to neutralize extracellular bacteria, viruses, toxins, or to antiparasitic responses (Sallusto and Lanzavecchia, 2009). Tissue-destructive responses are required to combat chronic virus infections and cancers and originate in lymph nodes as a tripartite meeting of type 1 CD4 T cells (Th1), CD8 T cells and antigen-carrying APC, usually a DC. The help by CD4 T cells during the priming phase is thought to exist of APC activation via the CD40–CD40L axis (Toes *et al.*, 1998a), thereby bridging APC with CD8 T cells. CD8 T-cell responses to cell-associated antigens elicited in the absence of CD4 T cells are blunted in their secondary expansion capacity needed for the memory phase, indicating that CD4 T cells confer instructions during the priming phase that are important for later on in the life of killer T cells (Janssen *et al.*, 2003). Moreover, CD4 T cells are important in the effector phase of the immune response, for instance, by providing growth factors like IL-2. These general notes also apply to the immunity to tumors (Ossendorp *et al.*, 2000; Toes *et al.*, 1999). Recent work suggests that the importance of tissue-infiltrating antigen-specific CD4 T cells exceeds the production of the growth factor IL-2 and actively promotes the recruitment and lytic functions of virus- or tumor-directed CD8 T cells, thereby shaping the microenvironment (Bos and Sherman, 2010; Nakanishi *et al.*, 2009; Wong *et al.*, 2008).

The impact of helper T cells in peptide vaccination is obvious in many model systems. The generation of protective T-cell responses is clearly improved after addition of T helper peptides (Bijker *et al.*, 2007a; Gritzapis *et al.*, 2010; Ossendorp *et al.*, 1998; Reiser *et al.*, 2011). Interestingly, a closer look at some of the SLPs used for vaccination revealed that the effectiveness of a LCMV 15-mer SLP to induce LCMV-specific CD8 T-cell reactivity depended on CD4 T-cell help (Fayolle *et al.*, 1991), suggesting that this longer peptide also comprised a helper epitope. Similarly, the HPV16 E7 SLP vaccine in IFA failed to induce strong peptide-specific CD8 T-cell responses in MHC-II knockout mice (Zwaveling *et al.*, 2002). The region covered by the HPV16 E7 SLPs indeed comprises a Th epitope that overlaps with the CTL epitope. These data imply that recruitment of antigen-specific helper cells by including peptides comprising helper-epitopes is an important parameter for successful peptide vaccines.

Subsequent studies on the LCMV peptide, however, revealed that immunization with short minimal peptides instead of the 15-mer SLP did *not* require CD4 T cells (Fayolle *et al.*, 1996) and also the HPV peptide can elicit CTL in the absence of CD4 T cells provided that strong DC-activating compounds are codelivered (Zwaveling *et al.*, 2002). Together with the results of other investigations, these data suggest that a number of SSPs are well capable of inducing protective CD8 T-cell responses without the help of CD4 T cells (Aichele *et al.*, 1995; Assudani *et al.*, 2008; Bijker *et al.*, 2008; Cho and Celis, 2009; Daftarian *et al.*, 2007; Kast *et al.*, 1993; Mansour *et al.*, 2007). Importantly, SSPs without helper epitopes might induce short-term CD8 T cells that vanish from the system in the memory phase, and most studies in which the capacity of SSP-induced CD8 T cells in the absence of help were tested for efficacy, relied on short-term experiments in which T cells were tested or challenged at the peak of the initial response. In the OVA model, we found that OVA SSPs in IFA can induce a strong effective CTL response at day 10 after vaccination. This response, however, was not detectable anymore at day 30 as analyzed *in vivo* and *in vitro* (Bijker *et al.*, 2007a). The addition of a T helper peptide-epitope to this OVA SSPs in IFA fully restored the long-term capacity of vaccine-induced OVA-specific CTL, showing that CD4 T cells are important to sustain good protective immunity (Bijker *et al.*, 2007a). Still, this role of helper cells can be replaced by a cocktail of powerful innate stimuli (Assudani *et al.*, 2008; Cho and Celis, 2009), and we conclude that SSPs can be effective vaccines under these conditions.

Agonistic CD40 antibody as APC-stimulating signal only partially substitutes for the lack of CD4 T-cell help. This aid is most important during priming of the CD8 T cells but fails to rescue CD8 T-cell reactivity at the long run (Bijker *et al.*, 2007a). This finding of poor CD8 T-cell memory formation and loss of cytolytic function following SSP vaccination with anti-CD40 was also observed for other antigenic models (den Boer *et al.*, 2001; Welters *et al.*, 2007). Based on these data, we conclude that real help is better than surrogate help in that installment of strong sustainable CD8 T-cell responses is reached by the inclusion of cognate T helper epitopes, whereas addition of single strong APC-stimulating adjuvant might not completely suffice. Quite often, helper peptides are included in clinical trials nowadays, either as common agonistic sequences (PADRE) or as specific antigen-derived peptides (reviews: Bijker *et al.*, 2007b; Cho and Celis, 2010; Melief and van der Burg, 2008; Perez *et al.*, 2010; Purcell *et al.*, 2007). In view of the local immunomodulatory function of CD4 T cells (Bos and Sherman, 2010; Nakanishi *et al.*, 2009; Wong *et al.*, 2008), it is anyway preferred to activate cognate help which is likely to be present in the target tissue, for example, derived from antigens of the targeted virus or tumor.

Interestingly, elongation of SSPs with their natural flanking sequences frequently results in inclusion of helper T-cell epitopes. The resulting

SLPs therefore automatically trigger helper T cells. Good examples are the earlier described peptides of LCMV and HPV, which comprise overlapping epitopes for CD8 and CD4 T cells. This antigenic linkage is often found in nature including viral structural and early proteins, but also tumor-associated antigens with naturally occurring linked CTL and Th epitope have been described (NY-ESO-1, HER-2/neu and CEA) (Perez *et al.*, 2010). Consequently, foreign antigens and even tumor-associated proteins often contain immunogenic stretches that function as hotspots for the immune system. Maybe this antigenic linkage is a design of nature to facilitate intimate interactions of APC, CD4, and CD8 T cells for the induction of optimal and protective CD8 T-cell responses.

3.4. Right time, right dose.....

Quick peptide spread from the site of administration creates a circumstance in which peptides can be presented outside the context of danger. As argued before, this will rather lead to tolerance than immunity, as nicely illustrated by the induction of regulatory T cells when peptides are continuously fed to the system using osmotic minipumps (Daniel *et al.*, 2011). It has been shown that short peptides of the same length but differing in amino acid contents are distributed in mice with completely distinct pharmacokinetics (Weijzen *et al.*, 2001). A clear example of extremely different biodistributions was revealed using radioactive labeled short peptides from Ad5E1 and HPV16 E7. The Ad5E1 SSP, which induces T-cell tolerance when administered in IFA, spreads from the subcutaneous IFA depot at a high rate. The first peptide already arrives in the spleen after as little as 1 h, whereas it takes at least a day before the HPV16-E7 SSPs can be detected in the spleen (Weijzen *et al.*, 2001). Although weak, the mineral oil IFA displays adjuvant activity (Jensen *et al.*, 1998) allowing nearby DCs to become activated. At longer distances, however, the quick spreading peptide is more likely to be presented by APC in an immature status, causing T-cell tolerance as a result. This was substantiated by a study in which repeated intraperitoneal injections with high doses of a LCMV-SSPs resulted in T-cell tolerance, whereas local administration—injection of lower doses in IFA under the skin—primed peptide-specific T cells (Aichele *et al.*, 1995).

Most probably, the influences of the mode of administration on the immune outcome depend on underlying parameters like MHC-I-binding affinity, the rate of spreading, the distance of spreading, and the presenting cell. First of all, due to their design, SSPs can bind exogenously to MHC-I and these molecules are present on virtually every cell type they encounter (e.g., professional APC, nonprofessional APC, T cells, endothelial cells). Peptides with high MHC-I affinity generally display high on-rates and low off-rates (van der Burg *et al.*, 1996) not only allowing them to compete with already bound peptides in MHC-I at the surface of the cell they encounter—thereby rescuing it from clearance from the system—but also allowing them to be presented for a long time by this cell. Quick spreading peptides translate in higher doses of peptide at any given time and point in the body. In combination with a high MHC-I affinity, this will result in strong peptide presentation to T cells by nonprofessional APC or by professional APC that are "immature" and have not received instructions to become activated (Bijker *et al.*, 2008). So, SSPs with such pharmacokinetics and SSPs that are systemically applied are very likely to tolerize T cells, especially when danger signals are not systemically available. In contrast, when peptides are slowly released or do not spread too far to be presented outside the area of inflammation or have less strong affinity for MHC-I, the threshold for T-cell recognition in a nonstimulatory context will not be met. Our own experiments in which we compared the OVA SSP (SIINFEKL) that binds with high affinity to MHC-I with the OVA variant SSP (SIINFEKI) which binds with intermediate affinity to MHC-I corroborate this notion as we showed that the variant peptide was rapidly cleared and failed to gain access to MHC-I molecules *in vivo* at stimulatory levels. In contrast, the 30-mer low-affinity OVA (SIINFEKI) was still capable to drain to the local lymph node and to induce CD8 T cells. Obviously, the design of elongated peptides (15–35mers) does not allow them to get exogenous access to MHC-I and thus prevents the presentation of CTL epitopes by any cell in locations that are in homeostasis and not inflamed. SLP presentation requires uptake and intracellular processing, a process that is most efficient in APCs. The sheer fact that SLPs are too long for direct MHC-I binding is one of the mechanistic explanations of their better performance in vaccination protocols.

Another peculiar characteristic of IFA is the extended duration of peptide release, for which it is known as a "slow release depot." Strikingly, the short Ad5E1 peptide still leaks from the IFA depot at day 200 (den Boer *et al.*, 2001, 2004) and the OVA SSP does this for at least 60 days (Bijker *et al.*, 2007a). The reason that the agonistic CD40 antibody only prevents tolerance induction in the early phase, but not in the memory phase may well lie in the fact that peptide presentation ensues for a long time in the absence of DC activation after the antibody has been cleared allowing T cells to interact in the context of tolerogenic APC (Bijker *et al.*, 2007a; den Boer *et al.*, 2001, 2004). The same simple argument can be used for experiments in which TLR agonists are used: the SSP is still present long after the TLR agonist has been cleared. Indeed, some TLR agonists are present in a stimulatory fashion only for short periods of time (Welters *et al.*, 2007).

Further proof for this hypothesis is delivered by experiments in which peptide was administered in saline without IFA. This obviously resulted in a fast biodistribution but also a faster clearance of the peptides. This indeed prevented tolerance induction by SSPs in the memory phase (Bijker *et al.*,

2007a). However, administration in saline also carries the disadvantage that SSPs with weak binding capacity to MHC-I are too quickly removed from the system to be presented long enough for naïve CD8 T cells to encounter the APC presenting the peptide at stimulating concentrations (Bijker *et al.*, 2008). Interestingly, long peptides injected in saline seem to end up in a good profile in that their presentation endures up to day 10, but not much longer than that (Bijker *et al.*, 2008; Blair *et al.*, 2011). Moreover, long synthetic peptides were found not to become systemically distributed throughout the mice but are specifically drained to local lymph nodes, irrespective of the constituent of the depot (Bijker *et al.*, 2007a, 2008; Ly *et al.*, 2010).

Thus, optimal peptide vaccines predominantly drain to local activated lymph nodes where they are presented for a sufficient amount of time and at sufficient concentrations to allow T-cell priming. One way to prevent systemic spread is the attachment of lipid tails to peptides as pioneered by the group of Rammensee (Deres *et al.*, 1989), but this is not effective for all peptides (Toes *et al.*, 1998b). Alternatively, one could physically link APC activating compounds and antigen as this would ensure ideal peptide presentation both in time and in location (see chapter 7 by Khan and Ossendorp). Another solution would be to include separate peptides comprising T helper epitopes or to use linkers between CTL and helper peptides (Sette *et al.*, 2002). The release of the OVA T helper peptide from IFA is as long as that of the OVA SSPs (Bijker *et al.*, 2007a) and as such should provide DC activation on the spot.

Investigations on new delivery systems for peptide vaccines are important to help reaching the ideal kinetics and biodistribution of antigen in combination with APC activating compounds. Recently, the FDA-approved biodegradable poly-lactic-*co*-glycolic acid (PLGA) microparticles were shown to properly shuttle antigens to the immune system, which resulted in good T-cell responses (Mueller *et al.*, 2011; Schliehe *et al.*, 2011). When these PLGA particles are pressurized to form a small disk, they interestingly behave as an immune scaffold when placed under the skin, mimicking a lymph node (Ali *et al.*, 2011, 2009). The replacement of mineral oil by these novel delivery systems or, alternatively, direct lymph node injections with peptide (Ribas *et al.*, 2011) will also solve the problem of itching granuloma formation under the skin, which is a negative long-term side effect of montanide ISA 51.

3.5. ......and right place!

A so-far-underexposed virtue of SLP vaccines is that the frequency and function of peptide-specific CD8 T-cell responses they induce were better than that of SSPs even when strong DC-activating TRL-agonists were provided (Bijker *et al.*, 2007a, 2008; Zwaveling *et al.*, 2002). Importantly, this superiority was sustained in the absence of helper T cells, as evidenced by antibody-mediated depletion of CD4 T cells and by vaccinations in MHC-II and CD40 knockout mice. Interestingly, the long OVA peptide is released from IFA for similar long periods of time as SSP OVA but does not coincide with loss of T-cell function (Bijker *et al.*, 2007a). These results pointed out that simply the increased length of a peptide was advantageous, which was not explained by providing help or creating a different biodistribution. The lacking parameter turned out to be targeting to professional APC, as will be discussed in this section.

In order to be presented, long peptides need to be taken up and intracellularly processed before they can arrive in MHC-I molecules to become presented at the outside of cells to CD8 T lymphocytes. Most studies assessing the immunogenicity of SLPs made use of 20–35mers in which the CTL epitope is situated more or less in the middle region, implying that N- and C-terminal cleavages are required before the epitope can be loaded in MHC-I. Several proteolytic enzymes have been reported that possesses endopeptidase activity, of which the proteasome constitutes the most important one for generating peptides for MHC-I binding. In addition, trimming enzymes are present in the cytosol and ER that shorten peptides by nibbling off single or small sets of amino acids. Thus, the full antigen processing equipment that is in place to process endogenous proteins can be used for processing of internalized long peptides. The routing of exogenous antigens to MHC-I loading and surface display is called cross-presentation and is predominantly active in DC. This process is the basis of priming CD8 T-cell immunity and, therefore, obviously attracted considerable interest in the vaccine field. Vaccinations aiming at T-cell-mediated protection strongly depend on optimal targeting of DC *in vivo*. When tested *in vitro*, SLPs are preferentially internalized by DC when compared to B cells and monocytes (Hambach *et al.*, 2010), whereas SSPs are equally well presented by all these cell types. An *in vivo* comparison of the immunogenicity of OVA SSPs and OVA SLPs revealed that SSPs were presented by all APC cell types and even by T cells after injection in mice (Bijker *et al.*, 2008). Moreover, experiments in B-cell knockout mice revealed that the T-cell stimulatory capacity of OVA SSPs was almost completely gone (Bijker *et al.*, 2008), suggesting that in contrast to SLPs, the *in vivo* presentation of SSPs largely relies on the semiprofessional APC, predominantly the abundant B cells. In contrast, 15–30mer long peptides were found to reside selectively in $CD11c^{+}$ DC (Bijker *et al.*, 2008; Kitamura *et al.*, 2010). This striking difference suggests that targeting professional APC, preferably DC, is an important factor in the design of peptide vaccines. Interestingly, SLPs are well treated by DCs in that they are stored in long-lasting compartments from which the antigen can be retrieved for MHC-I presentation for several days (Faure *et al.*, 2009). In contrast, DCs pulsed with SSPs failed to stimulate CD8 T cells after the initial loading in MHC-I molecules at the cell surface, the presentation time of which is likely to depend on the off-rate of each particular SSP (van der Burg *et al.*, 1996). Further, elongation of nominal peptides at the N-terminus resulted in improved cross-presentation by DC, suggesting that processing-dependence converts peptides into better immunogens (Wei and Sherman, 2007). Importantly, SLPs are superior to proteins in eliciting protective CD8 T-cell responses. Proteins primarily induced antigen-specific CD4 T cells but were much less efficiently cross-presented (Zhang *et al.*, 2009). Thus, targeting of peptides to DC might be advantageous for many different peptides. Indeed, the "tolerizing" Ad5E1-derived SSP leads to protective T-cell responses if loaded on DC *in vitro* before injection (Toes *et al.*, 1998b). In addition, very strong uptake and storage in special storage compartments were observed when SSPs or SLPs were physically coupled to TLR ligands (Khan *et al.*, 2007). Encapsulation of peptides in formulations that target uptake receptors on DC might also increase their immunogenicity. *In vivo* targeted delivery of antigens to DC clearly constitutes the next step forward in vaccinology (Tacken *et al.*, 2007; Unger and van Kooyk, 2011; van Montfoort *et al.*, 2009). Together, these data show that for the stimulation of CD8 T-cell responses, peptides preferentially should be presented in MHC-I molecules of DC, but not other APC.

4. VACCINE-INDUCED HYPER REACTIVITY

4.1. Cytokine release syndrome

Peptide vaccines thus should obey a number of rules in order to become strong immune stimuli. To circumvent some of the deficits or to crank up the immune response to an even higher level, strong immunostimulatory agents have been applied in mouse models. Injection of SSPs in MPL admixed with IL-12 resulted in TNF-induced shock and death of mice within 24h (Bilsborough *et al.*, 2002). Similarly, vaccination of animals at the top of a virus-induced T-cell response with SSPs of virus epitopes in saline also resulted in a TNF-mediated lethal shock (Liu *et al.*, 2006). Most likely, this is the result of quick and wide spread biodistribution of these short peptides, leading to massive synchronous T-cell activation and strong cytokine release and/or to overwhelming systemic immune stimulation (Bilsborough *et al.*, 2002; Liu *et al.*, 2006). These adverse effects represented on-target toxicity and were reminiscent of the disaster of the agonistic antibody to CD28 that was applied to young volunteers, a study known as TGN1412 (Suntharalingam *et al.*, 2006). In relation to this, systemic administration of agonistic antibodies to CD40 is used to provide a strong APC activation signal for the boosting of T-cell responses. However, at the same time, this systemic application leads to antigen-independent cytokine release syndrome and splenomegaly (Fransen *et al.*, 2011; Vonderheide *et al.*, 2007). Spleen sizes roughly triple due to massive B cell proliferation. Interestingly, these symptoms can be curtailed by local administration of the antibody near the antigen site in a slow release depot without affecting its capacity to support the induction of antitumor T cells (Fransen *et al.*, 2011) and as such may safely support the immunogenicity of peptide vaccines. These results teach us that peptide vaccines should aim at providing a strong but localized immune stimulus.

Recently, two studies reported on the emergence of severe adverse events in mouse models for melanoma after vaccination with SLPs (Kitamura *et al.*, 2010; Ly *et al.*, 2010). Peptide vaccination in both systems resulted in cytokine release syndrome starting a few hours after peptide administration. The high blood levels of cytokines, including TNFα and IFNγ, led to multiorgan failure and death of the animals. These dramatic symptoms resulted from a synchronous and massive activation of peptide-specific T cells, pointing to the highly efficient activation by SLPs. However, the side effects in the animal models were only observed after adoptively transferred transgenic T cells that were stimulated with multiple injections of SLP vaccines. Although the use of transgenic T cells is artificial and comparable findings have not been described yet with endogenous T-cell repertoires, these data demonstrate that the power of SLP vaccines can be detrimental. Clearly, the potency of currently available vaccines requires careful considerations to harness the destructive strength of T-cell immunity. Interestingly, in one study, the adverse events were prevented when the 20-mer SLP—aiming to induce a strong CD8 T-cell response—was administered in an IFA depot, which slowly distributed their constituents in the animal and thereby prevented systemic and synchronous T-cell activation (Ly *et al.*, 2010). As such, these findings were alike previous observations with SSP vaccines that also quickly released peptides in an immune system with specific T cells in high frequency (Bilsborough *et al.*, 2002; Liu *et al.*, 2006). We like to emphasize that long peptides are commonly released to the local lymph nodes only and are loaded on professional APCs. However, increased doses may result in more wide spread of the peptide and the described adverse effects, thus pointing at the importance of dose–response studies with peptide vaccines (Ly *et al.*, 2010). The other study made use of a 50-mer SLP comprising a CTL and T helper epitope, which systemically activated highly frequent peptide-specific TCR-transgenic CD4 T cells. These findings are one of this kind, as SLPs of this length have not widely been studied. Notably, the 50-mer SLP was mixed with the strong TLR agonist CpG and injected intraperitoneally. In view of the other studies and what we know concerning the important role of keeping the stimulation localized, it does not come as a surprise that systemic stimulation with peptide and

CpG in the context of a vast number of antigen-specific CD4 T cells results in cytokine release syndrome. This notion is sustained by another study in which a 98-mer SLP was used to stimulate CD8 T-cell responses from the endogenous T-cell repertoire of mice. Vaccination with this 98-mer SLP in combination with CpG induced strong CD8 T-cell responses which exceeded that of the responses induced by a 35-mer SLP plus CpG (Welters *et al.*, 2004). In both cases, no adverse effects were found. Similarly, the injection of malaria LSA3-based SLPs of lengths ranging from 74 to over 100 amino acids were capable of inducing strong T-cell responses from the normal repertoire without serious effects (Perlaza *et al.*, 2001). Interestingly, no cytokine release syndrome was triggered in the aforementioned study when TCR-transgenic CD8 T cells were injected. This may be explained by the fact that the 50-mer SLP first has to be ingested and processed before it can be presented in MHC-I, and this process will lower the effective dose of peptides being presented via MHC-I. It is likely that the processing of the 50-mer SLP is much less efficient than the 20-mer SLP used in the mouse melanoma model where the 20-mer SLP did induce CD8 T-cell-mediated shock (Ly *et al.*, 2010). Of note, the 50-mer SLP can bind directly in the groove of MHC-II as this has two open ends explaining why it may trigger an efficient response by the CD4 TCR-transgenic mice (Kitamura *et al.*, 2010). In addition, the 50-mer long peptide might have evoked strong antibody responses, leading to formation of immunocomplexes *in vivo*, which are strong immunogens and activators of DCs (Schuurhuis *et al.*, 2000, 2006; van Montfoort *et al.*, 2009). This idea is supported by the fact that B-cell knockout animals did not display cytokine release syndrome after vaccination (Kitamura *et al.*, 2010). This explanation would also substantiate recent findings on the induction of peptide-specific antibody responses by SLPs.

4.2. Induction of anaphylactic shock by SLPs-specific antibodies

One recent paper reported the occurrence of systemic anaphylaxis after application of SLPs (Smith *et al.*, 2011). Analysis of the vaccine-induced immune response revealed the efficient generation of CD4 T helper cells and the generation of peptide-specific IgG and IgE antibodies. Serum titers were high at time of the booster vaccination and mice responded within minutes with anaphylaxis, accompanied with quick increase of blood histamine levels (Smith *et al.*, 2011). These detrimental effects were only observed when strong underlying CD4 T-cell responses were present and most peptides were coupled to KLH, a strong hapten that elicits strong CD4 T-cell immunity and is often coupled to proteins with the intention to evoke strong antibody responses (Ragupathi *et al.*, 2005). One peptide displayed similar features even without the KLH coupling, and moreover, we recently identified several other free long peptides with this allergenic capacity able to induce anaphylaxis within minutes (E. Quakkelaar and C. Melief, unpublished observations). Again, no adverse reactions were found when the booster vaccination was performed in slow release IFA depots. Finally, vaccine-induced antibodies to long peptides were detected in blood of patients who were treated with the HPV long peptide vaccine (our own unpublished data), whereas we never observed anaphylaxis in our patients, suggesting that it is not the presence of SLPs-specific antibodies *per se* that is associated with adverse events.

5. THE HALLMARKS OF PEPTIDE VACCINATION

The finding that an overlapping HPV16 SLP vaccine covering the amino acid sequence of the two HPV16 oncoproteins E6 and E7 admixed with the IFA-like mineral oil Montanide-51 was robust and installed vaccine-induced T-cell immunity in almost all injected patients at different stages of disease was satisfying and certainly functions as a solid stepping stone allowing the development of peptide vaccines for the treatment of cancer (van der Burg and Melief, 2011; van der Burg *et al.*, 2011). The strong immunogenicity of this type of vaccines is not restricted to viral antigens *per se* as phase I/II trials in patients with colorectal cancer and ovarian cancer have shown that SLP vaccines comprising "self"-p53 sequences display the capacity to induce T-cell responses with similar robustness (Leffers *et al.*, 2009, 2012; Speetjens *et al.*, 2009).

An aspect which so far has not been touched upon concerns the breadth of the induced T-cell response by peptide vaccines. Although the number of T-cell epitopes targeted within a peptide vaccine is not a parameter that influences the success of peptide vaccine to induce a T-cell response, it may impact, however, the clinical success of the whole approach. On the one hand, inducing T-cell immunity against an array of epitopes may suppress complete escape of tumor when the presentation of one or more epitopes is downregulated. On the other, attack of chronic diseases may require the full strength of the immune system in order to reinforce the protective arms of immunity which have been successfully deregulated during the establishment of disease. Vaccine-induced increases of the breadth of the T-cell response against murine cytomegalovirus enhanced the level of protection with each increase in the number of antigens injected to finally a complete protection against viral replication (Morello *et al.*, 2002). Also our own studies on immune correlates of vaccine-induced regression of HPV-induced premalignant lesions in vaccinated patients revealed that success was correlated with the breadth of the induced T-cell response (Kenter *et al.*, 2009; Welters *et al.*, 2010).

We discussed seven different parameters in the design of peptide vaccines which all bear impact on the outcome of peptide vaccines,

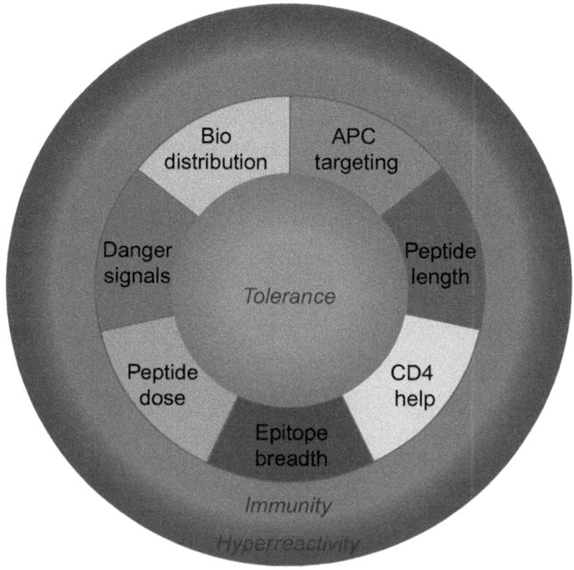

FIGURE 3.1 Diagram representing the hallmarks of peptide vaccination. Seven independent parameters have decisive influence on the immunological outcome of peptide vaccination. Steering on these parameters in the design of peptide vaccines guides toward protective T-cell-mediated immunity. Vaccine-induced tolerance or hyperreactivity is unwanted outcomes that can be prevented by adjustments in one of the seven parameters. In analogy to the hallmarks of cancer of Hanahan and Weinberg, we adapted the figure to represent the hallmarks of peptide vaccination. (See Color Insert.)

which can be protective immunity, induction of tolerance or, in some situations, even an overshoot of T-cell reactivity. Each of these individual hallmarks (Fig. 3.1) has to be carefully considered in the design of a peptide vaccine as each choice may have direct consequences on the influence of one of the other parameters.

ACKNOWLEDGMENTS

Financial support for our vaccination studies was provided by the Dutch Cancer Society (2009–4400 and 2010–4785) and the Netherlands Organization for Scientific Research Zon/Mw (917.56.311; 920.03.425 and 40.008.12.98.09012).

REFERENCES

Aichele, P., Hengartner, H., Zinkernagel, R. M., and Schulz, M. (1990). Antiviral cytotoxic T cell response induced by in vivo priming with a free synthetic peptide. *J. Exp. Med.* **171** (5), 1815–1820.

Aichele, P., Brduscha-Riem, K., Zinkernagel, R. M., Hengartner, H., and Pircher, H. (1995). T cell priming versus T cell tolerance induced by synthetic peptides. *J. Exp. Med.* **182**(1), 261–266.

Ali, O. A., Emerich, D., Dranoff, G., and Mooney, D. J. (2009). In situ regulation of DC subsets and T cells mediates tumor regression in mice. *Sci. Transl. Med.* **1**(8), 8ra19.

Ali, O. A., Doherty, E., Bell, W. J., Fradet, T., Hudak, J., Laliberte, M. T., Mooney, D. J., and Emerich, D. F. (2011). Biomaterial-based vaccine induces regression of established intracranial glioma in rats. *Pharm. Res.* **28**(5), 1074–1080.

Amoscato, A. A., Prenovitz, D. A., and Lotze, M. T. (1998). Rapid extracellular degradation of synthetic class I peptides by human dendritic cells. *J. Immunol.* **161**(8), 4023–4032.

Anderson, M. S., and Su, M. A. (2011). Aire and T cell development. *Curr. Opin. Immunol.* **23** (2), 198–206.

Anderson, C. C., Carroll, J. M., Gallucci, S., Ridge, J. P., Cheever, A. W., and Matzinger, P. (2001). Testing time-, ignorance-, and danger-based models of tolerance. *J. Immunol.* **166** (6), 3663–3671.

Assudani, D., Cho, H. I., DeVito, N., Bradley, N., and Celis, E. (2008). In vivo expansion, persistence, and function of peptide vaccine-induced CD8 T cells occur independently of CD4 T cells. *Cancer Res.* **68**(23), 9892–9899.

Bennett, S. R., Carbone, F. R., Toy, T., Miller, J. F., and Heath, W. R. (1998). B cells directly tolerize CD8(+) T cells. *J. Exp. Med.* **188**(11), 1977–1983.

Bijker, M. S., van den Eeden, S. J., Franken, K. L., Melief, C. J., Offringa, R., and van der Burg, S. H. (2007a). CD8+ CTL priming by exact peptide epitopes in incomplete Freund's adjuvant induces a vanishing CTL response, whereas long peptides induce sustained CTL reactivity. *J. Immunol.* **179**(8), 5033–5040.

Bijker, M. S., Melief, C. J., Offringa, R., and van der Burg, S. H. (2007b). Design and development of synthetic peptide vaccines: Past, present and future. *Expert Rev. Vaccines* **6**(4), 591–603.

Bijker, M. S., van den Eeden, S. J., Franken, K. L., Melief, C. J., van der Burg, S. H., and Offringa, R. (2008). Superior induction of anti-tumor CTL immunity by extended peptide vaccines involves prolonged, DC-focused antigen presentation. *Eur. J. Immunol.* **38**(4), 1033–1042.

Bilsborough, J., Uyttenhove, C., Colau, D., Bousso, P., Libert, C., Weynand, B., Boon, T., and van den Eynde, B. J. (2002). TNF-mediated toxicity after massive induction of specific CD8+ T cells following immunization of mice with a tumor-specific peptide. *J. Immunol.* **169**(6), 3053–3060.

Bjorkman, P. J., Saper, M. A., Samraoui, B., Bennett, W. S., Strominger, J. L., and Wiley, D. C. (1987a). Structure of the human class I histocompatibility antigen, HLA-A2. *Nature* **329** (6139), 506–512.

Bjorkman, P. J., Saper, M. A., Samraoui, B., Bennett, W. S., Strominger, J. L., and Wiley, D. C. (1987b). The foreign antigen binding site and T cell recognition regions of class I histocompatibility antigens. *Nature* **329**(6139), 512–518.

Blair, D. A., Turner, D. L., Bose, T. O., Pham, Q. M., Bouchard, K. R., Williams, K. J., McAleer, J. P., Cauley, L. S., Vella, A. T., and Lefrancois, L. (2011). Duration of antigen availability influences the expansion and memory differentiation of T cells. *J. Immunol.* **187**(5), 2310–2321.

Bos, R., and Sherman, L. A. (2010). CD4+ T-cell help in the tumor milieu is required for recruitment and cytolytic function of CD8+ T lymphocytes. *Cancer Res.* **70**(21), 8368–8377.

Carbone, F. R., Kurts, C., Bennett, S. R., Miller, J. F., and Heath, W. R. (1998). Cross-presentation: A general mechanism for CTL immunity and tolerance. *Immunol. Today* **19**(8), 368–373.

Cho, H. I., and Celis, E. (2009). Optimized peptide vaccines eliciting extensive CD8 T-cell responses with therapeutic antitumor effects. *Cancer Res.* **69**(23), 9012–9019.

Cho, H. I., and Celis, E. (2010). Overcoming doubts and other obstacles in the development of effective peptide-based therapeutic vaccines against cancer. *Expert Rev. Vaccines* **9**(4), 343–345.

Daftarian, P. M., Mansour, M., Pohajdak, B., Fuentes-Ortega, A., Korets-Smith, E., Macdonald, L., Weir, G., Brown, R. G., and Kast, W. M. (2007). Rejection of large HPV-16 expressing tumors in aged mice by a single immunization of VacciMax encapsulated CTL/T helper peptides. *J. Transl. Med.* **5,** 26.

Daniel, C., Weigmann, B., Bronson, R., and von Boehmer, H. (2011). Prevention of type 1 diabetes in mice by tolerogenic vaccination with a strong agonist insulin mimetope. *J. Exp. Med.* **208**(7), 1501–1510.

den Boer, A. T., Diehl, L., van Mierlo, G. J., van der Voort, E. I., Fransen, M. F., Krimpenfort, P., Melief, C. J., Offringa, R., and Toes, R. E. (2001). Longevity of antigen presentation and activation status of APC are decisive factors in the balance between CTL immunity versus tolerance. *J. Immunol.* **167**(5), 2522–2528.

den Boer, A. T., van Mierlo, G. J., Fransen, M. F., Melief, C. J., Offringa, R., and Toes, R. E. (2004). The tumoricidal activity of memory CD8+ T cells is hampered by persistent systemic antigen, but full functional capacity is regained in an antigen-free environment. *J. Immunol.* **172**(10), 6074–6079.

Deres, K., Schild, H., Wiesmuller, K. H., Jung, G., and Rammensee, H. G. (1989). In vivo priming of virus-specific cytotoxic T lymphocytes with synthetic lipopeptide vaccine. *Nature* **342**(6249), 561–564.

Diehl, L., den Boer, A. T., Schoenberger, S. P., van der Voort, E. I., Schumacher, T. N., Melief, C. J., Offringa, R., and Toes, R. E. (1999). CD40 activation in vivo overcomes peptide-induced peripheral cytotoxic T-lymphocyte tolerance and augments anti-tumor vaccine efficacy. *Nat. Med.* **5**(7), 774–779.

Diehl, L., Den Boer, A. T., van der Voort, E. I., Melief, C. J., Offringa, R., and Toes, R. E. (2000). The role of CD40 in peripheral T cell tolerance and immunity. *J. Mol. Med.* **78**(7), 363–371.

Diehl, L., van Mierlo, G. J., den Boer, A. T., van der Voort, E., Fransen, M., van Bostelen, L., Krimpenfort, P., Melief, C. J., Mittler, R., Toes, R. E., and Offringa, R. (2002). In vivo triggering through 4-1BB enables Th-independent priming of CTL in the presence of an intact CD28 costimulatory pathway. *J. Immunol.* **168**(8), 3755–3762.

Duthie, M. S., Windish, H. P., Fox, C. B., and Reed, S. G. (2011). Use of defined TLR ligands as adjuvants within human vaccines. *Immunol. Rev.* **239**(1), 178–196.

Falo, L. D., Jr., Colarusso, L. J., Benacerraf, B., and Rock, K. L. (1992). Serum proteases alter the antigenicity of peptides presented by class I major histocompatibility complex molecules. *Proc. Natl. Acad. Sci. USA* **89**(17), 8347–8350.

Faure, F., Mantegazza, A., Sadaka, C., Sedlik, C., Jotereau, F., and Amigorena, S. (2009). Long-lasting cross-presentation of tumor antigen in human DC. *Eur. J. Immunol.* **39**(2), 380–390.

Fayolle, C., Deriaud, E., and Leclerc, C. (1991). In vivo induction of cytotoxic T cell response by a free synthetic peptide requires CD4+ T cell help. *J. Immunol.* **147**(12), 4069–4073.

Fayolle, C., Abdel-Motal, U. M., Berg, L., Deriaud, E., Jondal, M., and Leclerc, C. (1996). Induction of cytotoxic T-cell response by optimal-length peptides does not require CD4+ T-cell help. *Immunology* **89**(1), 41–45.

Feltkamp, M. C., Smits, H. L., Vierboom, M. P., Minnaar, R. P., de Jongh, B. M., Drijfhout, J. W., ter Schegget, J., Melief, C. J., and Kast, W. M. (1993). Vaccination with cytotoxic T lymphocyte epitope-containing peptide protects against a tumor induced by human papillomavirus type 16-transformed cells. *Eur. J. Immunol.* **23**(9), 2242–2249.

Feltkamp, M. C., Vreugdenhil, G. R., Vierboom, M. P., Ras, E., van der Burg, S. H., ter Schegget, J., Melief, C. J., and Kast, W. M. (1995). Cytotoxic T lymphocytes raised against a subdominant epitope offered as a synthetic peptide eradicate human papillomavirus type 16-induced tumors. *Eur. J. Immunol.* **25**(9), 2638–2642.

Fransen, M. F., Sluijter, M., Morreau, H., Arens, R., and Melief, C. J. (2011). Local activation of CD8 T cells and systemic tumor eradication without toxicity via slow release and local delivery of agonistic CD40 antibody. *Clin. Cancer Res.* **17**(8), 2270–2280.

Gao, X. M., Zheng, B., Liew, F. Y., Brett, S., and Tite, J. (1991). Priming of influenza virus-specific cytotoxic T lymphocytes vivo by short synthetic peptides. *J. Immunol.* **147**(10), 3268–3273.

Gritzapis, A. D., Voutsas, I. F., Lekka, E., Papamichail, M., and Baxevanis, C. N. (2010). Peptide vaccination breaks tolerance to HER-2/neu by generating vaccine-specific FasL (+) CD4(+) T cells: first evidence for intratumor apoptotic regulatory T cells. *Cancer Res.* **70**(7), 2686–2696.

Hambach, L., Aghai, Z., Pool, J., Kroger, N., and Goulmy, E. (2010). Peptide length extension skews the minor HA-1 antigen presentation toward activated dendritic cells but reduces its presentation efficiency. *J. Immunol.* **185**(8), 4582–4589.

Heath, W. R., and Carbone, F. R. (2001). Cross-presentation, dendritic cells, tolerance and immunity. *Annu. Rev. Immunol.* **19,** 47–64.

Janeway, C. A., Jr., and Medzhitov, R. (2002). Innate immune recognition. *Annu. Rev. Immunol.* **20,** 197–216.

Janssen, E. M., Lemmens, E. E., Wolfe, T., Christen, U., von Herrath, M. G., and Schoenberger, S. P. (2003). CD4+ T cells are required for secondary expansion and memory in CD8+ T lymphocytes. *Nature* **421**(6925), 852–856.

Jensen, F. C., Savary, J. R., Diveley, J. P., and Chang, J. C. (1998). Adjuvant activity of incomplete Freund's adjuvant. *Adv. Drug Deliv. Rev.* **32**(3), 173–186.

Jung, S., Unutmaz, D., Wong, P., Sano, G., De los Santos, K., Sparwasser, T., Wu, S., Vuthoori, S., Ko, K., Zavala, F., Pamer, E. G., Littman, D. R., *et al.* (2002). In vivo depletion of CD11c+ dendritic cells abrogates priming of CD8+ T cells by exogenous cell-associated antigens. *Immunity* **17**(2), 211–220.

Kast, W. M., Roux, L., Curren, J., Blom, H. J., Voordouw, A. C., Meloen, R. H., Kolakofsky, D., and Melief, C. J. (1991). Protection against lethal Sendai virus infection by in vivo priming of virus-specific cytotoxic T lymphocytes with a free synthetic peptide. *Proc. Natl. Acad. Sci. USA* **88**(6), 2283–2287.

Kast, W. M., Brandt, R. M., and Melief, C. J. (1993). Strict peptide length is not required for the induction of cytotoxic T lymphocyte-mediated antiviral protection by peptide vaccination. *Eur. J. Immunol.* **23**(5), 1189–1192.

Kenter, G. G., Welters, M. J., Valentijn, A. R., Lowik, M. J., Berends-van der Meer, D. M., Vloon, A. P., Drijfhout, J. W., Wafelman, A. R., Oostendorp, J., Fleuren, G. J., Offringa, R., van der Burg, S. H., *et al.* (2008). Phase I immunotherapeutic trial with long peptides spanning the E6 and E7 sequences of high-risk human papillomavirus 16 in end-stage cervical cancer patients shows low toxicity and robust immunogenicity. *Clin. Cancer Res.* **14**(1), 169–177.

Kenter, G. G., Welters, M. J., Valentijn, A. R., Lowik, M. J., Berends-van der Meer, D. M., Vloon, A. P., Essahsah, F., Fathers, L. M., Offringa, R., Drijfhout, J. W., Wafelman, A. R., Oostendorp, J., *et al.* (2009). Vaccination against HPV-16 oncoproteins for vulvar intraepithelial neoplasia. *N. Engl. J. Med.* **361**(19), 1838–1847.

Khan, S., Bijker, M. S., Weterings, J. J., Tanke, H. J., Adema, G. J., van Hall, T., Drijfhout, J. W., Melief, C. J., Overkleeft, H. S., van der Marel, G. A., Filippov, D. V., van der Burg, S. H., *et al.* (2007). Distinct uptake mechanisms but similar intracellular processing of two different toll-like receptor ligand-peptide conjugates in dendritic cells. *J. Biol. Chem.* **282** (29), 21145–21159.

Kitamura, H., Sedlik, C., Jacquet, A., Zaragoza, B., Dusseaux, M., Premel, V., Sastre-Garau, X., and Lantz, O. (2010). Long peptide vaccination can lead to lethality through CD4+ T cell-mediated cytokine storm. *J. Immunol.* **185**(2), 892–901.

Klein, L., Hinterberger, M., Wirnsberger, G., and Kyewski, B. (2009). Antigen presentation in the thymus for positive selection and central tolerance induction. *Nat. Rev. Immunol.* **9** (12), 833–844.

Kyburz, D., Aichele, P., Speiser, D. E., Hengartner, H., Zinkernagel, R. M., and Pircher, H. (1993). T cell immunity after a viral infection versus T cell tolerance induced by soluble viral peptides. *Eur. J. Immunol.* **23**(8), 1956–1962.

Larsen, S. L., Pedersen, L. O., Buus, S., and Stryhn, A. (1996). T cell responses affected by aminopeptidase N (CD13)-mediated trimming of major histocompatibility complex class II-bound peptides. *J. Exp. Med.* **184**(1), 183–189.

Leffers, N., Lambeck, A. J., Gooden, M. J., Hoogeboom, B. N., Wolf, R., Hamming, I. E., Hepkema, B. G., Willemse, P. H., Molmans, B. H., Hollema, H., Drijfhout, J. W., Sluiter, W. J., *et al.* (2009). Immunization with a P53 synthetic long peptide vaccine induces P53-specific immune responses in ovarian cancer patients, a phase II trial. *Int. J. Cancer* **125**(9), 2104–2113.

Leffers, N., Vermeij, R., Hoogeboom, B. N., Schulze, U. R., Wolf, R., Hamming, I. E., van der Zee, A. G., Melief, K. J., van der Burg, S. H., Daemen, T., and Nijman, H. W. (2012). Long-term clinical and immunological effects of p53-SLP(R) vaccine in patients with ovarian cancer. *Int. J. Cancer* **130**(1), 105–112. doi: 10.1002/ijc.25980.

Liu, F., Feuer, R., Hassett, D. E., and Whitton, J. L. (2006). Peptide vaccination of mice immune to LCMV or vaccinia virus causes serious CD8 T cell-mediated, TNF-dependent immunopathology. *J. Clin. Invest.* **116**(2), 465–475.

Luckashenak, N., Schroeder, S., Endt, K., Schmidt, D., Mahnke, K., Bachmann, M. F., Marconi, P., Deeg, C. A., and Brocker, T. (2008). Constitutive crosspresentation of tissue antigens by dendritic cells controls CD8+ T cell tolerance in vivo. *Immunity* **28**(4), 521–532.

Ly, L. V., Sluijter, M., Versluis, M., Luyten, G. P., van Stipdonk, M. J., van der Burg, S. H., Melief, C. J., Jager, M. J., and van Hall, T. (2010). Peptide vaccination after T-cell transfer causes massive clonal expansion, tumor eradication, and manageable cytokine storm. *Cancer Res.* **70**(21), 8339–8346.

Mandelboim, O., Vadai, E., Fridkin, M., Katz-Hillel, A., Feldman, M., Berke, G., and Eisenbach, L. (1995). Regression of established murine carcinoma metastases following vaccination with tumour-associated antigen peptides. *Nat. Med.* **1**(11), 1179–1183.

Mansour, M., Pohajdak, B., Kast, W. M., Fuentes-Ortega, A., Korets-Smith, E., Weir, G. M., Brown, R. G., and Daftarian, P. (2007). Therapy of established B16-F10 melanoma tumors by a single vaccination of CTL/T helper peptides in VacciMax. *J. Transl. Med.* **5,** 20.

Matzinger, P. (1994). Tolerance, danger, and the extended family. *Annu. Rev. Immunol.* **12,** 991–1045.

Matzinger, P. (2002). The danger model: A renewed sense of self. *Science* **296**(5566), 301–305.

Melief, C. J., and van der Burg, S. H. (2008). Immunotherapy of established (pre)malignant disease by synthetic long peptide vaccines. *Nat. Rev. Cancer* **8**(5), 351–360.

Mocellin, S., Mandruzzato, S., Bronte, V., Lise, M., and Nitti, D. (2004). Part I: Vaccines for solid tumours. *Lancet Oncol.* **5**(11), 681–689.

Morello, C. S., Ye, M., and Spector, D. H. (2002). Development of a vaccine against murine cytomegalovirus (MCMV), consisting of plasmid DNA and formalin-inactivated MCMV, that provides long-term, complete protection against viral replication. *J. Virol.* **76**(10), 4822–4835.

Mueller, M., Schlosser, E., Gander, B., and Groettrup, M. (2011). Tumor eradication by immunotherapy with biodegradable PLGA microspheres—An alternative to incomplete Freund's adjuvant. *Int. J. Cancer* **129**(2), 407–416.

Nakanishi, Y., Lu, B., Gerard, C., and Iwasaki, A. (2009). CD8(+) T lymphocyte mobilization to virus-infected tissue requires CD4(+) T-cell help. *Nature* **462**(7272), 510–513.

Noguchi, Y., Chen, Y. T., and Old, L. J. (1994). A mouse mutant p53 product recognized by CD4+ and CD8+ T cells. *Proc. Natl. Acad. Sci. USA* **91**(8), 3171–3175.

Ossendorp, F., Mengede, E., Camps, M., Filius, R., and Melief, C. J. (1998). Specific T helper cell requirement for optimal induction of cytotoxic T lymphocytes against major histocompatibility complex class II negative tumors. *J. Exp. Med.* **187**(5), 693–702.

Ossendorp, F., Toes, R. E., Offringa, R., van der Burg, S. H., and Melief, C. J. (2000). Importance of CD4(+) T helper cell responses in tumor immunity. *Immunol. Lett.* **74**(1), 75–79.

Perez, S. A., von Hofe, E., Kallinteris, N. L., Gritzapis, A. D., Peoples, G. E., Papamichail, M., and Baxevanis, C. N. (2010). A new era in anticancer peptide vaccines. *Cancer* **116**(9), 2071–2080.

Perlaza, B. L., Sauzet, J. P., Balde, A. T., Brahimi, K., Tall, A., Corradin, G., and Druilhe, P. (2001). Long synthetic peptides encompassing the Plasmodium falciparum LSA3 are the target of human B and T cells and are potent inducers of B helper, T helper and cytolytic T cell responses in mice. *Eur. J. Immunol.* **31**(7), 2200–2209.

Piccinini, A. M., and Midwood, K. S. (2010). DAMPening inflammation by modulating TLR signalling. *Mediators Inflamm.* **2010,** 1–21. doi: 10.1155/2010/672395.

Purcell, A. W., McCluskey, J., and Rossjohn, J. (2007). More than one reason to rethink the use of peptides in vaccine design. *Nat. Rev. Drug Discov.* **6**(5), 404–414.

Ragupathi, G., Gathuru, J., and Livingston, P. (2005). Antibody inducing polyvalent cancer vaccines. *Cancer Treat. Res.* **123,** 157–180.

Reinholdsson-Ljunggren, G., Ramqvist, T., Ahrlund-Richter, L., and Dalianis, T. (1992). Immunization against polyoma tumors with synthetic peptides derived from the sequences of middle- and large-T antigens. *Int. J. Cancer* **50**(1), 142–146.

Reiser, M., Wieland, A., Plachter, B., Mertens, T., Greiner, J., and Schirmbeck, R. (2011). The immunodominant CD8 T cell response to the human cytomegalovirus tegument phosphoprotein pp65(495–503) epitope critically depends on CD4 T cell help in vaccinated HLA-A*0201 transgenic mice. *J. Immunol.* **187**(5), 2172–2180.

Ribas, A., Weber, J. S., Chmielowski, B., Comin-Anduix, B., Lu, D., Douek, M., Ragavendra, N., Raman, S., Seja, E., Rosario, D., Miles, S., Diamond, D. C., *et al.* (2011). Intra-lymph node prime-boost vaccination against Melan A and tyrosinase for the treatment of metastatic melanoma: Results of a phase 1 clinical trial. *Clin. Cancer Res.* **17**(9), 2987–2996.

Rosenberg, S. A., Yang, J. C., and Restifo, N. P. (2004). Cancer immunotherapy: Moving beyond current vaccines. *Nat. Med.* **10**(9), 909–915.

Rotzschke, O., Falk, K., Deres, K., Schild, H., Norda, M., Metzger, J., Jung, G., and Rammensee, H. G. (1990a). Isolation and analysis of naturally processed viral peptides as recognized by cytotoxic T cells. *Nature* **348**(6298), 252–254.

Rotzschke, O., Falk, K., Wallny, H. J., Faath, S., and Rammensee, H. G. (1990b). Characterization of naturally occurring minor histocompatibility peptides including H-4 and H-Y. *Science* **249**(4966), 283–287.

Salek-Ardakani, S., Moutaftsi, M., Sette, A., and Croft, M. (2011a). Targeting OX40 promotes lung-resident memory CD8 T cell populations that protect against respiratory poxvirus infection. *J. Virol.* **85**(17), 9051–9059.

Salek-Ardakani, S., Flynn, R., Arens, R., Yagita, H., Smith, G. L., Borst, J., Schoenberger, S. P., and Croft, M. (2011b). The TNFR family members OX40 and CD27 link viral virulence to protective T cell vaccines in mice. *J. Clin. Invest.* **121**(1), 296–307.

Sallusto, F., and Lanzavecchia, A. (2009). Heterogeneity of CD4+ memory T cells: Functional modules for tailored immunity. *Eur. J. Immunol.* **39**(8), 2076–2082.

Schliehe, C., Redaelli, C., Engelhardt, S., Fehlings, M., Mueller, M., van Rooijen, N., Thiry, M., Hildner, K., Weller, H., and Groettrup, M. (2011). CD8− dendritic cells and macrophages cross-present poly(D, L-lactate-co-glycolate) acid microsphere-encapsulated antigen in vivo. *J. Immunol.* **187**(5), 2112–2121.

Schulz, M., Zinkernagel, R. M., and Hengartner, H. (1991). Peptide-induced antiviral protection by cytotoxic T cells. *Proc. Natl. Acad. Sci. USA* **88**(3), 991–993.

Schuurhuis, D. H., Laban, S., Toes, R. E., Ricciardi-Castagnoli, P., Kleijmeer, M. J., van der Voort, E. I., Rea, D., Offringa, R., Geuze, H. J., Melief, C. J., and Ossendorp, F. (2000). Immature dendritic cells acquire CD8(+) cytotoxic T lymphocyte priming capacity upon activation by T helper cell-independent or -dependent stimuli. *J. Exp. Med.* **192**(1), 145–150.

Schuurhuis, D. H., van Montfoort, N., Ioan-Facsinay, A., Jiawan, R., Camps, M., Nouta, J., Melief, C. J., Verbeek, J. S., and Ossendorp, F. (2006). Immune complex-loaded dendritic cells are superior to soluble immune complexes as antitumor vaccine. *J. Immunol.* **176**(8), 4573–4580.

Sette, A., Newman, M., Livingston, B., McKinney, D., Sidney, J., Ishioka, G., Tangri, S., Alexander, J., Fikes, J., and Chesnut, R. (2002). Optimizing vaccine design for cellular processing, MHC binding and TCR recognition. *Tissue Antigens* **59**(6), 443–451.

Smith, C. M., Bradding, P., Neill, D. R., Baxendale, H., Felici, F., and Andrew, P. W. (2011). Novel immunogenic peptides elicit systemic anaphylaxis in mice: Implications for Peptide vaccines. *J. Immunol.* **187**(3), 1201–1206.

Speetjens, F. M., Kuppen, P. J., Welters, M. J., Essahsah, F., Voet van den Brink, A. M., Lantrua, M. G., Valentijn, A. R., Oostendorp, J., Fathers, L. M., Nijman, H. W., Drijfhout, J. W., van de Velde, C. J., *et al.* (2009). Induction of p53-specific immunity by a p53 synthetic long peptide vaccine in patients treated for metastatic colorectal cancer. *Clin. Cancer Res.* **15**(3), 1086–1095.

Suntharalingam, G., Perry, M. R., Ward, S., Brett, S. J., Castello-Cortes, A., Brunner, M. D., and Panoskaltsis, N. (2006). Cytokine storm in a phase 1 trial of the anti-CD28 monoclonal antibody TGN1412. *N. Engl. J. Med.* **355**(10), 1018–1028.

Tacken, P. J., de Vries, I. J., Torensma, R., and Figdor, C. G. (2007). Dendritic-cell immunotherapy: From ex vivo loading to in vivo targeting. *Nat. Rev. Immunol.* **7**(10), 790–802.

Toes, R. E., Blom, R. J., Offringa, R., Kast, W. M., and Melief, C. J. (1996a). Enhanced tumor outgrowth after peptide vaccination. Functional deletion of tumor-specific CTL induced by peptide vaccination can lead to the inability to reject tumors. *J. Immunol.* **156**(10), 3911–3918.

Toes, R. E., Offringa, R., Blom, R. J., Melief, C. J., and Kast, W. M. (1996b). Peptide vaccination can lead to enhanced tumor growth through specific T-cell tolerance induction. *Proc. Natl. Acad. Sci. USA* **93**(15), 7855–7860.

Toes, R. E., Schoenberger, S. P., van der Voort, E. I., Offringa, R., and Melief, C. J. (1998a). CD40-CD40 ligand interactions and their role in cytotoxic T lymphocyte priming and anti-tumor immunity. *Semin. Immunol.* **10**(6), 443–448.

Toes, R. E., van der Voort, E. I., Schoenberger, S. P., Drijfhout, J. W., van Bloois, L., Storm, G., Kast, W. M., Offringa, R., and Melief, C. J. (1998b). Enhancement of tumor outgrowth through CTL tolerization after peptide vaccination is avoided by peptide presentation on dendritic cells. *J. Immunol.* **160**(9), 4449–4456.

Toes, R. E., Ossendorp, F., Offringa, R., and Melief, C. J. (1999). CD4 T cells and their role in antitumor immune responses. *J. Exp. Med.* **189**(5), 753–756.

Townsend, A. R., Rothbard, J., Gotch, F. M., Bahadur, G., Wraith, D., and McMichael, A. J. (1986). The epitopes of influenza nucleoprotein recognized by cytotoxic T lymphocytes can be defined with short synthetic peptides. *Cell* **44**(6), 959–968.

Unger, W. W., and van Kooyk, Y. (2011). 'Dressed for success' C-type lectin receptors for the delivery of glyco-vaccines to dendritic cells. *Curr. Opin. Immunol.* **23**(1), 131–137.

van der Burg, S. H., and Melief, C. J. (2011). Therapeutic vaccination against human papilloma virus induced malignancies. *Curr. Opin. Immunol.* **23**(2), 252–257.

van der Burg, S. H., Visseren, M. J., Brandt, R. M., Kast, W. M., and Melief, C. J. (1996). Immunogenicity of peptides bound to MHC class I molecules depends on the MHC-peptide complex stability. *J. Immunol.* **156**(9), 3308–3314.

van der Burg, S. H., Bijker, M. S., Welters, M. J., Offringa, R., and Melief, C. J. (2006). Improved peptide vaccine strategies, creating synthetic artificial infections to maximize immune efficacy. *Adv. Drug Deliv. Rev.* **58**(8), 916–930.

van der Burg, S. H., Arens, R., and Melief, C. J. (2011). Immunotherapy for persistent viral infections and associated disease. *Trends Immunol.* **32**(3), 97–103.

van Montfoort, N., Camps, M. G., Khan, S., Filippov, D. V., Weterings, J. J., Griffith, J. M., Geuze, H. J., van Hall, T., Verbeek, J. S., Melief, C. J., and Ossendorp, F. (2009). Antigen storage compartments in mature dendritic cells facilitate prolonged cytotoxic T lymphocyte cross-priming capacity. *Proc. Natl. Acad. Sci. USA* **106**(16), 6730–6735.

Vonderheide, R. H., Flaherty, K. T., Khalil, M., Stumacher, M. S., Bajor, D. L., Hutnick, N. A., Sullivan, P., Mahany, J. J., Gallagher, M., Kramer, A., Green, S. J., O'Dwyer, P. J., *et al.* (2007). Clinical activity and immune modulation in cancer patients treated with CP-870,893, a novel CD40 agonist monoclonal antibody. *J. Clin. Oncol.* **25**(7), 876–883.

Wei, C. H., and Sherman, L. A. (2007). N-terminal trimer extension of nominal CD8 T cell epitopes is sufficient to promote cross-presentation to cognate CD8 T cells in vivo. *J. Immunol.* **179**(12), 8280–8286.

Weijzen, S., Meredith, S. C., Velders, M. P., Elmishad, A. G., Schreiber, H., and Kast, W. M. (2001). Pharmacokinetic differences between a T cell-tolerizing and a T cell-activating peptide. *J. Immunol.* **166**(12), 7151–7157.

Wells, J. W., Choy, K., Lloyd, C. M., and Noble, A. (2009). Suppression of allergic airway inflammation and IgE responses by a class I restricted allergen peptide vaccine. *Mucosal Immunol.* **2**(1), 54–62.

Welters, M. J., Filippov, D. V., van den Eeden, S. J., Franken, K. L., Nouta, J., Valentijn, A. R., van der Marel, G. A., Overkleeft, H. S., Lipford, G., Offringa, R., Melief, C. J., van Boom, J. H., *et al.* (2004). Chemically synthesized protein as tumour-specific vaccine: Immunogenicity and efficacy of synthetic HPV16 E7 in the TC-1 mouse tumour model. *Vaccine* **23**(3), 305–311.

Welters, M. J., Bijker, M. S., van den Eeden, S. J., Franken, K. L., Melief, C. J., Offringa, R., and van der Burg, S. H. (2007). Multiple CD4 and CD8 T-cell activation parameters predict vaccine efficacy in vivo mediated by individual DC-activating agonists. *Vaccine* **25**(8), 1379–1389.

Welters, M. J., Kenter, G. G., Piersma, S. J., Vloon, A. P., Lowik, M. J., Berends-van der Meer, D. M., Drijfhout, J. W., Valentijn, A. R., Wafelman, A. R., Oostendorp, J., Fleuren, G. J., Offringa, R., *et al.* (2008). Induction of tumor-specific CD4+ and CD8+ T-cell immunity in cervical cancer patients by a human papillomavirus type 16 E6 and E7 long peptides vaccine. *Clin. Cancer Res.* **14**(1), 178–187.

Welters, M. J., Kenter, G. G., de Vos van Steenwijk, P. J., Lowik, M. J., Berends-van der Meer, D. M., Essahsah, F., Stynenbosch, L. F., Vloon, A. P., Ramwadhdoebe, T. H., Piersma, S. J., van der Hulst, J. M., Valentijn, A. R., *et al.* (2010). Success or failure of vaccination for HPV16-positive vulvar lesions correlates with kinetics and phenotype of induced T-cell responses. *Proc. Natl. Acad. Sci. USA* **107**(26), 11895–11899.

Wong, S. B., Bos, R., and Sherman, L. A. (2008). Tumor-specific CD4+ T cells render the tumor environment permissive for infiltration by low-avidity CD8+ T cells. *J. Immunol.* **180**(5), 3122–3131.

Zhang, H., Hong, H., Li, D., Ma, S., Di, Y., Stoten, A., Haig, N., Di Gleria, K., Yu, Z., Xu, X. N., McMichael, A., and Jiang, S. (2009). Comparing pooled peptides with intact protein for accessing cross-presentation pathways for protective CD8+ and CD4+ T cells. *J. Biol. Chem.* **284**(14), 9184–9191.

Zinkernagel, R. M., and Doherty, P. C. (1974). Restriction of in vitro T cell-mediated cytotoxicity in lymphocytic choriomeningitis within a syngeneic or semiallogeneic system. *Nature* **248**(450), 701–702.

Zwaveling, S., Ferreira Mota, S. C., Nouta, J., Johnson, M., Lipford, G. B., Offringa, R., van der Burg, S. H., and Melief, C. J. (2002). Established human papillomavirus type 16-expressing tumors are effectively eradicated following vaccination with long peptides. *J. Immunol.* **169**(1), 350–358.

CHAPTER 4

Experience with Synthetic Vaccines for Cancer and Persistent Virus Infections in Nonhuman Primates and Patients

Esther D. Quakkelaar* and **Cornelis J.M. Melief***,†

Contents

* Department of Immunohematology, Leiden University Medical Center, Leiden, The Netherlands
† Immune System Activation (ISA) Pharmaceuticals, Leiden, The Netherlands

Advances in Immunology, Volume 114
ISSN 0065-2776, DOI: 10.1016/B978-0-12-396548-6.00004-4

Abstract

Synthetic vaccines, in particular long synthetic peptides of approximately 25–50 amino acids in length, are attractive for HIV vaccine development and for induction of therapeutic immune responses in patients with (pre-)malignant disorders. In the case of preventive vaccine development against HIV, no major success has been achieved, but the possibilities are by no means exhausted. A long peptide vaccine consisting of 13 overlapping peptides, which together cover the entire length of the two oncogenic proteins E6 and E7 of high-risk human papilloma virus type 16 (HPV16), caused complete regression of all lesions and eradication of virus in 9 out of 20 women with high-grade vulvar intraepithelial neoplasia, a therapy-resistant preneoplastic disorder. The nature and strength of the vaccine-prompted T cell responses were significantly correlated with the clinical response. Synthetic peptide vaccines are attractive, because they allow rational improvement of vaccine design and detailed pharmacokinetic and pharmacodynamic studies not possible with conventional vaccines. Improvements are possible by addition or conjugation of adjuvants, notably TLR ligands, to the synthetic peptides.

1. INTRODUCTION

For about one and a half century, vaccine strategies were concerned with prophylactic vaccines that induce neutralizing antibodies to prevent infectious diseases. Although these strategies have been remarkably successful, effective prophylactic vaccines are not yet available against many pathogens that still pose large disease burdens caused by among others HIV-1, HCV, tuberculosis, and malaria. These infectious diseases are a major health concern, especially in developing countries in which they are a leading cause of death (Piot *et al.*, 2009). HIV-1 and HCV can induce chronic infections that persist lifelong in infected individuals, often leading to death if not treated (Halliday *et al.*, 2011; Piot *et al.*, 2009). In addition, natural infection does not protect against re-infections, which is also the case for malaria and tuberculosis (Crompton *et al.*, 2010; Ottenhoff *et al.*, 2010). A vaccine that confers protection against infection should thus be different from natural infection and superior in inducing immune responses (Roestenberg *et al.*, 2011). Although antiviral and antiparasite drug therapies are currently available for HIV-1 and malaria, these do not sufficiently reach people in developing countries and the associated socioeconomic costs are rising. This underscores the need for preventive and/or therapeutic vaccines to effectively reduce these epidemics. Although prophylactic vaccination is widely accepted and recognized, therapeutic vaccination is only in its infancy, but under intensive study in patients with persistent infection or cancer (Kantoff *et al.*, 2010; Kenter *et al.*, 2009).

2. VACCINATION OF CANCER PATIENTS

Therapeutic vaccination, in contrast to prophylactic vaccination, is focused on the induction of T cell responses in patients with established disease, such as patients with (pre-)malignant disease caused by oncogenic viruses. Therapeutic vaccination also aims at eliciting and enhancing tumor-specific immune responses in nonviral cancer. In all of these patients, the host immune system does not mount an effective antitumor immune response for numerous reasons. First, persistently infecting viruses or tumors utilize numerous escape mechanisms, making it difficult for the immune system to recognize and eliminate tumor cells (Melief, 2008) (see also Chapter 9). These include downregulation of HLA class I and II (Cabrera *et al.*, 2003; Seliger *et al.*, 2008), immunosuppressive factors within the tumor microenvironment (Botti *et al.*, 1998; Gajewski *et al.*, 2011; Youn and Gabrilovich, 2010), defects in antigen processing and presentation (Lampen and van Hall, 2011; Marincola *et al.*, 2000; Restifo *et al.*, 1993), and induction of T cell dysfunction (Demotte *et al.*, 2010; Kiessling *et al.*, 1999). Further, cancer cells are derived from self-tissue and are thus not recognized as foreign. In addition, nonviral cancer cells generally lack powerful danger signals such as TLR, NOD, and RIG-I ligands characteristic of most virulent pathogens (Melief, 2008). Immunotherapy that induces a robust effector T cell response directed against the tumor cells is thus a promising approach in the treatment of cancer. Vaccination with tumor-associated antigens (TAAs) provides an opportunity to induce tumor-specific T cell responses that can eradicate tumors. In the past years, several TAAs have been described that provide a basis for vaccination (Cheever *et al.*, 2009). Five categories of tumor antigens have so far been used in immunotherapy: mutated antigens (p53 or Ras), overexpressed self-antigens (Her-2/neu or mucin-1), differentiation antigen (gp100 or tyrosinase), cancer testis antigens (MAGE, BAGE, or GAGE families, NY-ESO-1), and viral antigens (HPV16 E6 or E7, EBV and others) (Cheever *et al.*, 2009). The role of viruses as causative agent of several cancers provides the opportunity to control certain cancer types through effective vaccination against the virus, such as HPV-induced cervical cancer (Melief and van der Burg, 2008; van der Burg *et al.*, 2011). Both viral antigens and TAA can thus be used for vaccination to induce tumor-specific T cell responses that specifically target tumor cells without targeting healthy cells (Cheever *et al.*, 2009; Melief and van der Burg, 2008; van der Burg *et al.*, 2011).

3. VACCINATION AGAINST HIV-1

In the case of HIV, the foremost problem appears to be the tremendous variability of the viral envelope proteins, thus causing great difficulties in generating neutralizing antibodies for effective vaccination (see Chapter 2). Considerable demand exists for a prophylactic vaccine that would be able to induce both neutralizing antibodies and robust T cell responses to fully exploit the two major arms of the adaptive immune system (McMichael *et al.*, 2010; Pantaleo *et al.*, 2010). Studies over the past decades have shown a role for the cellular immune system in shaping the viral infection. In the case of HIV-1, for example, ample evidence exists that CD8+ T cell responses can play a role in the disease outcome of infected individuals (Goulder and Watkins, 2008; McMichael *et al.*, 2010; Pereyra *et al.*, 2010). Studies in HIV-1-infected patients have shown that natural control of viral load is associated with potent and broad cellular immune responses which are mainly directed against the conserved Gag protein (Edwards *et al.*, 2002; Kiepiela *et al.*, 2007). A major role is ascribed to HLA class I resistant alleles such as HLA-B57, a molecule that is supremely capable of presenting several conserved epitopes of HIV Gag (Pereyra *et al.*, 2010; Streeck *et al.*, 2007). This indicates that some HIV-1-infected patients can mount a broad T cell response against conserved regions of HIV-1. Both CD8+ and CD4+ T cells are needed to control chronic virus infections (Harari and Pantaleo, 2008; Hill *et al.*, 2010; McMichael *et al.*, 2010; Pantaleo *et al.*, 2010). The current successful prophylactic vaccines that provide sterilizing immunity against, for example, measles are fully dependent on the induction of neutralizing antibodies that prevent the infection of host cells by steric hindrance or complement binding (Burton, 2002). However, extensive evidence exists that for some pathogens causing chronic disease, induction of neutralizing antibodies is not sufficient. Once the disease has established itself, effector T cell immunity is clearly needed (van der Burg *et al.*, 2011).

4. VACCINATION STRATEGIES

4.1. Successful vaccination strategies

The first generation vaccines, attenuated or inactivated whole-organisms, have proven successful in the eradication of smallpox and polio, and in prophylactic vaccination against measles, rubella, and diphtheria

(Amanna and Slifka, 2011; Burton, 2002). The protection induced by these vaccines is mediated by neutralizing antibodies that prevent infection of host cells (Burton, 2002). A second successful strategy that induces neutralizing antibodies is subunit vaccines. These vaccines consist of purified protein antigens or recombinant proteins, such as the surface or capsid proteins and have reduced safety issues compared to attenuated or inactivated whole-organisms. Subunit vaccines are applied for vaccination against hepatitis B (Huang *et al.*, 2011) and human papilloma virus (Frazer *et al.*, 2007; Schiller and Lowy, 2010).

4.2. Vaccination strategies under development

Numerous vaccination strategies are under development. One of these is a DNA vaccine that encodes specific proteins or antigens. DNA vaccination alone is not suitable for vaccination to induce robust and sustained T cell responses (McConkey *et al.*, 2003; Mwau *et al.*, 2004). This is mainly due to the fact that in the end, all vaccination results in protein/peptide presentation. DNA vaccines have to travel the long road from DNA to RNA to protein/peptides. Nevertheless, DNA vaccination has been shown to be an excellent priming principle. DNA vaccination is currently tested in a number or preclinical and clinical studies, mostly in prime-boost combination with viral vectors expressing the same antigens (Hill *et al.*, 2010; Pantaleo *et al.*, 2010).

Viral vectors are recombinant viruses that contain genetic material of the antigen of interest that will be delivered into cells. Viral vectors are, in general, derived from live viruses but can be modified such as by deletion of genes that encode proteins involved in viral replication or immunomodulation (Gomez *et al.*, 2008; Quakkelaar *et al.*, 2011). A number of virus families are under intensive development as vaccine vectors for human or veterinary use, both replication competent and attenuated viruses (Draper and Heeney, 2010). Recently, attenuated recombinant CMV virus, incorporating SIV antigens, has been studied in macaques (Hansen *et al.*, 2011). This viral vector established a persistent, high-frequency, SIV-specific effector memory T cell response in rhesus macaques that was able to control highly pathogenic SIV_{mac239} infection early after mucosal challenge (Hansen *et al.*, 2011). Nevertheless, combating AIDS by establishing persistent CMV infection poses serious safety concerns.

The main disadvantage of viral vectors is the huge amount of vector sequences in relation to the insert sequence. In the case of attenuated poxviruses such as ALVAC, MVA, and NYVAC, the insert sequence is frequently less than 2–3% of the total amount of sequences, depending on the size of the insert (Gomez *et al.*, 2007, 2011). Adenoviruses, other viral vectors under intense preclinical study, have a smaller genome, but adenovirus sequences are still much more numerous than the insert sequences (~15% of the total vector depending on the size of the insert). As these vector sequences outnumber the insert sequences, this results in antigenic competition between the vector and the insert protein (Jing *et al.*, 2005; McShane and Hill, 2005; Pasquetto *et al.*, 2005; van der Burg *et al.*, 2001).

A potentially promising development in synthetic vaccination is the generation of synthetic viruses. Synthetic viruses have recently been proposed as vaccine candidates (Wimmer and Paul, 2010). In particular, recoding of poliovirus or influenza virus shows promise for rapid generation of effective designer vaccines. This strategy follows from the advances that have been made during the past decades in DNA technology. Synthetic biology and chemical synthesis result in the *de novo* generation of viral genomes. In combination with changes in codon bias that leads to attenuation of viruses, this generates a new class of live but attenuated vaccines (Wimmer and Paul, 2010). These vaccines can be devoid of the unpredictable performance of, for example, attenuated or heat-killed (recombinant) organisms. In the case of development of vaccines against seasonal influenza, this approach can theoretically reduce the time needed for the development of the appropriate influenza virus vaccine variant.

Dendritic cell (DC)-based therapeutic vaccination has recently been approved for patients with hormone-resistant prostate cancer (Thara *et al.*, 2011). DCs are professional antigen-presenting cells that are specialized in uptake and processing to induce proper T cell responses. Therefore, this therapy is based on loading autologous DCs *ex vivo* with TAA and subsequent administration to patients to induce tumor-specific T cell responses (Banchereau *et al.*, 2001; Steinman and Pope, 2002). These vaccines can be effective in subgroups of patients (Boudreau *et al.*, 2011; Figdor *et al.*, 2004; Melief, 2008; Romani *et al.*, 2010; Steinman and Pope, 2002), but correlates of induced immune responses with cancer microenvironment and clinical outcome are needed (Gajewski *et al.*, 2011; van der Burg *et al.*, 2011). Unfortunately, clinical efficacy of such vaccines is still limited (Figdor *et al.*, 2004; Lesterhuis *et al.*, 2008). The generation of DCs *ex vivo* is very labor intensive and this vaccine strategy is patient specific. Further, DC vaccines need to travel to the lymph node to induce robust CD8+ T cell responses, whereas only a very limited number of the administered DCs reaches the lymph nodes (Lesterhuis *et al.*, 2008, 2011).

The advantages of vaccines such as DNA, proteins, and peptides are the relative ease of production and the absence of major safety and regulatory issues (Parvanova *et al.*, 2011). Further, in contrast to the laborious and patient-specific DC-based vaccines, synthetic vaccines are much less expensive, less laborious, and applicable as standardized drugs to large groups of patients. Further, the absence of unrelated sequences such as viral sequences reduces the antigenic competition between antigen-specific and unrelated sequences for the induction of T cell responses.

5. SYNTHETIC LONG PEPTIDE VACCINE

Recent developments in vaccine research have described a new generation synthetic vaccines: synthetic long peptides (SLP). SLP are synthetic peptides of 25–50 amino acids that require internalization and processing and are thus predominantly processed by DCs (Bijker *et al.*, 2008; Melief and van der Burg, 2008; van der Burg and Melief, 2011). In contrast, all cell types that express MHC class I can present short peptides. Many of these cells do not provide costimulation, a crucial requirement for T cell stimulation. Maturation of DCs, associated with upregulation of costimulatory molecules, is crucial for proper induction of T cell responses. Indeed, inappropriately activated DCs induce tolerance rather than immunity (Bijker *et al.*, 2007; Schuurhuis *et al.*, 2000; Steinman *et al.*, 2003). The addition of strong adjuvants, such as TLR ligands, can partially overcome this problem (see also Chapter 3) (Celis, 2007). However, if the short peptides are distributed systemically after injection, the adjuvant also needs to be distributed systemically, creating a potentially dangerous situation when vaccine-induced T cells would reach high proportions of all T cells. Further, not all MHC class I expressing cells also express TLRs and thus still lack proper costimulation. Local vaccination without systemic distribution of small peptides is to be preferred, for example, in a slow-release adjuvant such as Montanide ISA-51. In the case of local vaccination with long peptides, addition of TLR ligands to synthetic peptide vaccines improves immunogenicity in both mouse models and patients (Welters *et al.*, 2007; Zwaveling *et al.*, 2002).

Overlapping SLP contain both CD4 and CD8 epitopes leading to a parallel stimulation of both CD4+ and CD8+ T cells resulting in a strong and more effective immune response (Hiranuma *et al.*, 1999; Knutson *et al.*, 2001; Shirai *et al.*, 1994; van der Burg and Melief, 2011; Widmann *et al.*, 1992; Zeng *et al.*, 2002). Further, as overlapping SLP contain all potential epitopes irrespective of an individual's MHC type, SLP vaccines are highly convenient in a polymorphic human population (Melief and van der Burg, 2008; van der Burg and Melief, 2011). The presence of a CD4 epitope in the SLP will induce DC activation via CD40–CD40L interaction (Bennett *et al.*, 1998; Schoenberger *et al.*, 1998; Zwaveling *et al.*, 2002) (Fig. 4.1). CD4+ T cell help is needed for the induction and maintenance of the CD8+ T cell response (Arens and Schoenberger, 2010; Schoenberger *et al.*, 1998). CD8+ T cells can be primed without CD4 help, but only if the CD4+ T cells are substituted by the crucial DC-activating signals CD40 agonist or TLR ligand triggering (Celis, 2007; Schuurhuis *et al.*, 2000).

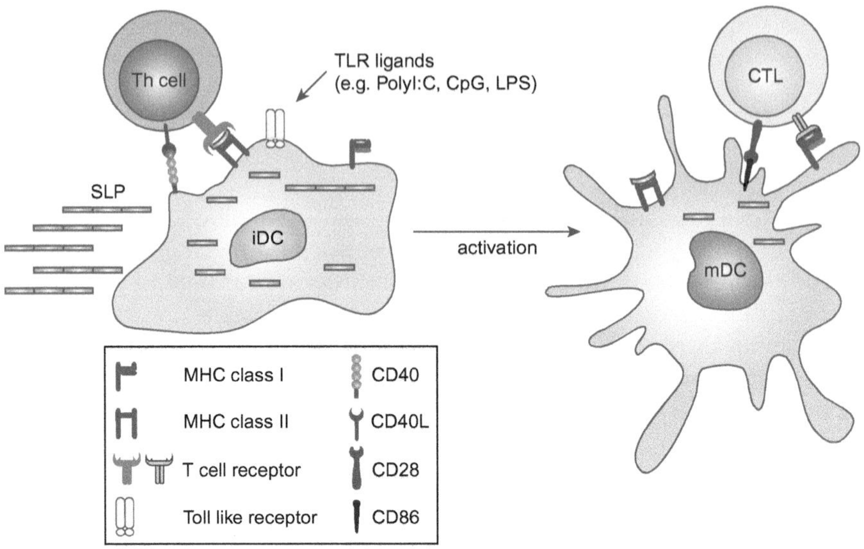

FIGURE 4.1 Synthetic long peptides (SLP) are internalized and processed by immature DC into minimal epitopes. CD8+ CTLs recognize the minimal epitope in MHC class I. The presence of helper epitopes in the SLP that are loaded into MHC class II molecules results in the stimulation of CD4+ T helper cells that CD40L, which interacts with CD40 on the immature DC, resulting in maturation of the DC and upregulation of costimulatory molecules, such as CD86. iDC, immature dendritic cell; mDC, mature dendritic cell. (See Color Insert.)

Optimal DC activation can be achieved by combining ligation of CD40 with TLR ligand triggering on the DC (Napolitani *et al.*, 2005).

Protein vaccination is very suitable for the induction of CD4+ T cell responses and antibodies, but it does not induce proper CD8+ T cell immunity in contrast to long peptides (Zhang *et al.*, 2009). Further, vaccination with protein will mainly induce responses against the dominant epitopes, whereas preprocessed SLP allow for the simultaneous induction of T cell responses against multiple dominant and subdominant epitopes and thus induce a broader T cell repertoire (Rosario *et al.*, 2010; Zhang *et al.*, 2009). Not only processing of SLP is more efficient compared to intact protein, but also uptake of SLP compared to protein is more efficient in DCs (Zhang *et al.*, 2009). Thereby, higher amounts of peptides will reach the class I and class II pathways, leading to improved antigen presentation.

Antigenic competition will always occur in cases in which more than one sequence is present, and thus antigenic competition will also occur between overlapping SLP. In a clinical study of Kenter *et al.*, overlapping SLP of the HPV16 E6 and E7 proteins induced only responses against the

E6 protein when all SLP were administered at one vaccination site. In contrast, responses against both E6 and E7 were detectable when the E6 and E7 SLP were separately injected at anatomically distant sites (Kenter *et al.*, 2008). Antigenic competition can thus be reduced by limiting the number of antigens delivered at one vaccination site. As discussed in paragraph 4.2, viral vectors can cause antigenic competition between vector sequences and the inserted antigen of choice. Bos *et al.* showed that immunization with a recombinant vector sequence can reduce the number of antigen-specific T cells against the inserted antigen (Bos *et al.*, 2007). This appears to be due to repeated vaccination with the much larger vector, after which an overwhelming vector-specific response apparently outcompetes the specific response against the insert antigen of choice. This problem can be overcome by heterologous prime/boosting, using a different vaccine to boost, most commonly priming with DNA and boosting with a viral vector. SLP can be used repeatedly or in combination with DNA priming or viral vector boosting to focus the immune response on the antigen of interest.

Different vaccine strategies that involve vaccination with DNA, antigen-loaded DCs, viral vectors, recombinant proteins, and synthetic peptides are extensively studied for therapeutic vaccination in cancer patients (Melief, 2008; Melief and van der Burg, 2008; Palucka *et al.*, 2011; van der Burg *et al.*, 2011). Advantages and pitfalls of these strategies are summarized in Table 4.1.

6. IMMUNE ESCAPE

As indicated above, tumors have several escape mechanisms. Antigen escape is one of these mechanisms, which is also frequently observed in virus infections, especially HIV-1 (Korber *et al.*, 2001). If only limited numbers of peptides are used for vaccination, there is considerable risk of antigen escape. This might result in subsequent outgrowth of a tumor or metastasis or increase in viral burden in the case of viruses. The use of overlapping peptides reduces the chance of immune escape, as an entire protein sequence is represented by the overlapping SLP. A different strategy is to focus the immune response on target molecules that are implicated in the malignant transformation such as the E6 and E7 viral oncogenes of high-risk HPV. Loss of these proteins would lead to loss of malignant transformation, because expression of these proteins is required for maintenance of the transformed state. Another escape mechanism of tumors is MHC class I down modulation or wholesale loss. This results in the lack of recognition of tumor cells by CD8+ T cells and thereby reduced killing. Recent evidence shows that this is not necessarily fatal, because if tumor antigens are cross-presented by stromal elements

TABLE 4.1 Vaccine strategies in clinical studies for HPV and their pitfalls

Vaccine	Strategy	Advantages	Pitfalls	References
TA-HPV	Viral vector (live recombinant vaccinia)	Presence of vaccinia virus-derived TLR ligands	Antigenic competition by vector sequences	Bos *et al*. (2007)
MVA	Viral vector (attenuated vaccinia)	Presence of vaccinia virus-derived TLR ligands	Antigenic competition by vector sequences	Bos *et al*. (2007)
DNA	DNA	Reduced antigenic competition	Inefficient to induce long-lived antigen expression in DCs	Sharma and Khuller (2001)
TA-CIN, E6E7 Iscomatrix	Protein	No antigenic competition	Inefficient CD8+ T cell induction	Zhang *et al*. (2009)
Peptide vaccines	Minimal MHC class I-binding peptides	No antigenic competition	Induction of tolerance, lack of CD4 help, not applicable in a diverse population	Melief and van der Burg (2008), Toes *et al*. (1996b)

such as endothelial cells, the tumor undergoes vascular strangulation, allowing bystander killing of MHC-negative cells (Schietinger *et al.*, 2010; Zhang *et al.*, 2008). Alternatively, loss of antigen presentation by tumors might be reverted by epigenetic modulation or, in the case of genetic loss, be targeted by natural killer cells or T cells specific for immune escape variants (Lampen and van Hall, 2011). Viruses have evolved comparable mechanisms of immune evasion, such as expression of genes that encode for proteins that downregulate or interfere with antiviral cytokines, apoptosis, or MHC expression (Alcami and Koszinowski, 2000; Horst *et al.*, 2011). Addition or combination therapy with certain cytokines, for example, IFN-α, can increase MHC class I expression on tumor or infected cells and thereby reduces escape from CD8+ T cells. Treatment of metastatic melanoma patients with IFN-α and immunotherapy resulted in regression of lesions that restored MHC class I expression (Carretero *et al.*, 2008). In addition, MHC class II negative tumors can start to express MHC class II, if infiltrated by tumor-specific CD4+ T cells that secrete IFN-γ. Under the right conditions, such CD4+ T cells can subsequently eradicate these tumors by direct cytolysis (Quezada *et al.*, 2010).

7. CLINICAL STUDIES WITH PEPTIDE VACCINES IN CANCER PATIENTS

7.1. Short peptides

Synthetic peptides have been the subject of numerous clinical trials. The majority of these studies have used minimal peptides derived from TAAs, the disadvantages of which have been described above. Clinical outcomes of these studies differ and have not always been the primary endpoint of the study, but in general, response rates following vaccination with short peptides were low (Rosenberg *et al.*, 2004). The use of minimal epitopes only allows for the induction of CD8+ T cell responses. Short peptides, not requiring peptide processing by professional APC, can bind exogenously to any cell type expressing MHC class I, and without proper costimulation, this will not result in the induction of cytotoxic CD8+ T cells but rather induce tolerance (Bijker *et al.*, 2007; Toes *et al.*, 1996a,b). Moreover because of the absence of CD4 help, CD8+ T cell responses can be induced but are not maintained over time (Bijker *et al.*, 2007). Indeed, in many of these studies, patients were given boost vaccinations for a long time to make up for the absence of memory CD8+ T cell responses (Rosenberg *et al.*, 2004; Schwartzentruber *et al.*, 2011). As shown by Bijker *et al.*, elongation of the short peptides into long peptides induces sustained CTL responses (Bijker *et al.*, 2007, 2008). Long peptides need uptake and processing before the minimal epitope is able to bind to MHC class I (Fig. 4.1) (Bijker *et al.*, 2008). Indeed, our experience with long peptide vaccination against HPV16 E6/E7 shows that the immunogenicity of long peptides is superior over that of vaccination with short peptides (Kenter *et al.*, 2008, 2009; Ressing *et al.*, 2000).

Another limitation of the use of a limited set of minimal epitopes, compared to a set of multiple SLP of 25–50 amino acids in length, is the induction of only a very restricted T cell response, presented by one or at best two HLA class I molecules (Melief and van der Burg, 2008). Such limited specificities might more easily induce escape of a tumor, which on the other hand indicates that an effector T cell response was induced (Marincola *et al.*, 2000). A broader T cell repertoire to a number of epitopes that are expressed by the tumor would be more effective and could prevent tumor escape and increase tumor eradication (Melief and van der Burg, 2008). This is supported by a study from Odunsi *et al.*, who studied vaccination in ovarian cancer patients with a 14-mer peptide of NY-ESO-1. This peptide was able to induce CD4+ T cell responses in all vaccinated patients and in a proportion of the patients also CD8+ T cell responses, however, up to 15 immunizations were administered (Odunsi *et al.*, 2007). Unfortunately, recurrent tumors in a subset of patients lacked expression of NY-ESO-1, suggesting immune escape by loss of antigen expression. Thus, incorporating multiple antigenic targets containing CD8+ and CD4+ T cell epitopes will induce a broader T cell repertoire directed at the tumor and thereby limiting immune escape.

Schwartzentruber *et al.* performed a clinical trial with a single HLA*A201 8-mer peptide from gp100 in combination with IL-2 or IL-2 alone. As expected based on the absence of a CD4 epitope, these patients need to receive repeated vaccinations, 1–10 vaccinations per patient with 8–80 doses of IL-2 (Schwartzentruber *et al.*, 2011). Although these patients received a huge number of IL-2 doses (8 per immunization), the proportion of patients that developed reactive T cells was small. Further, levels of circulating antigen-specific T cells did not always correlate with a clinical response. The authors suggest that T cells might have migrated to the tumor site. It is thus important not only to study presence of antigen-specific T cells in the periphery but, if possible, also to study the presence of antigen-specific T cells at the tumor or at the vaccination site. Moreover, although IL-2 may have been instrumental for the expansion of certain T cell populations, including nonspecific ones, the absence of CD4 helper epitopes in the vaccine may have caused insufficient CD8 expansion and memory.

Unfortunately, the consensus of most studies performed with short peptides is the absence of a clinical response and thus a lack of immune correlates with treatment efficacy. This is most likely the result of an insufficiently robust effector T cell response due to the absence of CD4 help and suboptimal pharmacokinetics of short peptides causing antigen loading of nonprofessional APC.

7.2. Long peptides

Several studies have been published by our group employing SLP from HPV16 E6 and E7 oncogenes in patients with cervical cancer or VIN lesions (Kenter *et al.*, 2008, 2009; Welters *et al.*, 2008, 2010). The SLP vaccine is more effective in inducing HPV16-specific immunity, compared to other studies with similar or larger group sizes. Based on IFN-γ production, an immunological response rate between 40% and 75% has been observed with other vaccine approaches (Baldwin *et al.*, 2003; de Jong *et al.*, 2002; Frazer *et al.*, 2004; Smyth *et al.*, 2004), whereas the SLP vaccine resulted in a 100% response rate (Welters *et al.*, 2008). Not only the response rate but also the breadth of the response is better after SLP vaccination when compared with vaccine trials in which TA-CIN, TA-HPV, or both were injected (Welters *et al.*, 2008). Although in a phase I/II SLP vaccination study of end-stage cervical cancer patients, only one of the patients showed long-term tumor regression. No obvious tumor regressions were seen in the other patients, although there was a tendency for the vaccinated patients to live longer. In a more recent study from our group, patients with premalignant VIN lesions were vaccinated with the overlapping SLP HPV16 vaccine. Half of the patients showed a complete regression of the lesions after three or four vaccinations. Complete regression was associated with a significantly stronger HPV16-specific immune response compared to noncomplete regression patients by multiple parameters, including lymphoproliferation, IFN-γ ELIspot, intracellular cytokine staining, and recall responses of HPV-specific $CD25^{hi}$, $FoxP3^{+}$ regulatory T cells (Kenter *et al.*, 2009; Welters *et al.*, 2010). Of note, these patients did not receive any other treatment such as surgical removal, in contrast to some of the other studies cited, in which either surgical removal of the tumor or previous chemo- or radiotherapy had been applied.

Two studies have been performed using overlapping SLP from the p53 protein. This vaccine has been studied in patients with colorectal cancer (Speetjens *et al.*, 2009) and ovarian cancer (Leffers *et al.*, 2009). The p53-SLP vaccine was able to induce strong and sustained p53-specific T cell reactivity in the majority of cases. Solely, p53-specific CD4+ T cells and no p53-specific CD8+ T cells were detected. This was not unexpected since in a murine model we observed that there is no demonstrable tolerance of p53-specific CD4+ T cells (Lauwen *et al.*, 2008), whereas the CD8+ T cell repertoire toward p53 is severely restricted by self-tolerance (Theobald *et al.*, 1997; Vierboom *et al.*, 1997) and is likely to consist only of lower-affinity p53-specific T cells. Surprisingly, colorectal and ovarian cancer patients have received the same p53-SLP vaccine, but there was a clear difference in the cytokine production by the CD4+ T cells. Whereas the colorectal cancer patients showed a Th1 profile with low IFN-γ production by CD4+ T cells (Speetjens *et al.*, 2009), the ovarian cancer patients showed both Th1 and Th2 cytokine production, of which the latter was more frequent (Leffers *et al.*, 2009). Which mechanism is responsible for the polarization of the induced p53-specific immune response? The question arises whether the number of immunizations could explain this. The ovarian cancer patients received four, whereas the colorectal cancer patients received two immunizations. However, there could be a role for the microenvironment of the tumor that can be characterized by either unfavorable inflammatory conditions or more favorable circumstances to influence the formation of a proper cytokine profile, including IFN-γ, to generate effector CD4+ T cells, in addition to effector CD8+ T cells to uncharacterized antigens (Coward *et al.*, 2011; Fridman *et al.*, 2011).

Kakimi *et al.* (2011) studied immunogenicity of a long peptide spanning a peptide region of NY-ESO-1 based on previous observation from our group and a study that showed that T cells induced by vaccination with short peptides had low affinity and did not recognize naturally processed NY-ESO-1 (Le Gal *et al.*, 2005). Next to T cells against NY-ESO-1, antibodies were also induced. The sera from NY-ESO-1 peptide-immunized patients reacted with NY-ESO-1 protein as well as the peptide, suggesting elicitation of an antibody response by a long peptide vaccine including a dominant B cell epitope (Kakimi *et al.*, 2011) in humans as was observed in nonhuman primates.

Speiser *et al.* (2010) performed a phase IIa study using a 20-mer peptide derived from Melan-A which was coupled to virus-like nanoparticles loaded with CpG G10, a completely unmodified A-type CpG. CD8+ T cell responses were detected in the majority of the patients both in early and in late clinical stages of metastatic melanoma. This vaccine regimen induced memory T cells that were present in significantly larger proportions compared to an earlier study (Lienard *et al.*, 2004) in which patients had been repetitively vaccinated with short peptide in IFA. It remains to be determined whether this is due to the long peptide or the vaccine formulation or both.

7.3. Correlates of protection

Although quite some studies have been performed with long or short synthetic peptides in humans, not all describe a correlation between immunogenicity and disease progression. As discussed above, Kenter *et al.* and Welters *et al.* have found statistically significant correlations between strength of vaccine-prompted T cell responses and clinical responses (Kenter *et al.*, 2009; Welters *et al.*, 2010). It would be attractive to link the higher levels of vaccine-prompted HPV-specific FoxP3-positive Tregs in VIN patients without a complete clinical response to the lower levels of vaccine-prompted effector T cells in these patients. This finding calls for more extensive investigation of the correlates of protection in cancer patients, including studies why there are more Tregs in some patients compared to others. It seems logical that with a vaccination modality that induces increasing amount of specific T cells, increased levels of Tregs are also induced to balance the specific effector T cell response as a natural feedback mechanism. It is interesting to note that Welters *et al.* observed a different Teff/Treg ratio between responders and nonresponders, with a high ratio predictive of clinical success (Welters *et al.*, 2010). This is most likely due to host factors that remain to be determined. In any case, future vaccination strategies should be aimed at fully exploiting the effector T cell repertoire while trying to limit the induction of Tregs.

In the case of p53-specific immunity, there is a priori CD8+ T cell tolerance, whereas in the case of virus-induced tumors, the CD8 and CD4 tolerance are acquired and appear to involve peripherally induced Tregs (Welters *et al.*, 2010) and potentially other inhibitory mechanisms operational in chronic virus infections such as PD-1/PD-L1-mediated suppression (van der Burg *et al.*, 2011). This difference may play a role in the success of the HPV16 SLP vaccine, as all virus-derived proteins in the tumor are nonself and are thus not limited by central tolerance. In the study by Speetjens *et al.*, only two vaccinations were given based on the results from our previous studies, that strong Th1 responses were observed after two vaccinations (Kenter *et al.*, 2008; Welters *et al.*, 2008). Here, two vaccinations were insufficient to activate a strong Th1 response. As the vaccine was composed of peptides in Montanide ISA-51 only, there is room for improvement by the addition of adjuvants with strong Th1-inducing activity such as poly I:C (Navabi *et al.*, 2009; Verdijk *et al.*, 1999), CpG (Vollmer and Krieg, 2009), and others.

Many studies have focused on IFN-γ production only, whereas it is now common knowledge that polyfunctionality, production of multiple cytokines, is associated with better protection (Darrah *et al.*, 2007) and in the case of HIV infection with better viral control (Owen *et al.*, 2010). It is likely that this is not only important in the control of HIV-1 infection but also in other infectious diseases and in cancer patients. However, the immunomonitoring techniques currently available are more elaborate and more sophisticated and are likely to reveal even more important correlates of protection.

8. SYNTHETIC PEPTIDE VACCINATION IN NONHUMAN PRIMATES

8.1. Long peptides

Several preclinical studies in nonhuman primates have explored peptide vaccination. In these studies, the peptides were 11–33 amino acids long. A number of these studies investigated the induction of neutralizing antibodies against HIV-1 (Hart *et al.*, 1990; Haynes *et al.*, 1993; Yasutomi *et al.*, 1993), whereas others have studied the induction of T cell responses (Azizi *et al.*, 2008; Belyakov *et al.*, 2001; Nehete *et al.*, 2001, 2008; Rosario *et al.*, 2010; Yasutomi *et al.*, 1993). Although these studies have shown induction of antibodies that were able to neutralize virus infection *in vitro* as determined by reverse transcriptase or syncytium inhibition assay, this was not observed for all monkeys (Haynes *et al.*, 1993). In more recent studies, vaccination with SLP was studied for the induction of T cell responses but also showed the induction of antibodies (Azizi *et al.*, 2008; Rosario *et al.*, 2010). Azizi *et al.* showed that some monkeys generated peptide-specific antibodies that also bind the envelope glycoprotein and were capable of neutralizing T-cell line adapted and primary isolates of subtypes D and E (Azizi *et al.*, 2008). This shows that linear sequences are able to induce neutralizing antibodies. The ongoing research and increasing knowledge on the epitopes of broadly neutralizing antibodies and vaccinology provide opportunities to optimize SLP vaccination for induction of broadly neutralizing antibodies.

In a more recent study from the group of Hanke, the induction of HIV-specific T cell responses was studied after a heterologous vaccination schedule using the most conserved regions of HIV-1 (HIVconsv) (Rosario *et al.*, 2010). In this study, macaques received a heterologous vaccination schedule consisting of DNA, different viral vectors, overlapping SLP, or virus-like particles, which all contained the same sequences (Letourneau *et al.*, 2007; Rosario *et al.*, 2010). The HIVconsv region comprised 46 overlapping SLP. To limit the antigenic competition at one vaccination site, SLP were divided into six pools that were administered at anatomically distinct sites, in contrast to the other vaccine formulations, that represented the HIVconsv sequence in one single open reading frame (ORF). The monkeys showed broadened T cell responses after HIV-SLP boosting but not after previous or subsequent boosting with single ORF viral vectors (Rosario *et al.*, 2010). These observations are supported by a recent study performed in collaboration with Mooij *et al.* (Biomedical Primate Research Centre BRPC, the Netherlands). Rhesus macaques that were previously vaccinated with the attenuated NYVAC poxvirus vector were boosted with overlapping HIV-SLP. These monkeys showed an enormous increase in the magnitude of the T cell response as well as in the breadth of the T cell response (Petra Mooij, Gerrit Koopman, and Willy Bogers (BPRC), personal communication). The question whether vaccination with SLP boosts an existing repertoire or induced new T cell responses is difficult to address. The study at the BPRC shows that the monkeys are able to mount a T cell response against HIV sequences that were only present in the SLP but not in the NYVAC vector that were used for the first two vaccinations. This suggests that SLP vaccination can boost as well as induce T cell responses from the naive repertoire. This argues for heterologous vaccination including SLP vaccines. However, the relative contribution of the different vaccine modalities in the heterologous prime/boost regimens remains unclear.

8.2. Correlates of protection

All approaches in macaques showed the induction of T cell responses, but antigen-specific CD4 and CD8 responses were not always determined. However, vaccination schemes were quite different and sometimes involved combination with other vaccine modalities such as DNA vaccination or peptide-pulsed DCs (Nehete *et al.*, 2001; Qin *et al.*, 2010). Some of these studies also challenged the vaccinated monkeys with SHIV (a chimeric simian/human immunodeficiency virus able to infect macaques) (Belyakov *et al.*, 2001; Nehete *et al.*, 2001, 2008). All monkeys in these studies became infected, but some vaccinated monkeys showed a lower viral load compared to the control groups. Only the group of Berzofsky used solely peptides for vaccination; however, the group that was intrarectally vaccinated had no detectable viral load, whereas the group vaccinated subcutaneously had detectable viral loads comparable to the control (Belyakov *et al.*, 2001). These studies provide evidence for the role of SLP in the induction of both T cell responses and antibodies. The improving knowledge on vaccinology and the increasing availability of adjuvants in recent years provide a window of opportunity to improve SLP vaccination because in the aforementioned studies only Freund's adjuvant, or in one case *Escherichia coli* labile toxin was used as an adjuvant (Belyakov *et al.*, 2001).

Unfortunately, the studies performed by Rosario *et al.* (2010) and Mooij *et al.* do not provide the opportunity to analyze the effect of the vaccine-induced T cell response on the infection. The animals in these studies cannot be challenged because HIV-1 does not replicate in rhesus macaques. For that reason, the BRPC has initiated a study in which overlapping SLP from the most conserved region of SIV have been generated and used for vaccination of rhesus macaques, either alone or in combination with DNA. T cell immunogenicity and protection or control of viral load will be studied.

Several differences exist between the different studies in macaques, which make it difficult to compare them. One of the striking differences between the studies performed in the earlier years compared to those performed more recently is the use of adjuvants and the increasing length of HIV sequence, thereby expanding the number of epitopes used for vaccination. Adjuvants are of major importance for optimal vaccination and can further enhance the results of synthetic peptide vaccination (Melief, 2008; Chapter 1). Therefore, huge efforts are currently spent on studying the mode of action of various adjuvants, and new or improved adjuvants have been described that are likely to further improve the results of SLP vaccination.

9. LONG PEPTIDES AS PROPHYLACTIC VACCINES

SLP vaccine as prophylactic vaccine in infectious disease should be able to induce both humoral and cell-mediated immune responses. Synthetic peptides have been described to be able to induce both antibodies and effector T cells (Agadjanyan *et al.*, 2005; Schellinger *et al.*, 2011) and therefore would be effective as a prophylactic vaccine. The antibody response to peptides, however, is limited to linear B cell epitopes. It would be very challenging if not impossible to generate long peptides with conformations that resemble the native protein for the induction of antibodies that are able to recognize conformational epitopes. However, the presence of antibodies that are able to recognize intact protein implies that antibodies can be induced by peptide vaccination and might have neutralizing capacity (Azizi *et al.*, 2008; Hart *et al.*, 1990; Haynes *et al.*, 1993; Yasutomi *et al.*, 1993). The approach to use peptides for the induction of sufficiently protective antibodies for prophylaxis of disease needs optimization.

10. IMPROVEMENT OF LONG PEPTIDE VACCINATION BY COMBINATION OF SYNTHETIC VACCINES WITH OTHER CANCER TREATMENT MODALITIES

As discussed before, SLP lack a danger signal and therefore need the addition of adjuvants. Adjuvants might also shape the immune response toward Th1 or Th2 responses, for example, depending on the goal of the vaccination (e.g., prophylactic of therapeutic). An attractive family of adjuvants is that of the TLR ligands that elicit their effects by binding to their receptor. These receptors are prominently expressed on subsets of DCs and therefore constitute excellent adjuvants, because TLR triggering causes DC activation and immune response initiation. Each TLR recognizes a distinct molecular pattern (see Chapter 1). The interaction of the TLR ligand with its receptor determines the type of immune response that is induced, as TLR ligands are specific for each pathogen and induce different types of immune response (Kawai and Akira, 2011; Schenten and Medzhitov, 2011). It is therefore important that SLP and the adjuvant used are directed at the same DC to obtain the best result (Khan *et al.*, 2007). For that reason, a number of groups have studied the coupling of SLP to adjuvants. In the earlier studies, lipid tails were added to the peptides to improve uptake by DCs since lipid tail more easily diffuses through the cell membrane (Gahery-Segard *et al.*, 2003). Studies from our group and others have shown that peptides covalently linked to the TLR-2 ligand Pam3Cys (Jackson *et al.*, 2004; Khan *et al.*, 2007) or the TLR-9 ligand CpG (Heit *et al.*, 2005; Khan *et al.*, 2007, 2009; Maurer *et al.*, 2002; Tighe *et al.*, 2000a,b) are superior in their ability to induce specific CD8+ T cells compared to a vaccine modality composed of a mixture of the free TLR ligand with the free antigen.

Combination with other (standard) treatments (e.g., chemo- or radiotherapy) with synthetic peptide vaccination is attractive and has already been tried in experimental models and occasionally in the clinic. A marked benefit of combined chemotherapy or irradiation with immunotherapy has been reported in rodent models (Lake and Robinson, 2005; Nowak *et al.*, 2006). A clinical study reported that patients with lung cancer showed no survival benefit following vaccination with a recombinant adenovirus expressing wild-type p53. However, subsequent chemotherapy provided a significant survival advantage for the vaccinated patients, whereas chemotherapy alone was of no benefit (Antonia *et al.*, 2006; Gabrilovich, 2007).

The first registered cancer vaccine, Sipuleucel (Provenge) for hormone-resistant late-stage prostate cancer, confers an average survival advantage for this category of patients of 4 months (Kantoff *et al.*, 2010). While this is encouraging, further improvement of this type of vaccine itself, as well as more prolonged survival by combination with other treatment modalities, is highly desirable. A first category of drugs that comes to mind is combination of standard chemotherapy with cancer vaccines. This is an excellent concept, particularly with those forms of chemotherapy that do not adversely affect T cell immunity and cause immunogenic cancer cell death (Zitvogel *et al.*, 2011). Next to chemotherapy, a variety of monoclonal antibodies with immunomodulatory effects can be expected to further augment the effector T cell generation mediated by vaccination alone (Melief, 2008). The checkpoint control blocking antibody Yervoy (Ipilimumab, CTLA-4 blocker) has now been registered as monotherapy for late-stage melanoma treatment and induces prolonged survival of a subgroup of patients (Robert *et al.*, 2011). It is very attractive to combine this drug for even more specific expansion of cancer-specific effector T cells in combination with robust synthetic vaccines. Other monoclonal antibodies to be explored in combination with cancer vaccines are antibodies against members of the TNF receptor family such as CD40, CD137 (4-1BB), CD27, and CD134 (OX40) (Melief, 2008). Implementation of combination therapies will require considerable effort, because each new drug manufacturer primarily wants to position its drug as a blockbuster monotherapy.

11. IMMUNOPHARMACOLOGY

One of the prime advantages of synthetic vaccines is that this approach allows more rational vaccine design. Instead of working with poorly understood complex dead or live (recombinant) microorganisms, synthetic vaccine design incorporates only those well-proven immunostimulants and antigens that have been proven to augment performance in a well-understood way. A second major advantage is that the vaccines now consist of relatively small biomolecules such as peptides that resemble other chemically well-defined small drugs, allowing pharmacokinetic and -dynamic studies on an unprecedented scale and with much greater precision than in the case of conventional vaccines. We therefore advocate the development of a new field of research, namely, development of the immunopharmacology of synthetic vaccines. It should now be studied (i) which cells are targeted by the synthetic vaccines, (ii) how the vaccines are metabolized, (iii) how long the crucially active components remain involved in antigen presentation by subsets of DCs, and (iv) how these vaccines optimally imprint T cell functions and expansions in the lymphoid architecture and in individual nonlymphoid tissues to subsequently generate circulating and tissue/cancer-homing effector T cells.

12. HURDLES TO SUCCESSFUL THERAPEUTIC VACCINATION

As alluded to before in this review, spectacular results of cancer vaccines cannot be expected in the case of cancers with a hostile microenvironment toward effector T cells, such as cancers producing the wrong chemokines for effector T cell attraction and instead chemokines attracting immunosuppressive myeloid derived suppressor cells producing nitric oxide (Condamine and Gabrilovich, 2011; Fridman *et al.*, 2011; Gajewski *et al.*, 2011; Sonda *et al.*, 2011) or granulocytes producing IL-10 (De Santo *et al.*, 2010). Selective measures specifically depleting myeloid-derived suppressor cells (MDSC) or FoxP3 regulatory T cells are not yet available, but in the case of IL-10-producing granulocytes, treatment with a strong NKT agonist appears to largely eliminate this type of immuno-down modulation (De Santo *et al.*, 2010). To an unknown extent, specific chemotherapeutic compounds can have immunomodulatory activity, but even in the case of such a well-known compound as cyclophosphamide, scientists do not agree as to its exact mode of action (Golovina and Vonderheide, 2010; Mkrtichyan *et al.*, 2011), although obviously it can be of use.

13. CONCLUSIONS AND PERSPECTIVE

The future for synthetic vaccines looks promising. Such vaccines, in particular SLP, have already shown clinical benefit in a therapeutic setting and might also be used to induce high levels of protective antibodies for preventive vaccination. In the near future, improved formulation with potent adjuvants such as TLR ligands can be expected to further improve the quality of the synthetic vaccine-induced immune responses. Further improvements by rational design of synthetic vaccines, such as peptide conjugation to TLR ligands or other immunostimulatory compounds, can drastically improve the performance of synthetic vaccines as already demonstrated in preclinical models. Major advantages of synthetic vaccines over conventional vaccines are the absence of antigenic competition and the defined chemical nature of the vaccine opening up the opportunity to conduct pharmacodynamic and pharmacokinetic studies unprecedented in vaccine research. This can then lead to further science-driven improvements in vaccine performance. Optimal effectiveness, particularly of therapeutic cancer vaccines, can be expected to require combination treatment with other compounds such as chemotherapeutics, checkpoint control antibodies (CTLA-4 blocker, PD-1 blocker), and agonistic antibodies against members of the TNF receptor family of molecules, in particular, CD40, CD27, CD134, and CD137.

ACKNOWLEDGMENTS

The authors would like to thank Drs. van Hall and Arens for critical reading of the chapter. Financial support to E.D.Q. is received from The Aids Fonds Netherlands (Grant 2010017).

REFERENCES

Agadjanyan, M. G., Ghochikyan, A., Petrushina, I., Vasilevko, V., Movsesyan, N., Mkrtichyan, M., Saing, T., and Cribbs, D. H. (2005). Prototype Alzheimer's disease vaccine using the immunodominant B cell epitope from beta-amyloid and promiscuous T cell epitope Pan HLA DR-binding peptide. *J. Immunol.* **174,** 1580–1586.

Alcami, A., and Koszinowski, U. H. (2000). Viral mechanisms of immune evasion. *Immunol. Today* **21,** 447–455.

Amanna, I. J., and Slifka, M. K. (2011). Contributions of humoral and cellular immunity to vaccine-induced protection in humans. *Virology* **411,** 206–215.

Antonia, S. J., Mirza, N., Fricke, I., Chiappori, A., Thompson, P., Williams, N., Bepler, G., Simon, G., Janssen, W., Lee, J. H., Menander, K., Chada, S., *et al.* (2006). Combination of p53 cancer vaccine with chemotherapy in patients with extensive stage small cell lung cancer. *Clin. Cancer Res.* **12,** 878–887.

Arens, R., and Schoenberger, S. P. (2010). Plasticity in programming of effector and memory CD8 T-cell formation. *Immunol. Rev.* **235,** 190–205.

Azizi, A., Anderson, D. E., Torres, J. V., Ogrel, A., Ghorbani, M., Soare, C., Sandstrom, P., Fournier, J., and Diaz-Mitoma, F. (2008). Induction of broad cross-subtype-specific HIV-1 immune responses by a novel multivalent HIV-1 peptide vaccine in cynomolgus macaques. *J. Immunol.* **180,** 2174–2186.

Baldwin, P. J., van der Burg, S. H., Boswell, C. M., Offringa, R., Hickling, J. K., Dobson, J., Roberts, J. S., Latimer, J. A., Moseley, R. P., Coleman, N., Stanley, M. A., and Sterling, J. C. (2003). Vaccinia-expressed human papillomavirus 16 and 18 E6 and E7 as a therapeutic vaccination for vulval and vaginal intraepithelial neoplasia. *Clin. Cancer Res.* **9,** 5205–5213.

Banchereau, J., Schuler-Thurner, B., Palucka, A. K., and Schuler, G. (2001). Dendritic cells as vectors for therapy. *Cell* **106,** 271–274.

Belyakov, I. M., Hel, Z., Kelsall, B., Kuznetsov, V. A., Ahlers, J. D., Nacsa, J., Watkins, D. I., Allen, T. M., Sette, A., Altman, J., Woodward, R., Markham, P. D., *et al.* (2001). Mucosal AIDS vaccine reduces disease and viral load in gut reservoir and blood after mucosal infection of macaques. *Nat. Med.* **7,** 1320–1326.

Bennett, S. R. M., Carbone, F. R., Karamalis, F., Flavell, R. A., Miller, J. F. A. P., and Heath, W. R. (1998). Help for cytotoxic-T-cell responses is mediated by CD40 signalling. *Nature* **393,** 478–480.

Bijker, M. S., van den Eeden, S. J., Franken, K. L., Melief, C. J., Offringa, R., and van der Burg, S. H. (2007). CD8+ CTL priming by exact peptide epitopes in incomplete Freund's adjuvant induces a vanishing CTL response, whereas long peptides induce sustained CTL reactivity. *J. Immunol.* **179,** 5033–5040.

Bijker, M. S., van den Eeden, S. J., Franken, K. L., Melief, C. J., van der Burg, S. H., and Offringa, R. (2008). Superior induction of anti-tumor CTL immunity by extended peptide vaccines involves prolonged, DC-focused antigen presentation. *Eur. J. Immunol.* **38,** 1033–1042.

Bos, R., van, D. S., van, H. T., Lauwen, M. M., Parrington, M., Berinstein, N. L., McNeil, B., Melief, C. J., Verbeek, J. S., van der Burg, S. H., and Offringa, R. (2007). Characterization of antigen-specific immune responses induced by canarypox virus vaccines. *J. Immunol.* **179,** 6115–6122.

Botti, C., Seregni, E., Ferrari, L., Martinetti, A., and Bombardieri, E. (1998). Immunosuppressive factors: Role in cancer development and progression. *Int. J. Biol. Markers* **13,** 51–69.

Boudreau, J. E., Bonehill, A., Thielemans, K., and Wan, Y. (2011). Engineering dendritic cells to enhance cancer immunotherapy. *Mol. Ther.* **19,** 841–853.

Burton, D. R. (2002). Antibodies, viruses and vaccines. *Nat. Rev. Immunol.* **2,** 706–713.

Cabrera, T., Lopez-Nevot, M. A., Gaforio, J. J., Ruiz-Cabello, F., and Garrido, F. (2003). Analysis of HLA expression in human tumor tissues. *Cancer Immunol. Immunother.* **52,** 1–9.

Carretero, R., Romero, J., Ruiz-Cabello, F., Maleno, I., Rodriguez, F., Camacho, F., Real, L., Garrido, F., and Cabrera, T. (2008). Analysis of HLA class I expression in progressing and regressing metastatic melanoma lesions after immunotherapy. *Immunogenetics* **60,** 439–447.

Celis, E. (2007). Toll-like receptor ligands energize peptide vaccines through multiple paths. *Cancer Res.* **67,** 7945–7947.

Cheever, M. A., Allison, J. P., Ferris, A. S., Finn, O. J., Hastings, B. M., Hecht, T. T., Mellman, I., Prindiville, S. A., Viner, J. L., Weiner, L. M., and Matrisian, L. M. (2009).

The prioritization of cancer antigens: A national cancer institute pilot project for the acceleration of translational research. *Clin. Cancer Res.* **15,** 5323–5337.

Condamine, T., and Gabrilovich, D. I. (2011). Molecular mechanisms regulating myeloid-derived suppressor cell differentiation and function. *Trends Immunol.* **32,** 19–25.

Coward, J., Kulbe, H., Chakravarty, P., Leader, D. A., Vassileva, V., Leinster, D. A., Thompson, R., Schioppa, T., Nemeth, J. A., Vermeulin, J., Singh, N., Avril, N. E., *et al.* (2011). Interleukin-6 as a therapeutic target in human ovarian cancer. *Clin. Cancer Res.* **17,** 6083–6096.

Crompton, P. D., Pierce, S. K., and Miller, L. H. (2010). Advances and challenges in malaria vaccine development. *J. Clin. Invest.* **120,** 4168–4178.

Darrah, P. A., Patel, D. T., De Luca, P. M., Lindsay, R. W. B., Davey, D. F., Flynn, B. J., Hoff, S. T., Andersen, P., Reed, S. G., Morris, S. L., Roederer, M., and Seder, R. A. (2007). Multifunctional TH1 cells define a correlate of vaccine-mediated protection against Leishmania major. *Nat. Med.* **13,** 843–850.

de Jong, A., O'Neill, T., Khan, A. Y., Kwappenberg, K. M. C., Chisholm, S. E., Whittle, N. R., Dobson, J. A., Jack, L. C., St Clair Roberts, J., Offringa, R., van der Burg, S. H., and Hickling, J. K. (2002). Enhancement of human papillomavirus (HPV) type 16 E6 and E7-specific T-cell immunity in healthy volunteers through vaccination with TA-CIN, an HPV16 L2E7E6 fusion protein vaccine. *Vaccine* **20,** 3456–3464.

De Santo, C., Arscott, R., Booth, S., Karydis, I., Jones, M., Asher, R., Salio, M., Middleton, M., and Cerundolo, V. (2010). Invariant NKT cells modulate the suppressive activity of IL-10-secreting neutrophils differentiated with serum amyloid A. *Nat. Immunol.* **11,** 1039–1046.

Demotte, N., Wieërs, G., Van Der Smissen, P., Moser, M., Schmidt, C., Thielemans, K., Squifflet, J. L., Weynand, B., Carrasco, J., Lurquin, C., Courtoy, P. J., and van der Bruggen, P. (2010). A galectin-3 ligand corrects the impaired function of human CD4 and CD8 tumor-infiltrating lymphocytes and favors tumor rejection in mice. *Cancer Res.* **70,** 7476–7488.

Draper, S. J., and Heeney, J. L. (2010). Viruses as vaccine vectors for infectious diseases and cancer. *Nat. Rev. Microbiol.* **8,** 62–73.

Edwards, B. H., Bansal, A., Sabbaj, S., Bakari, J., Mulligan, M. J., and Goepfert, P. A. (2002). Magnitude of functional CD8+ T-cell responses to the gag protein of human immunodeficiency virus type 1 correlates inversely with viral load in plasma. *J. Virol.* **76,** 2298–2305.

Figdor, C. G., de Vries, I. J., Lesterhuis, W. J., and Melief, C. J. (2004). Dendritic cell immunotherapy: Mapping the way. *Nat. Med.* **10,** 475–480.

Frazer, I. H., Quinn, M., Nicklin, J. L., Tan, J., Perrin, L. C., Ng, P., O'Connor, V. M., White, O., Wendt, N., Martin, J., Crowley, J. M., Edwards, S. J., *et al.* (2004). Phase 1 study of HPV16-specific immunotherapy with E6E7 fusion protein and ISCOMATRIX(TM) adjuvant in women with cervical intraepithelial neoplasia. *Vaccine* **23,** 172–181.

Frazer, I. H., Lowy, D. R., and Schiller, J. T. (2007). Prevention of cancer through immunization: Prospects and challenges for the 21st century. *Eur. J. Immunol.* **37**(Suppl. 1), S148–S155.

Fridman, W. H., Mlecnik, B., Bindea, G., Pages, F., and Galon, J. (2011). Immunosurveillance in human non-viral cancers. *Curr. Opin. Immunol.* **23,** 272–278.

Gabrilovich, D. I. (2007). Combination of chemotherapy and immunotherapy for cancer: A paradigm revisited. *Lancet Oncol.* **8,** 2–3.

Gahery-Segard, H., Pialoux, G., Figueiredo, S., Igea, C., Surenaud, M., Gaston, J., Gras-Masse, H., Levy, J. P., and Guillet, J. G. (2003). Long-term specific immune responses induced in humans by a human immunodeficiency virus type 1 lipopeptide vaccine: Characterization of CD8+−T-cell epitopes recognized. *J. Virol.* **77,** 11220–11231.

Gajewski, T. F., Fuertes, M., Spaapen, R., Zheng, Y., and Kline, J. (2011). Molecular profiling to identify relevant immune resistance mechanisms in the tumor microenvironment. *Curr. Opin. Immunol.* **23,** 286–292.

Golovina, T. N., and Vonderheide, R. H. (2010). Regulatory T cells: Overcoming suppression of T-cell immunity. *Cancer J.* **16,** 342–347.

Gomez, C. E., Najera, J. L., Jimenez, V., Bieler, K., Wild, J., Kostic, L., Heidari, S., Chen, M., Frachette, M. J., Pantaleo, G., Wolf, H., Liljestrom, P., *et al.* (2007). Generation and immunogenicity of novel HIV/AIDS vaccine candidates targeting HIV-1 Env/Gag-Pol-Nef antigens of clade C. *Vaccine* **25,** 1969–1992.

Gomez, C. E., Najera, J. L., Krupa, M., and Esteban, M. (2008). The poxvirus vectors MVA and NYVAC as gene delivery systems for vaccination against infectious diseases and cancer. *Curr. Gene Ther.* **8,** 97–120.

Gomez, C. E., Najera, J. L., Krupa, M., Perdiguero, B., and Esteban, M. (2011). MVA and NYVAC as vaccines against emergent infectious diseases and cancer. *Curr. Gene Ther.* **11,** 189–217.

Goulder, P. J. R., and Watkins, D. I. (2008). Impact of MHC class I diversity on immune control of immunodeficiency virus replication. *Nat. Rev. Immunol.* **8,** 619–630.

Halliday, J., Klenerman, P., and Barnes, E. (2011). Vaccination for hepatitis C virus: Closing in on an evasive target. *Expert Rev. Vaccines* **10,** 659–672.

Hansen, S. G., Ford, J. C., Lewis, M. S., Ventura, A. B., Hughes, C. M., Coyne-Johnson, L., Whizin, N., Oswald, K., Shoemaker, R., Swanson, T., Legasse, A. W., Chiuchiolo, M. J., *et al.* (2011). Profound early control of highly pathogenic SIV by an effector memory T-cell vaccine. *Nature* **473,** 523–527.

Harari, A., and Pantaleo, G. (2008). HIV-1-specific immune response. *In* "Advances in Pharmacology; HIV-1: Molecular Biology and Pathogenesis", (K. T. Jeang, ed.). Academic Press, Amsterdam.

Hart, M. K., Palker, T. J., Matthews, T. J., Langlois, A. J., Lerche, N. W., Martin, M. E., Scearce, R. M., McDanal, C., Bolognesi, D. P., and Haynes, B. F. (1990). Synthetic peptides containing T and B cell epitopes from human immunodeficiency virus envelope gp120 induce anti-HIV proliferative responses and high titers of neutralizing antibodies in rhesus monkeys. *J. Immunol.* **145,** 2677–2685.

Haynes, B. F., Torres, J. V., Langlois, A. J., Bolognesi, D. P., Gardner, M. B., Palker, T. J., Scearce, R. M., Jones, D. M., Moody, M. A., McDanal, C., *et al.* (1993). Induction of HIVMN neutralizing antibodies in primates using a prime-boost regimen of hybrid synthetic gp120 envelope peptides. *J. Immunol.* **151,** 1646–1653.

Heit, A., Schmitz, F., O'Keeffe, M., Staib, C., Busch, D. H., Wagner, H., and Huster, K. M. (2005). Protective CD8 T cell immunity triggered by CpG-protein conjugates competes with the efficacy of live vaccines. *J. Immunol.* **174,** 4373–4380.

Hill, A. V., Reyes-Sandoval, A., O'Hara, G., Ewer, K., Lawrie, A., Goodman, A., Nicosia, A., Folgori, A., Colloca, S., Cortese, R., Gilbert, S. C., and Draper, S. J. (2010). Prime-boost vectored malaria vaccines: Progress and prospects. *Hum. Vaccin.* **6,** 78–83.

Hiranuma, K., Tamaki, S., Nishimura, Y., Kusuki, S., Isogawa, M., Kim, G., Kaito, M., Kuribayashi, K., Adachi, Y., and Yasutomi, Y. (1999). Helper T cell determinant peptide contributes to induction of cellular immune responses by peptide vaccines against hepatitis C virus. *J. Gen. Virol.* **80,** 187–193.

Horst, D., Verweij, M. C., Davison, A. J., Ressing, M. E., and Wiertz, E. J. (2011). Viral evasion of T cell immunity: Ancient mechanisms offering new applications. *Curr. Opin. Immunol.* **23,** 96–103.

Huang, L. M., Lu, C. Y., and Chen, D. S. (2011). Hepatitis B virus infection, its sequelae, and prevention by vaccination. *Curr. Opin. Immunol.* **23,** 237–243.

Jackson, D. C., Lau, Y. F., Le, T., Suhrbier, A., Deliyannis, G., Cheers, C., Smith, C., Zeng, W., and Brown, L. E. (2004). A totally synthetic vaccine of generic structure that targets Toll-like receptor 2 on dendritic cells and promotes antibody or cytotoxic T cell responses. *Proc. Natl. Acad. Sci. USA* **101,** 15440–15445.

Jing, L., Chong, T. M., McClurkan, C. L., Huang, J., Story, B. T., and Koelle, D. M. (2005). Diversity in the acute CD8 T cell response to vaccinia virus in humans. *J. Immunol.* **175,** 7550–7559.

Kakimi, K., Isobe, M., Uenaka, A., Wada, H., Sato, E., Doki, Y., Nakajima, J., Seto, Y., Yamatsuji, T., Naomoto, Y., Shiraishi, K., Takigawa, N., *et al.* (2011). A phase I study of vaccination with NY-ESO-1f peptide mixed with Picibanil OK-432 and Montanide ISA-51 in patients with cancers expressing the NY-ESO-1 antigen. *Int. J. Cancer* **129,** 2836–2846.

Kantoff, P. W., Higano, C. S., Shore, N. D., Berger, E. R., Small, E. J., Penson, D. F., Redfern, C. H., Ferrari, A. C., Dreicer, R., Sims, R. B., Xu, Y., Frohlich, M. W., *et al.* (2010). Sipuleucel-T immunotherapy for castration-resistant prostate cancer. *N. Engl. J. Med.* **363,** 411–422.

Kawai, T., and Akira, S. (2011). Toll-like receptors and their crosstalk with other innate receptors in infection and immunity. *Immunity* **34,** 637–650.

Kenter, G. G., Welters, M. J., Valentijn, A. R., Lowik, M. J., Berends-van der Meer, D. M., Vloon, A. P., Drijfhout, J. W., Wafelman, A. R., Oostendorp, J., Fleuren, G. J., Offringa, R., van der Burg, S. H., *et al.* (2008). Phase I immunotherapeutic trial with long peptides spanning the E6 and E7 sequences of high-risk human papillomavirus 16 in end-stage cervical cancer patients shows low toxicity and robust immunogenicity. *Clin. Cancer Res.* **14,** 169–177.

Kenter, G. G., Welters, M. J. P., Valentijn, A. R., Lowik, M. J. G., Berends-van der Meer, D., Vloon, A. P. G., Essahsah, F., Fathers, L. M., Offringa, R., Drijfhout, J. W., Wafelman, A. R., Oostendorp, J., *et al.* (2009). Vaccination against HPV-16 oncoproteins for vulvar intraepithelial neoplasia. *N. Engl. J. Med.* **361,** 1838–1847.

Khan, S., Bijker, M. S., Weterings, J. J., Tanke, H. J., Adema, G. J., van, H. T., Drijfhout, J. W., Melief, C. J., Overkleeft, H. S., van der Marel, G. A., Filippov, D. V., van der Burg, S. H., *et al.* (2007). Distinct uptake mechanisms but similar intracellular processing of two different toll-like receptor ligand-peptide conjugates in dendritic cells. *J. Biol. Chem.* **282,** 21145–21159.

Khan, S., Weterings, J. J., Britten, C. M., de Jong, A. R., Graafland, D., Melief, C. J. M., van der Burg, S. H., van der Marel, G., Overkleeft, H. S., Filippov, D. V., and Ossendorp, F. (2009). Chirality of TLR-2 ligand Pam3CysSK4 in fully synthetic peptide conjugates critically influences the induction of specific CD8+ T-cells. *Mol. Immunol.* **46,** 1084–1091.

Kiepiela, P., Ngumbela, K., Thobakgale, C., Ramduth, D., Honeyborne, I., Moodley, E., Reddy, S., de Pierres, C., Mncube, Z., Mkhwanazi, N., Bishop, K., van der Stok, M., *et al.* (2007). CD8+ T-cell responses to different HIV proteins have discordant associations with viral load. *Nat. Med.* **13,** 46–53.

Kiessling, R., Wasserman, K., Horiguchi, S., Kono, K., Sjoberg, J., Pisa, P., and Petersson, M. (1999). Tumor-induced immune dysfunction. *Cancer Immunol. Immunother.* **48,** 353–362.

Knutson, K. L., Schiffman, K., and Disis, M. L. (2001). Immunization with a HER-2/neu helper peptide vaccine generates HER-2/neu CD8 T-cell immunity in cancer patients. *J. Clin. Invest.* **107,** 477–484.

Korber, B., Gaschen, B., Yusim, K., Thakallapally, R., Kesmir, C., and Detours, V. (2001). Evolutionary and immunological implications of contemporary HIV-1 variation. *Br. Med. Bull.* **58,** 19–42.

Lake, R. A., and Robinson, B. W. S. (2005). Immunotherapy and chemotherapy—A practical partnership. *Nat. Rev. Cancer* **5,** 397–405.

Lampen, M. H., and van Hall, T. (2011). Strategies to counteract MHC-I defects in tumors. *Curr. Opin. Immunol.* **23,** 293–298.

Lauwen, M. M., Zwaveling, S., de, Q. L., Ferreira Mota, S. C., Grashorn, J. A., Melief, C. J., van der Burg, S. H., and Offringa, R. (2008). Self-tolerance does not restrict the CD4+ T-helper response against the p53 tumor antigen. *Cancer Res.* **68,** 893–900.

Le Gal, F. A., Ayyoub, M., Dutoit, V., Widmer, V., Jager, E., Cerottini, J. C., Dietrich, P. Y., and Valmori, D. (2005). Distinct structural TCR repertoires in naturally occurring versus vaccine-induced CD8+ T-cell responses to the tumor-specific antigen NY-ESO-1. *J. Immunother.* **28,** 252–257.

Leffers, N., Lambeck, A. J., Gooden, M. J., Hoogeboom, B. N., Wolf, R., Hamming, I. E., Hepkema, B. G., Willemse, P. H., Molmans, B. H., Hollema, H., Drijfhout, J. W., Sluiter, W. J., *et al.* (2009). Immunization with a P53 synthetic long peptide vaccine induces P53-specific immune responses in ovarian cancer patients, a phase II trial. *Int. J. Cancer* **125,** 2104–2113.

Lesterhuis, W. J., Aarntzen, E. H., de Vries, I. J., Schuurhuis, D. H., Figdor, C. G., Adema, G. J., and Punt, C. J. (2008). Dendritic cell vaccines in melanoma: From promise to proof? *Crit. Rev. Oncol. Hematol.* **66,** 118–134.

Lesterhuis, W. J., de Vries, I. J., Schreibelt, G., Lambeck, A. J., Aarntzen, E. H., Jacobs, J. F., Scharenborg, N. M., van de Rakt, M. W., de Boer, A. J., Croockewit, S., van Rossum, M. M., Mus, R., *et al.* (2011). Route of administration modulates the induction of dendritic cell vaccine-induced antigen-specific T cells in advanced melanoma patients. *Clin. Cancer Res.* **17,** 5725–5735.

Letourneau, S., Im, E. J., Mashishi, T., Brereton, C., Bridgeman, A., Yang, H., Dorrell, L., Dong, T., Korber, B., McMichael, A. J., and Hanke, T. (2007). Design and pre-clinical evaluation of a universal HIV-1 vaccine. *PLoS One* **2,** e984.

Lienard, D., Rimoldi, D., Marchand, M., Dietrich, P. Y., van, B. N., Geldhof, C., Batard, P., Guillaume, P., Ayyoub, M., Pittet, M. J., Zippelius, A., Fleischhauer, K., *et al.* (2004). Ex vivo detectable activation of melan-a-specific T cells correlating with inflammatory skin reactions in melanoma patients vaccinated with peptides in IFA. *Cancer Immun.* **4,** 4.

Marincola, F. M., Jaffee, E. M., Hicklin, D. J., and Ferrone, S. (2000). Escape of human solid tumors from T-cell recognition: Molecular mechanisms and functional significance. *Adv. Immunol.* **74,** 181–273.

Maurer, T., Heit, A., Hochrein, H., Ampenberger, F., O'Keeffe, M., Bauer, S., Lipford, G. B., Vabulas, R. M., and Wagner, H. (2002). CpG-DNA aided cross-presentation of soluble antigens by dendritic cells. *Eur. J. Immunol.* **32,** 2356–2364.

McConkey, S. J., Reece, W. H., Moorthy, V. S., Webster, D., Dunachie, S., Butcher, G., Vuola, J. M., Blanchard, T. J., Gothard, P., Watkins, K., Hannan, C. M., Everaere, S., *et al.* (2003). Enhanced T-cell immunogenicity of plasmid DNA vaccines boosted by recombinant modified vaccinia virus Ankara in humans. *Nat. Med.* **9,** 729–735.

McMichael, A. J., Borrow, P., Tomaras, G. D., Goonetilleke, N., and Haynes, B. F. (2010). The immune response during acute HIV-1 infection: Clues for vaccine development. *Nat. Rev. Immunol.* **10,** 11–23.

McShane, H., and Hill, A. (2005). Prime-boost immunisation strategies for tuberculosis. *Microbes Infect.* **7,** 962–967.

Melief, C. J. M. (2008). Cancer immunotherapy by dendritic cells. *Immunity* **29,** 372–383.

Melief, C. J., and van der Burg, S. H. (2008). Immunotherapy of established (pre)malignant disease by synthetic long peptide vaccines. *Nat. Rev. Cancer* **8,** 351–360.

Mkrtichyan, M., Najjar, Y. G., Raulfs, E. C., Abdalla, M. Y., Samara, R., Rotem-Yehudar, R., Cook, L., and Khleif, S. N. (2011). Anti-PD-1 synergizes with cyclophosphamide to induce potent anti-tumor vaccine effects through novel mechanisms. *Eur. J. Immunol.* **41,** 2977–2986.

Mwau, M., Cebere, I., Sutton, J., Chikoti, P., Winstone, N., Wee, E. G., Beattie, T., Chen, Y. H., Dorrell, L., McShane, H., Schmidt, C., Brooks, M., *et al.* (2004). A human immunodeficiency virus 1 (HIV-1) clade a vaccine in clinical trials: Stimulation of HIV-specific T-cell responses by DNA and recombinant modified vaccinia virus Ankara (MVA) vaccines in humans. *J. Gen. Virol.* **85,** 911–919.

Napolitani, G., Rinaldi, A., Bertoni, F., Sallusto, F., and Lanzavecchia, A. (2005). Selected Toll-like receptor agonist combinations synergistically trigger a T helper type 1-polarizing program in dendritic cells. *Nat. Immunol.* **6,** 769–776.

Navabi, H., Jasani, B., Reece, A., Clayton, A., Tabi, Z., Donninger, C., Mason, M., and Adams, M. (2009). A clinical grade poly I:C-analogue (Ampligen) promotes optimal DC maturation and Th1-type T cell responses of healthy donors and cancer patients in vitro. *Vaccine* **27,** 107–115.

Nehete, P. N., Chitta, S., Hossain, M. M., Hill, L., Bernacky, B. J., Baze, W., Arlinghaus, R. B., and Sastry, K. J. (2001). Protection against chronic infection and AIDS by an HIV envelope peptide-cocktail vaccine in a pathogenic SHIV-rhesus model. *Vaccine* **20,** 813–825.

Nehete, P. N., Nehete, B. P., Hill, L., Manuri, P. R., Baladandayuthapani, V., Feng, L., Simmons, J., and Sastry, K. J. (2008). Selective induction of cell-mediated immunity and protection of rhesus macaques from chronic SHIV(KU2) infection by prophylactic vaccination with a conserved HIV-1 envelope peptide-cocktail. *Virology* **370,** 130–141.

Nowak, A. K., Lake, R. A., and Robinson, B. W. S. (2006). Combined chemoimmunotherapy of solid tumours: Improving vaccines? *Adv. Drug Deliv. Rev.* **58,** 975–990.

Odunsi, K., Qian, F., Matsuzaki, J., Mhawech-Fauceglia, P., Andrews, C., Hoffman, E. W., Pan, L., Ritter, G., Villella, J., Thomas, B., Rodabaugh, K., Lele, S., *et al.* (2007). Vaccination with an NY-ESO-1 peptide of HLA class I/II specificities induces integrated humoral and T cell responses in ovarian cancer. *Proc. Natl. Acad. Sci. USA* **104,** 12837–12842.

Ottenhoff, T. H., Doherty, T. M., van Dissel, J. T., Bang, P., Lingnau, K., Kromann, I., and Andersen, P. (2010). First in humans: A new molecularly defined vaccine shows excellent safety and strong induction of long-lived Mycobacterium tuberculosis-specific Th1-cell like responses. *Hum. Vaccin.* **6,** 1007–1015.

Owen, R. E., Heitman, J. W., Hirschkorn, D. F., Lanteri, M. C., Biswas, H. H., Martin, J. N., Krone, M. R., Deeks, S. G., and Norris, P. J. (2010). HIV+ elite controllers have low HIV-specific T-cell activation yet maintain strong, polyfunctional T-cell responses. *AIDS* **24,** 1095–1105.

Palucka, K., Ueno, H., and Banchereau, J. (2011). Recent developments in cancer vaccines. *J. Immunol.* **186,** 1325–1331.

Pantaleo, G., Esteban, M., Jacobs, B., and Tartaglia, J. (2010). Poxvirus vector-based HIV vaccines. *Curr. Opin. HIV AIDS* **5,** 391–396.

Parvanova, I., Rettig, L., Knuth, A., and Pascolo, S. (2011). The form of NY-ESO-1 antigen has an impact on the clinical efficacy of anti-tumor vaccination. *Vaccine* **29,** 3832–3836.

Pasquetto, V., Bui, H. H., Giannino, R., Mirza, F., Sidney, J., Oseroff, C., Tscharke, D. C., Irvine, K., Bennink, J. R., Peters, B., Southwood, S., Cerundolo, V., *et al.* (2005). HLA-a*0201, HLA-a*1101, and HLA-B*0702 transgenic mice recognize numerous poxvirus determinants from a wide variety of viral gene products. *J. Immunol.* **175,** 5504–5515.

Pereyra, F., Jia, X., McLaren, P. J., Telenti, A., de Bakker, P. I., Walker, B. D., Ripke, S., Brumme, C. J., Pulit, S. L., Carrington, M., Kadie, C. M., Carlson, J. M., *et al.* (2010). The major genetic determinants of HIV-1 control affect HLA class I peptide presentation. *Science* **330,** 1551–1557.

Piot, P., Kazatchkine, M., Dybul, M., and Lob-Levyt, J. (2009). AIDS: Lessons learnt and myths dispelled. *Lancet* **374,** 260–263.

Qin, H., Nehete, P. N., He, H., Nehete, B., Buchl, S., Cha, S. C., Sastry, J. K., and Kwak, L. W. (2010). Prime-boost vaccination using chemokine-fused gp120 DNA and HIV envelope peptides activates both immediate and long-term memory cellular responses in rhesus macaques. *J. Biomed. Biotechnol.* **2010,** 860160.

Quakkelaar, E. D., Redeker, A., Haddad, E. K., Harari, A., McCaughey, S. M., Duhen, T., Filali-Mouhim, A., Goulet, J. P., Loof, N. M., Ossendorp, F., Perdiguero, B., Heinen, P., *et al.* (2011). Improved innate and adaptive immunostimulation by genetically modified HIV-1 protein expressing NYVAC vectors. *PLoS One* **6,** e16819.

Quezada, S. A., Simpson, T. R., Peggs, K. S., Merghoub, T., Vider, J., Fan, X., Blasberg, R., Yagita, H., Muranski, P., Antony, P. A., Restifo, N. P., and Allison, J. P. (2010). Tumor-reactive CD4(+) T cells develop cytotoxic activity and eradicate large established melanoma after transfer into lymphopenic hosts. *J. Exp. Med.* **207,** 637–650.

Ressing, M. E., van Driel, W. J., Brandt, R. M., Kenter, G. G., de Jong, J. H., Bauknecht, T., Fleuren, G. J., Hoogerhout, P., Offringa, R., Sette, A., Celis, E., Grey, H., *et al.* (2000). Detection of T helper responses, but not of human papillomavirus-specific cytotoxic T lymphocyte responses, after peptide vaccination of patients with cervical carcinoma. *J. Immunother.* **23,** 255–266.

Restifo, N. P., Esquivel, F., Kawakami, Y., Yewdell, J. W., Mule, J. J., Rosenberg, S. A., and Bennink, J. R. (1993). Identification of human cancers deficient in antigen processing. *J. Exp. Med.* **177,** 265–272.

Robert, C., Thomas, L., Bondarenko, I., O'Day, S., Jeffrey, W., Garbe, C., Lebbe, C., Baurain, J. F., Testori, A., Grob, J. J., Davidson, N., Richards, J., *et al.* (2011). Ipilimumab plus dacarbazine for previously untreated metastatic melanoma. *N. Engl. J. Med.* **364,** 2517–2526.

Roestenberg, M., Teirlinck, A. C., McCall, M. B., Teelen, K., Makamdop, K. N., Wiersma, J., Arens, T., Beckers, P., van Gemert, G., van de Vegte-Bolmer, M., van der Ven, A. J., Luty, A. J., *et al.* (2011). Long-term protection against malaria after experimental sporozoite inoculation: An open-label follow-up study. *Lancet* **377,** 1770–1776.

Romani, N., Thurnher, M., Idoyaga, J., Steinman, R. M., and Flacher, V. (2010). Targeting of antigens to skin dendritic cells: Possibilities to enhance vaccine efficacy. *Immunol. Cell Biol.* **88,** 424–430.

Rosario, M., Bridgeman, A., Quakkelaar, E. D., Quigley, M. F., Hill, B. J., Knudsen, M. L., Ammendola, V., Ljungberg, K., Borthwick, N., Im, E. J., McMichael, A. J., Drijfhout, J. W., *et al.* (2010). Long peptides induce polyfunctional T cells against conserved regions of HIV-1 with superior breadth to single-gene vaccines in macaques. *Eur. J. Immunol.* **40,** 1973–1984.

Rosenberg, S. A., Yang, J. C., and Restifo, N. P. (2004). Cancer immunotherapy: Moving beyond current vaccines. *Nat. Med.* **10,** 909–915.

Schellinger, J. G., Danan-Leon, L. M., Hoch, J. A., Kassa, A., Srivastava, I., Davis, D., and Gervay-Hague, J. (2011). Synthesis of a trimeric gp120 epitope mimic conjugated to a T-helper peptide to improve antigenicity. *J. Am. Chem. Soc.* **133,** 3230–3233.

Schenten, D., and Medzhitov, R. (2011). The control of adaptive immune responses by the innate immune system. *Adv. Immunol.* **109,** 87–124.

Schietinger, A., Philip, M., Liu, R. B., Schreiber, K., and Schreiber, H. (2010). Bystander killing of cancer requires the cooperation of CD4(+) and CD8(+) T cells during the effector phase. *J. Exp. Med.* **207,** 2469–2477.

Schiller, J. T., and Lowy, D. R. (2010). Vaccines to prevent infections by oncoviruses. *Annu. Rev. Microbiol.* **64,** 23–41.

Schoenberger, S. P., Toes, R. E., van der Voort, E. I., Offringa, R., and Melief, C. J. (1998). T-cell help for cytotoxic T lymphocytes is mediated by CD40-CD40L interactions. *Nature* **393,** 480–483.

Schuurhuis, D. H., Laban, S., Toes, R. E., Ricciardi-Castagnoli, P., Kleijmeer, M. J., van der Voort, E. I., Rea, D., Offringa, R., Geuze, H. J., Melief, C. J., and Ossendorp, F. (2000). Immature dendritic cells acquire CD8(+) cytotoxic T lymphocyte priming capacity upon activation by T helper cell-independent or -dependent stimuli. *J. Exp. Med.* **192,** 145–150.

Schwartzentruber, D. J., Lawson, D. H., Richards, J. M., Conry, R. M., Miller, D. M., Treisman, J., Gailani, F., Riley, L., Conlon, K., Pockaj, B., Kendra, K. L., White, R. L., *et al.* (2011). gp100 peptide vaccine and interleukin-2 in patients with advanced melanoma. *N. Engl. J. Med.* **364,** 2119–2127.

Seliger, B., Ruiz-Cabello, F., and Garrido, F. (2008). IFN inducibility of major histocompatibility antigens in tumors. *In* "Advances in Cancer Research", (G. Vande Woude and G. Klein, eds.), pp. 249–276. Academic Press, New York (Chapter 7).

Sharma, A. K., and Khuller, G. K. (2001). DNA vaccines: Future strategies and relevance to intracellular pathogens. *Immunol. Cell Biol.* **79,** 537–546.

Shirai, M., Pendleton, C. D., Ahlers, J., Takeshita, T., Newman, M., and Berzofsky, J. A. (1994). Helper-cytotoxic T lymphocyte (CTL) determinant linkage required for priming of anti-HIV CD8+ CTL in vivo with peptide vaccine constructs. *J. Immunol.* **152,** 549–556.

Smyth, L. J. C., van Poelgeest, M. I., Davidson, E. J., Kwappenberg, K. M. C., Burt, D., Sehr, P., Pawlita, M., Man, S., Hickling, J. K., Fiander, A. N., Tristram, A., Kitchener, H. C., *et al.* (2004). Immunological responses in women with human papillomavirus type 16 (HPV-16)-associated anogenital intraepithelial neoplasia induced by heterologous prime-boost HPV-16 oncogene vaccination. *Clin. Cancer Res.* **10,** 2954–2961.

Sonda, N., Chioda, M., Zilio, S., Simonato, F., and Bronte, V. (2011). Transcription factors in myeloid-derived suppressor cell recruitment and function. *Curr. Opin. Immunol.* **23,** 279–285.

Speetjens, F. M., Kuppen, P. J., Welters, M. J., Essahsah, F., Voet van den Brink, A. M., Lantrua, M. G., Valentijn, A. R., Oostendorp, J., Fathers, L. M., Nijman, H. W., Drijfhout, J. W., van de Velde, C. J., *et al.* (2009). Induction of p53-specific immunity by a p53 synthetic long peptide vaccine in patients treated for metastatic colorectal cancer. *Clin. Cancer Res.* **15,** 1086–1095.

Speiser, D. E., Schwarz, K., Baumgaertner, P., Manolova, V., Devevre, E., Sterry, W., Walden, P., Zippelius, A., Conzett, K. B., Senti, G., Voelter, V., Cerottini, J. P., *et al.* (2010). Memory and effector CD8 T-cell responses after nanoparticle vaccination of melanoma patients. *J. Immunother.* **33,** 848–858.

Steinman, R. M., and Pope, M. (2002). Exploiting dendritic cells to improve vaccine efficacy. *J. Clin. Invest.* **109,** 1519–1526.

Steinman, R. M., Hawiger, D., and Nussenzweig, M. C. (2003). Tolerogenic dendritic cells. *Annu. Rev. Immunol.* **21,** 685–711.

Streeck, H., Lichterfeld, M., Alter, G., Meier, A., Teigen, N., Yassine-Diab, B., Sidhu, H. K., Little, S., Kelleher, A., Routy, J. P., Rosenberg, E. S., Sekaly, R. P., *et al.* (2007). Recognition of a defined region within p24 Gag by CD8+ T cells during primary human immunodeficiency virus type 1 infection in individuals expressing protective HLA class I alleles. *J. Virol.* **81,** 7725–7731.

Thara, E., Dorff, T. B., Pinski, J. K., and Quinn, D. I. (2011). Vaccine therapy with sipuleucel-T (Provenge) for prostate cancer. *Maturitas* **69,** 296–303.

Theobald, M., Biggs, J., Hernandez, J., Lustgarten, J., Labadie, C., and Sherman, L. A. (1997). Tolerance to p53 by A2.1-restricted cytotoxic T lymphocytes. *J. Exp. Med.* **185,** 833–841.

Tighe, H., Takabayashi, K., Schwartz, D., Marsden, R., Beck, L., Corbeil, J., Richman, D. D., Eiden, J. J., Jr., Spiegelberg, H. L., and Raz, E. (2000a). Conjugation of protein to immunostimulatory DNA results in a rapid, long-lasting and potent induction of cell-mediated and humoral immunity. *Eur. J. Immunol.* **30,** 1939–1947.

Tighe, H., Takabayashi, K., Schwartz, D., Van, N. G., Tuck, S., Eiden, J. J., Kagey-Sobotka, A., Creticos, P. S., Lichtenstein, L. M., Spiegelberg, H. L., and Raz, E. (2000b). Conjugation of immunostimulatory DNA to the short ragweed allergen amb a 1 enhances its immunogenicity and reduces its allergenicity. *J. Allergy Clin. Immunol.* **106,** 124–134.

Toes, R. E., Blom, R. J., Offringa, R., Kast, W. M., and Melief, C. J. (1996a). Enhanced tumor outgrowth after peptide vaccination. Functional deletion of tumor-specific CTL induced by peptide vaccination can lead to the inability to reject tumors. *J. Immunol.* **156,** 3911–3918.

Toes, R. E., Offringa, R., Blom, R. J., Melief, C. J., and Kast, W. M. (1996b). Peptide vaccination can lead to enhanced tumor growth through specific T-cell tolerance induction. *Proc. Natl. Acad. Sci. USA* **93,** 7855–7860.

van der Burg, S. H., and Melief, C. J. (2011). Therapeutic vaccination against human papilloma virus induced malignancies. *Curr. Opin. Immunol.* **23,** 252–257.

van der Burg, S. H., Kwappenberg, K. M. C., O'Neill, T., Brandt, R. M. P., Melief, C. J. M., Hickling, J. K., and Offringa, R. (2001). Pre-clinical safety and efficacy of TA-CIN, a recombinant HPV16 L2E6E7 fusion protein vaccine, in homologous and heterologous prime-boost regimens. *Vaccine* **19,** 3652–3660.

van der Burg, S. H., Arens, R., and Melief, C. J. (2011). Immunotherapy for persistent viral infections and associated disease. *Trends Immunol.* **32,** 97–103.

Verdijk, R. M., Mutis, T., Esendam, B., Kamp, J., Melief, C. J., Brand, A., and Goulmy, E. (1999). Polyriboinosinic polyribocytidylic acid (poly(I:C)) induces stable maturation of functionally active human dendritic cells. *J. Immunol.* **163,** 57–61.

Vierboom, M. P., Nijman, H. W., Offringa, R., van der Voort, E. I., van, H. T., van den Broek, L., Fleuren, G. J., Kenemans, P., Kast, W. M., and Melief, C. J. (1997). Tumor eradication by wild-type p53-specific cytotoxic T lymphocytes. *J. Exp. Med.* **186,** 695–704.

Vollmer, J., and Krieg, A. M. (2009). Immunotherapeutic applications of CpG oligodeoxynucleotide TLR9 agonists. *Adv. Drug Deliv. Rev.* **61,** 195–204.

Welters, M. J. P., Bijker, M. S., van den Eeden, S. J. F., Franken, K. L. M. C., Melief, C. J. M., Offringa, R., and van der Burg, S. H. (2007). Multiple CD4 and CD8 T-cell activation parameters predict vaccine efficacy in vivo mediated by individual DC-activating agonists. *Vaccine* **25,** 1379–1389.

Welters, M. J., Kenter, G. G., Piersma, S. J., Vloon, A. P., Lowik, M. J., Berends-van der Meer, D. M., Drijfhout, J. W., Valentijn, A. R., Wafelman, A. R., Oostendorp, J., Fleuren, G. J., Offringa, R., *et al.* (2008). Induction of tumor-specific CD4+ and CD8+ T-cell immunity in cervical cancer patients by a human papillomavirus type 16 E6 and E7 long peptides vaccine. *Clin. Cancer Res.* **14,** 178–187.

Welters, M. J., Kenter, G. G., de Vos van Steenwijk, P. J., Lowik, M. J., Berends-van der Meer, D. M., Essahsah, F., Stynenbosch, L. F., Vloon, A. P., Ramwadhdoebe, T. H., Piersma, S. J., van der Hulst, J. M., Valentijn, A. R., *et al.* (2010). Success or failure of vaccination for HPV16-positive vulvar lesions correlates with kinetics and phenotype of induced T-cell responses. *Proc. Natl. Acad. Sci. USA* **107,** 11895–11899.

Widmann, C., Romero, P., Maryanski, J. L., Corradin, G., and Valmori, D. (1992). T helper epitopes enhance the cytotoxic response of mice immunized with MHC class I-restricted malaria peptides. *J. Immunol. Methods* **155,** 95–99.

Wimmer, E., and Paul, A. V. (2010). Synthetic poliovirus and other designer viruses: What have we learned from them? *Annu. Rev. Microbiol.* **65,** 583–609.

Yasutomi, Y., Palker, T. J., Gardner, M. B., Haynes, B. F., and Letvin, N. L. (1993). Synthetic peptide in mineral oil adjuvant elicits simian immunodeficiency virus-specific CD8+ cytotoxic T lymphocytes in rhesus monkeys. *J. Immunol.* **151,** 5096–5105.

Youn, J. I., and Gabrilovich, D. I. (2010). The biology of myeloid-derived suppressor cells: The blessing and the curse of morphological and functional heterogeneity. *Eur. J. Immunol.* **40,** 2969–2975.

Zeng, G., Li, Y., El-Gamil, M., Sidney, J., Sette, A., Wang, R. F., Rosenberg, S. A., and Robbins, P. F. (2002). Generation of NY-ESO-1-specific CD4+ and CD8+ T cells by a single peptide with dual MHC class I and class II specificities. *Cancer Res.* **62,** 3630–3635.

Zhang, B., Karrison, T., Rowley, D. A., and Schreiber, H. (2008). IFN-gamma- and TNF-dependent bystander eradication of antigen-loss variants in established mouse cancers. *J. Clin. Invest.* **118,** 1398–1404.

Zhang, H., Hong, H., Li, D., Ma, S., Di, Y., Stoten, A., Haig, N., Di, G. K., Yu, Z., Xu, X. N., McMichael, A., and Jiang, S. (2009). Comparing pooled peptides with intact protein for accessing cross-presentation pathways for protective CD8+ and CD4+ T cells. *J. Biol. Chem.* **284,** 9184–9191.

Zitvogel, L., Kepp, O., and Kroemer, G. (2011). Immune parameters affecting the efficacy of chemotherapeutic regimens. *Nat. Rev. Clin. Oncol.* **8,** 151–160.

Zwaveling, S., Mota, S. C. F., Nouta, J., Johnson, M., Lipford, G. B., Offringa, R., van der Burg, S. H., and Melief, C. J. M. (2002). Established human papillomavirus type 16-expressing tumors are effectively eradicated following vaccination with long peptides. *J. Immunol.* **169,** 350–358.

CHAPTER 5

Malaria Vaccine Development Using Synthetic Peptides as a Technical Platform

Giampietro Corradin,* Nora Céspedes,*,† Antonio Verdini,* Andrey V. Kajava,‡ Myriam Arévalo-Herrera,† and **Sócrates Herrera†**

Contents

* Biochemstry Department, University of Lausanne, Epalinges, Switzerland
† Malaria Vaccine and Drug Development Center/Immunology Institute, Universidad del Valle, Cali, Colombia
‡ CRBM, CNRS, University of Montpellier, Montpellier, France

Advances in Immunology, Volume 114
ISSN 0065-2776, DOI: 10.1016/B978-0-12-396548-6.00005-6

Abstract The review covers the development of synthetic peptides as vaccine candidates for *Plasmodium falciparum*- and *Plasmodium vivax*-induced malaria from its beginning up to date and the concomitant progress of solid phase peptide synthesis (SPPS) that enables the production of long peptides in a routine fashion. The review also stresses the development of other complementary tools and actions in order to achieve the long sought goal of an efficacious malaria vaccine.

1. INTRODUCTION

Malaria remains the most important parasitic infection in the world. Up to 40% of the world population is estimated to be at risk of contracting malaria. The majority of over one million annual deaths is the result of *Plasmodium falciparum* (*P. falciparum*) infection, the most prevalent (80%) and lethal *Plasmodium* species, occurring among young children and pregnant women living in sub-Saharan Africa (Hay *et al.*, 2010). A second species *Plasmodium vivax* causes most of the remaining cases (~20%), particularly, in Southeast and East Asia, the Eastern Mediterranean and Central, and South America regions in which it coexists with *P. falciparum* (World Health Organization, 2010).

Even though *P. vivax* is considered to be a more benign parasite, its relapsing pattern and recent studies demonstrating a growing number of severe and complicated cases confer to *P. vivax* malaria infection increasing importance (Kochar *et al.*, 2009a,b; Price *et al.*, 2009; Tjitra *et al.*, 2008).

As reported by a former collaborator, Sope Olugbile, who grew up in a malaria-endemic region of South-West Nigeria and also treated malaria cases as a "doctor," "what is frequently overlooked is the pain and suffering young children living in malaria-endemic areas go through, often every month, sometimes more frequently, till they reach early adulthood when they achieve partial immunity against the debilitating symptoms of malaria. The impact is so immense, that as child he used to miss two to three school days almost every month due to malaria. The joint pains and the high fever were most distressing and equally harsh were the bitter medications, which on their own induce vomiting thus delaying the onset of drug action. So, frequently each episode had to be 'extinguished' by parenteral antimalarials, while another one was only a few weeks away. The majority of children that report to health facilities are also a result of malaria and its complications. Not uncommon were complications due to

P. falciparum infections that arose from treatments given at home before presentation at the hospital. These complications might be side-effects of orthodox medications or bizarre herbal concoctions 'prescribed' by neighbors and older family members. So, the impact of malaria in its entirety is the sum of the mortality mostly in young children and the frequent periodic morbidities that extend up into early adulthood (Verdini *et al.*, 2010)." In areas of low transmission intensity like those of Latin America, clinical manifestations and complications occur later in adolescents and young adults. Moreover, travelers may suffer of *P. vivax* malaria for several years after they have returned from endemic areas due to reactivation of parasite dormant forms (hypnozoites) that may remain in the liver for several years.

Although the classical measures to control malaria, that is, early diagnosis, effective treatment and mosquito control, have significantly contributed to shrink the malaria map (Feachem *et al.*, 2009), it is currently considered that the development of an efficacious antimalaria vaccine is a cost effective approach to reduce deaths, clinical complications and transmission to other members of the community, and is expected to accelerate malaria elimination and to free economic and social resources for other society needs (Alonso *et al.*, 2011).

A malaria vaccine seems to be possible because children from highly endemic areas become effectively protected from disease and death risk after several years of exposure to repeated infections, even though occasional clinical manifestations occur throughout the individual life span (Aponte *et al.*, 2007; Baird *et al.*, 1991, 1998). It is common to find children and adults that conduct a normal, healthy life who present an asymptomatic, and low level parasitemic infection (Branch *et al.*, 2005; Bruce *et al.*, 2000). Additionally, immunization of humans with *P. falciparum* and *P. vivax* radiation-attenuated sporozoites (RAS) or live *P. falciparum* sporozoites together with antimalarial drugs confers protection (Nussenzweig, 1980; Roestenberg *et al.*, 2009). Moreover, passive transfer of purified immunoglobulins from immune donors to malaria patients has shown to reduce parasitemia and confers clinical protection, clearly indicating that antibodies are involved in malaria protection (Bouharoun-Tayoun *et al.*, 1990; McGregor, 1964; McGregor *et al.*, 1968). Likewise, experiments in mice have demonstrated that the transfer of specific T-cell is also playing a role in protection (Overstreet *et al.*, 2008; Romero *et al.*, 1990).

As seen from Fig. 5.1, which describes the host cycle of the malaria parasite, prophylactic vaccines can target two different stages of the parasite: the preerythrocytic (sporozoite and liver stages) and the asexual erythrocytic stage based on their capability of stimulating both humoral and cellular immune responses. It has been shown that T-cells and antibodies are both mediators of protection through different mechanisms depending on the stage of the parasite to be targeted. During the preerythrocytic phase, antibodies can inhibit liver invasion by sporozoites (Jones *et al.*, 1993; Sinnis and Nussenzweig, 1996) and therefore prevent

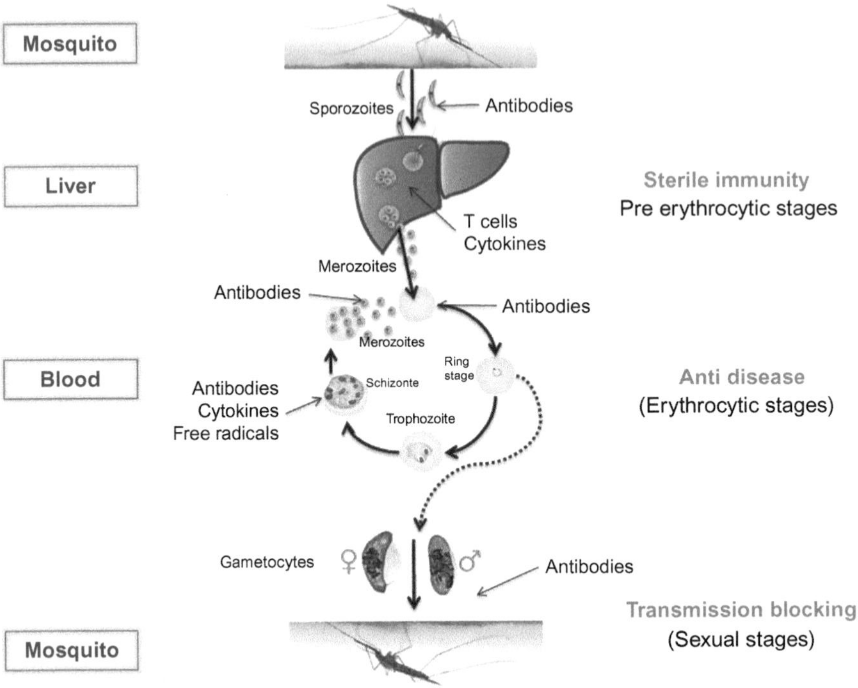

FIGURE 5.1 Plasmodium life cycle. Plasmodium sporozoites are injected intradermally during a blood meal of an infected female Anopheles mosquito. Once in circulation, sporozoites arrest in the liver, invade hepatocytes, and develop into EEFs, which, when mature, release merozoites that initiate blood stage infection. Each merozoite can infect a red blood cell. Within the red cell, the merozoite matures either into a uninucleate gametocyte, the sexual stage, or into a schizont containing multiple merozoites. Rupture of the schizont releases these merozoites, which infect other red cells. If a mosquito ingests nature gametocytes, the gametocytes develop into oocysts in the mosquito gut containing numerous sporozoites. (See Color Insert.)

further intracellular multiplication. If parasites develop in the liver to mature schizonts, merozoites are released into the blood stream. Then they would have to face the presence of antibodies that prevent parasite invasion into the erythrocytes by direct inhibition of merozoite attachment to the red blood cells (Hollingdale *et al.*, 1984; Lyon *et al.*, 1989) or through cytolytic IgG isotopes in the presence of monocytes (Antibody Dependent Cell Inhibition, ADCI; Bouharoun-Tayoun *et al.*, 1990, 1995) or other not yet defined mechanisms. Moreover, antibodies are able to block parasite transmission from humans to mosquitos by preventing the fertilization process in the mosquito stomach (Carter and Chen, 1976).

The destruction of parasites developing inside host cells can also be mediated by CD4+ and CD8+ T-cells producing cytokines and reactive radicals (Doolan *et al.*, 2009). During the preerythrocytic phase, cytokines such as IFN-γ released by both CD4+ and CD8+ T-cells are able to arrest the intracellular development of liver schizonts (Schofield *et al.*, 1987; Sedegah *et al.*, 1992). During the asexual parasite development in the red cells, oxygen radicals are able to destroy intracellular parasites (Golenser *et al.*, 1992; Kharazmi *et al.*, 1987). Furthermore, it appears that cytokines are also related to the blockage of parasite transmission to mosquitos (Carter and Mendis, 1992; Mendis *et al.*, 1987).

Under field conditions the development of clinical immunity is likely to involve a combination of these and other mechanisms, which by an unknown reason are incapable to produce sterile immunity (Doolan *et al.*, 2009; Marsh *et al.*, 1989). Surprisingly, repeated experimental vaccination with whole, live RAS induced solid sterile immunity (Clyde *et al.*, 1973; Herrington *et al.*, 1991). Although this protection was observed in a murine model (Nussenzweig *et al.*, 1967) and has been since reproduced for human malaria as well as for several other *Plasmodium* species, it is not yet clear which immune mechanisms and target antigens are involved in sterile protection (Good and Doolan, 2010). Sterile immunity requires that preerythrocytic vaccines achieve 100%, efficacy. In addition, protection ideally has to be lifelong or at least long lasting (several years). Vaccination against yellow fever for instance is recommended every 10 years (Poland *et al.*, 1981). Both of these two requisites have been shown to be quite demanding in malaria.

It appears more feasible to achieve clinical immunity. Individuals continuously exposed to malaria in endemic areas eventually develop reduced levels of parasitemia and asymptomatic infections. This could in theory be achieved by the use of highly effective vaccines based on erythrocytic stage derived antigens, or based on combinations of both partially protective preerythrocytic and asexual blood stage antigens.

Unfortunately, there is as yet a limited understanding on the specificity of antibodies and antibody-mediated mechanisms that limit liver invasion by sporozoites, as well as failure to detect a correlation between protection and the T-cell response to preerythrocytic antigens in individuals living in endemic areas. This may due to the fact that such a correlation does not exist, and the presence of many asymptomatic, infected individuals may support this hypothesis. However, it could also be that individuals from malaria-endemic regions develop partially protective responses, that limit the burden of preerythrocytic parasites, that is, sporozoites and liver schizonts leading to lower and easier to handle asexual parasitemia. In rural areas of Burkina Faso where malaria transmission is seasonal, the percentage of adult parasite carriers is 50% and 25% during high and low transmission seasons, respectively (I. Nebie, personal communication).

Additionally, at the present status of technology and basic knowledge, failure to detect a disease–immune response correlation is due in part to the extensive polymorphism of the MHC molecules and the weak T-cell responses usually seen. Therefore no effective selection procedure exists to identify protective antigens from a large number of possible vaccine candidates.

On the other hand, in our opinion, it is easier to apply a rigorous selection procedure to erythrocytic antigens based on their reactivity with antibodies. IgG obtained from immune individuals are known to be mediators of protection (McGregor, 1964; Perignon and Druilhe, 1994).

A last consideration to be made is that determination of efficacy for malaria vaccines is less difficult than for other infectious diseases (HIV, TB). In fact, for preerythrocytic and erythrocytic vaccine antigens, a reliable experimental parasite-challenge model exists that allow assessment of protective efficacy in a limited number of subjects (Herrera *et al.*, 2011b; Sauerwein *et al.*, 2011). Phase 2 clinical trials require only hundreds of volunteers and can be limited in time (6–12 months).

In spite of all of these considerations, the preerythrocytic antigen, circumsporozoite protein (CSP) of *P. falciparum*, has been the most used protein in malaria vaccine development in the last 25 years. This is due to the fact that it was the first protein to be sequenced (Dame *et al.*, 1984; Enea *et al.*, 1984), and initial results obtained in mice using the *Plasmodium berghei* model were quite spectacular (Zavala *et al.*, 1987). In fact, at that time, everybody expected to have a vaccine around the corner.

Several strategies from the use of whole malaria parasites to subunit vaccines based on recombinant technology, naked DNA and peptide synthesis have been envisaged, and the use of multistage and multispecies vaccine would have the advantage of simultaneous priming of synergistic immune mechanisms targeting the main parasite species circulating in a given region.

This brings us to the beginning of malaria clinical trials and the scope of this review, which is to focus on the use of synthetic peptides as a platform for the development of an effective malaria vaccine. The first part is a brief history and future perspectives of this technology followed by the most salient events in synthetic vaccine development against malaria caused by *P. falciparum* and *P. vivax* parasites.

2. PEPTIDE SYNTHESIS

2.1. Historical notes and future progress

Initial studies on synthetic peptides were based on the assumption that the amino acids constituting the protein molecule are linked together via amide bonds. Experimental research involved the condensation of aspartic acid and asparagine to a complex mixture of polymeric products, difficult to characterize, and with only a superficial resemblance to the protein molecules (Grimaux, 1882; Schaal, 1871).

The true beginning of peptide chemistry is considered to be the synthesis of benzoylglycylglycine as demonstrated by Curtius (1882) and that of glycylglycine by Fischer and Fourneau (1901).

The intensive work of these German chemists led, in the early 1900s, to the development of the first practical methods for peptide synthesis (Curtius, 1902; Fischer, 1903). The azide-coupling method was successfully employed by Curtius in the preparation of benzoylglycine oligopeptides, while the development of the acylchloride method enabled Fischer to synthesize several short peptides and complete in 1907 the synthesis of the octadecapeptide LGGGLGGGLGGGGGGGGG (Fischer, 1907).

Both approaches suffered from serious side reactions, such as racemization, the rearrangement of acyl azides and the practical impossibility to use amino acids with side-chain functionality. In addition, difficulties in obtaining enantiomerically pure amino acids and the lack of an easily removable group for the temporary protection of the amino group hampered, at that time and for years, any serious attempts to synthesize more complex peptides.

The introduction in 1932 of the carbobenzoxy group (Z) by Bergmann and Zervas (the abbreviated designation Z was chosen to honor Zervas in his lifetime) marks the origin of modern peptide synthesis (Bergman and Zervas, 1932).

The 30-year search for a satisfactory amino blocking group finally produced a protecting moiety readily removable without inducing breakdown of the labile peptide bond and with the important additional property to preserve the integrity of the amino acid chiral carbon upon "activation" (i.e., the attachment of a leaving group to the acyl carbon) of the carboxyl group.

Since then, peptide bond formation has been carried out by condensation of a Z-protected and activated amino acid with a second amino acid carrying a masked carboxyl group. The ready removal of Z allowed peptide chemists to assemble complex peptide sequences by addition of one residue at a time ("stepwise synthesis") proceeding from the esterified or amidated C-terminal amino acid to the N-terminal amino acid or by the conjunction of protected sequences of amino acids ("fragment condensation"). The desired free peptides were obtained at the end of the synthesis by removal of Z and all other protecting groups (Fig. 5.2).

After about 20years from the introduction of Z in peptide synthesis, du Vigneaud accomplished the formidable task of synthesizing the active hormone oxytocin, a nonapeptide amide with a disulfide bridge that forms a 20-atom ring containing six of the nine residues present in the molecule, with an overall yield well under 1% (du Vigneaud *et al.*, 1954). For his landmark work, du Vigneaud was awarded the 1955 Nobel Prize in chemistry.

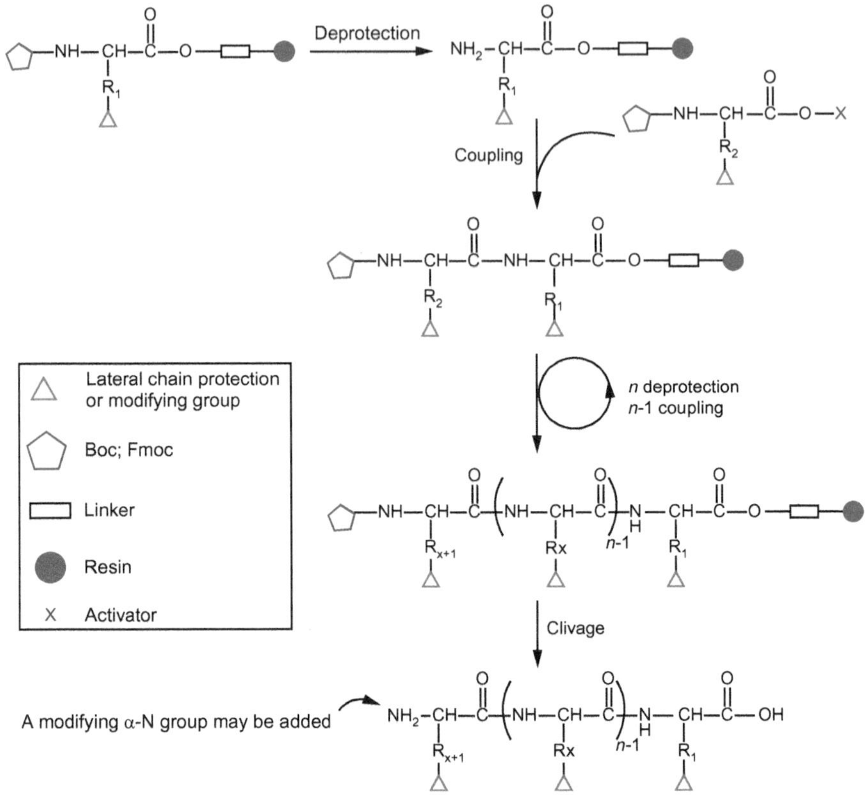

FIGURE 5.2 General scheme of the Boc-benzyl and Fmoc–*t*-butyl methods of stepwise solid-phase synthesis of linear peptides. Deprotection of the α-amino protecting group of the resin-linked growing peptide chain and coupling of the next protected amino acid constitute the repetitive cycle of the synthesis. X indicates the coupling reagent for amide bond formation. Both the α-amino group and the ε-amino group on lysine side chains can be modified for various purposes. The use of an insoluble support (resin) in a single reaction vessel allows for automation of the process. The crude peptide is obtained by resin-peptide acidolysis (liquid HF for Boc-benzyl and TFA for Fmoc–*t*-butyl methods) in the presence of scavengers. X: for example, diisopropylcarbodiimide–*N*-hydroxybenzotriazole; preformed symmetrical anhydrides; active esters; aminium salts such as HBTU [2-(1H-benzotriazole-1-yl)-1,1,3,3-tetramethylaminium hexafluorophosphate], TBTU [2-(1H-benzotriazole-1-yl)-1,1,3,3-tetramethylaminiumtetrafluoroborate], BOP [benzotriazole-1-yl-oxy-*tris*-(dimethylamino)-phosphoniumhexafluorophosphate], PyBOP (benzotriazole-1-yl-oxy-*tris*-pyrrolidino-phosphonium hexafluorophosphate), or HCTU [2-(6-chloro-1H-benzotriazole-1-yl)-1,1,3,3-tetramethylaminium hexafluorophosphate] in the presence of a tertiary base. (See Color Insert.)

Between 1932 and 1963, Z as well as new amino protecting groups, preeminent among them the acid-labile *tert*-butyloxycarbonyl group (Boc) introduced in 1957 (Carpino, 1957; Mckay and Albertson, 1957) and more efficient coupling methods such as dicyclohexylcarbodiimide (DCCI) and active esters (Bodanszky, 1955; Schwyzer, 1953; Sheehan and Hess, 1955) were used for the synthesis of many small- and medium-size biologically active peptides in solution, the most spectacular example being the synthesis of the 39-residue porcine β-corticotropin adrenocorticotrophic hormone (ACTH) by Schwyzer and Sieber (1963).

Chinese scientists wishing to accomplish a task on a grandiose scale started in 1958 the synthesis of bovine insulin. The total synthesis of the complex molecule (two linear A and B chains with 21 and 30aa residues, respectively, and three disulfide bridges between A6A11, A7B7, and A19B20) was fully accomplished in 1965 (Du *et al.*, 1961; Kung *et al.*, 1965). Crystalline bovine insulin was obtained by co-oxidation of separately prepared A and B chains and represents the first protein ever synthesized *in vitro*. In a recent personal reminiscence of the synthesis of insulin Zhang (2010), one of the many contributors, wrote: "when the final paper was published in 1966, the world scientific community was astonished, unable to imagine how such an important achievement was accomplished in China, a developing country not very advanced in science."

The general strategy of peptide synthesis in solution includes: (1) selection of main-chain and side-chain protective groups, (2) choice of the activation method, (3) careful selection of segments to avoid or minimize racemization during segment condensation, and (4) solubility considerations. Solution-based methods offer the chemist the attractive opportunity to isolate and characterize the intermediates after each reaction. Perhaps the most frustrating problem faced during actual synthesis is the unpredictable solubility of the growing peptide chain. Furthermore, peptide synthesis in solution is a very labor intensive and time-consuming procedure requiring the skills of experienced peptide chemists.

In an effort to overcome many of the problems encountered in solution synthesis, Merrifield introduced the concept of stepwise peptide synthesis on an insoluble matrix by describing the first successful synthesis of the tetrapeptide Leu-Ala-Gly-Val at the Federation of American Societies for Experimental Biology (FASEB) in 1962 (Merrifield, 1962) with a full paper appearing in 1963 (Merrifield, 1963).

The historic 1963 paper represents a second major breakthrough in peptide chemistry after the introduction of the Bergman and Zervas carbobenzoxy protecting group.

In this approach, the C-terminal amino acid is bound covalently through its carboxyl group to an insoluble support and synthesis is then carried out by the successive addition of amino acids in the desired sequence. In contrast to solution synthesis, all of the intermediate steps of purification are reduced to simple resin filtration and washings. Being a rapid, cyclic process (deprotection, washing, coupling, washing, deprotection, etc.) occurring in a single vessel, the method has been automated early on in its implementation (Merrifield *et al.*, 1966). At the end of the assembly, the peptide is released from the solid support and freed from the amino acid side-chain protecting groups (Fig. 5.2).

The original method of solid phase peptide synthesis (SPPS) was rapidly improved by Merrifield by replacement of $N^{\alpha}Z$ with N^{α}Boc-protecting groups and use of 2% cross-linked polystyrene resin in place of the nitropolystyrene support. A benzyl ester linkage to the cross-linked polystyrene remaining stable throughout the chain assembly, benzyl-based side-chain protection, *in situ* activation with DCCI and cleavage of the assembled peptides from the resin with HF secured a rapid step-wise synthesis of a series of biologically active peptides culminating with the total synthesis of a 124-residue enzyme with ribonuclease A activity in early 1969 (Gutte and Merrifield, 1969).

The difference in effort required between the SPPS and solution phase methods for the synthesis of ribonuclease A, attracted global attention in the scientific community. The synthesis based on the solid phase procedure was fully described in a single communication and involved only Merrifield and his first postdoctoral fellow Gutte; the synthesis in solution of ribonuclease S (which consists of residues 21–124 of ribonuclease A) was reported in detail by chemists working at the Merck laboratories in a series of communications, and involved over twenty people (Denkewalter *et al.*, 1969).

Nevertheless, the concept of a multistep synthesis without the isolation and purification of intermediates was an anathema to most synthetic chemists. Wünsch *et al.* (1968) described the first synthesis in solution, by classical fragment condensation, of fully active and crystalline mammalian glucagon, a 29-aa peptide hormone secreted by the pancreas. The preparation of the hormone required the efforts of a large, skilled team over a period of several years. In 1971, he reviewed the synthesis of peptides and concluded that SPPS was "unsuitable for the satisfactory synthesis of higher natural peptides (with more than 15aa residues)" (Wünsch, 1971).

This firm belief was demolished within a few years by Mojsov (a graduate student in the Merrifield laboratory) who prepared glucagon by SPPS in a few months and, after improving the synthetic protocol, obtained crystalline glucagon in an overall yield higher than that reported by Wünsch (Mojsov and Merrifield, 1984). By 2006, over 200 analogues (agonists and antagonists) of glucagon have been synthesized by SPPS (Unson, 2007).

As a consequence of these differences in effort and after reexamination and improvement of virtually every aspect of SPPS in Merrifield's laboratory (Merrifield, 1993), the solid phase methodology has become the more widely adopted. In 1984, Merrifield was awarded the Nobel Prize in chemistry for his invention.

The advantages of SPPS had become apparent to all but a few determined skeptics. The synthesis in solution of pure, crystalline ribonuclease A with full enzymatic activity achieved in 1981 by Yajima and Fujii marks the end of an era and represents the culmination of classical peptide synthesis in solution (Yajima and Fujii, 1981).

Sheppard and his group in Cambridge (UK) have taken the Merrifield basic concept and remodeled it very successfully with alternative chemistry (Atherton and Sheppard, 1989). The Sheppard method of SPPS has rapidly gained in popularity for the milder conditions of the synthesis protocol which uses the Fmoc group (9-fluorenylmethoxycarbonyl) for α-amino protection and ether, ester and urethane derivatives based on *t*-butanol for side-chain (ω) protection. The α/ω-protection is absolutely orthogonal as opposed to nearly orthogonal of the standard Merrifield approach. Fmoc is usually removed with piperidine in *N,N*-dimethylformamide. The final resin cleavage with simultaneous removal of mild, acid-labile side-chains protecting groups can be carried out under much gentler conditions with trifluoroacetic acid (TFA) in the presence of suitable scavengers (Fig. 5.2).

Improved chemistries, solid supports and protocols, incessantly developed over the years for both the Boc-benzyl and Fmoc–*t*-butyl methods, have been utilized in the stepwise assembly of many long peptides and small proteins containing 50–90 and even more than 100aa residues (Nilsson *et al.*, 2005). For example, the Boc method has been used by Kent and coworkers for the stepwise assembly of both L and D enantiomers of the 99-residue HIV-1 protease (1–99). The natural 198-residue HIV-1 protease obtained by the association of the monomers into an active, noncovalently bound homodimer is considered a landmark achievement in SPPS (Schneider and Kent, 1988). The stepwise synthesis (on an automatic peptide synthesizer) of the 99-residue monomer has been systematically optimized to reach a rate of synthesis of 75 residues per day and the assembly of the protected peptide in 33h! All but two couplings proceeded in >99.8%. As discussed by Kent, an extraordinary synthetic efficiency of each coupling step (99.9%) is necessary for preparing a 100-residue peptide in 90% overall yield; a 97.0% efficiency provides only a 5% overall yield (Kent, 1980).

Peptides control many of the processes involved in the immune system response. Since the late-1970, synthetic peptides obtained by stepwise SPPS have become increasingly important in almost all areas of immunological research. Designing new peptide vaccine candidates is one of the hottest challenges of the twenty-first century science. Vaccines based on chemically synthesized peptides offer implicit safety due to the absence of such contaminants as DNA and other viral or cellular debris. Since small peptides can hardly reproduce the secondary and tertiary structures of native protein molecules, today the best approach consists in chemically preparing by SPPS long, linear peptides (from about 50 to 100aa residues or more), which are safe and immunogenic when formulated with various adjuvants and suitable for eliciting an antibody response in humans (Corradin *et al.*, 2004, 2010; Olugbile *et al.*, 2010). These long peptides can mimic native structural epitopes when isolated from the context of the whole protein and can be identified in the proteomes by using bioinformatics approaches (Corradin *et al.*, 2007, 2010). Recently, this structure-based bioinformatics/peptide synthesis approach has been successfully applied to the identification of new malaria vaccine candidates (Olugbile *et al.*, 2009, 2011; Villard *et al.*, 2007).

Despite the significant gain made in advancing the technology of SPPS, most proteins cannot be synthesized by the stepwise assembly of amino acids. One successful approach used to access a protein with 238 residues (*Aequorea* green fluorescent protein) consisted in the assembly in solution of 26 protected peptide segments prepared by SPPS (Nishiuchi *et al.*, 1998).

Currently, the most common approach for the total chemical synthesis of proteins is native chemical ligation (NCL) (Schnolzer and Kent, 1992). In this approach, two fragments are initially assembled stepwise on the solid phase, one with an N-terminal Cys residue and the other with a C-terminal thioacid (Fig. 5.3). After resin cleavage, side chain deblocking and purification, the thioacid is converted to a thioester, allowing the two fragments to react in aqueous solution (transthioesterification) to form a thioester bond between them. Spontaneous rearrangement of this bond results in a native amide bond between the fragments with regeneration of the free sulfhydryl on the Cys residue (Fig. 5.3). The process can then be repeated to link additional peptide fragments. The cumulative effects of stepwise synthetic errors are minimized due to the coupling of highly purified fragments in water. Examples of proteins prepared via NCL are the 116-residues anticoagulant microprotein S (Hackeng *et al.*, 2000) and a 166-residues polyethylene glycol-modified erythropoiesis protein (Kochendoerfer *et al.*, 2003).

Long peptides and proteins can be also synthesized by solid phase NCL as described in 1999 by Kent and Dawson (Brik *et al.*, 2000; Canne *et al.*, 1999). This protocol allows to assemble the polypeptide chains either in the N→C or in the C→N direction. Human group V secretory phospholipase A_2 (118aa and six disulfide bonds) has been successfully prepared by three solid phase NCL reactions using purified, water-soluble peptide segments ranging from 25 to 33aa residues (Brik *et al.*, 2000).

An additional method for the synthesis of proteins, the expressed protein ligation (EPL) introduced in 1998 by Muir and Evans, is an amalgamation of SPPS (chemistry) and ribosomal peptide synthesis (Evans *et al.*, 1998; Muir *et al.*, 1998). Recombinant DNA technology is used to produce large protein fragments that after purification and

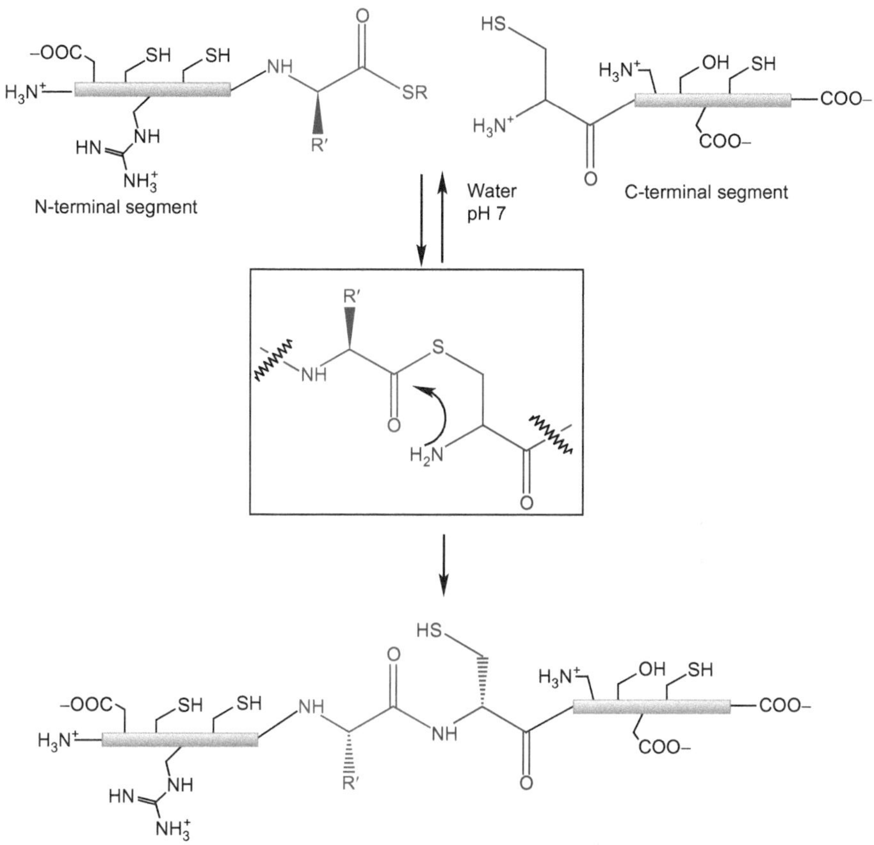

FIGURE 5.3 Chemical ligation. The method involves a thioester-mediated condensation of two unprotected peptide segments in aqueous solution at neutral pH resulting in the ligation of the terminal cysteine of one peptide segment to the other via a native amide bond. (See Color Insert.)

characterization are ligated by NCL to peptide segments prepared by SPPS. The size of proteins that are accessible by this semi synthetic technology is thus greatly increased. EPL has been used extensively for protein structure–function analyses and to produce a functional single-chain antibody with a C-terminal thioester (Sydor *et al.*, 2002).

Chemical peptide synthesis has enormously progressed from the time of Curtius and Fischer. As Fischer envisaged in his Nobel Prize Lecture on December 12, 1902, a century later enzymes and other proteins with full biological activity are generally considered accessible targets for synthetic chemistry (Kent, 2009).

2.2. Why to choose synthetic peptides as vaccines

The main reasons to use SPPS about 20 years ago for the discovery and development of malaria vaccines were the versatility of peptide synthesis, the speed of production and purity of the final product devoid of DNA or unrelated proteins, and the difficulty to express malarial recombinant proteins, especially the CSP from *P. falciparum*. These considerations not only are still valid today but increased availability of special amino acid reagents, resins, catalysts, and state of the art instrumentations has rendered peptide synthesis even more attractive and cheaper (see Section 2.1). Since the peptide length we felt comfortable to synthesize was around 100 aa residues, we were quite careful to choose domains whose structure as it appears in the native protein could be predicted or was already determined. Using our chain assembly and folding protocols biologically active, commercially available chemokines were produced (Thierry *et al.*, 2001; Verdini *et al.*, 2008);

Mimicry of the correct antigen structure is of extreme importance for antigens from the sporozoite or the erythrocytic stage against which specific antibodies need to exert the protective function. On the other hand, for liver stage antigens against which elicitation of a specific T cell response is needed, linear peptides of limited length (8–15 aa residues) are required. These short peptide segments can be used as such or inserted colinearly into a long peptide chain with interposed nonimmunogenic spacers $NH(CH_2CH_2O)_nCO$ to prevent the formation of neoepitopes (Olugbile *et al.*, 2011).

One can argue that domains or multi subunit polyepitopes of 100 or more aa may not be sufficient to confer protection against a complicated disease such as malaria, and only larger proteins may activate the immune response to obtain a protective response. Our approach is that properly targeted epitopes or domains can indeed be effective in preventing malaria. A well-documented example is the spectacular success of monoclonal antibodies against a variety of diseases including cancer. In addition, using well-defined domains it is possible to avoid the presence of polymorphic regions, which are present in most of the antigens developed in the last 25 years and, possibly, the consequence of their failure. Furthermore, once nonpolymorphic domains are identified, recombinant DNA technology can be used to produce multivalent constructs. In addition, large constructs can also be produced by peptide synthesis; polypeptides of 150 and more aa have been prepared in our laboratory (Perlaza *et al.*, 2001, unpublished data).

We have always adopted the Fmoc–*t*-butyl solid phase stepwise method to synthesize long peptides. This procedure does not require a highly skilled operator and is easy to learn. Even a high school student, well trained and supervised, is able to accurately follow the synthetic protocol. Purification of the crude material is, generally, first performed through a size exclusion chromatography, usually a Sephadex G50 resin, which very effectively eliminates smaller truncated peptides which occur most of the time in the first 10–40 aa. This size exclusion chromatography usually yields a good product (≥70% purity) to be used for T-cell proliferation and ELISA. Better quality products (>90%) for animal model immunization can be obtained by reverse phase high performance liquid chromatography (RP-HPLC) (Regnier, 1983).

3. PREERYTHROCYTIC *P. FALCIPARUM* SYNTHETIC VACCINES

3.1. CSP–NANP-based trials

As mentioned above the CSP was the first *P. falciparum* protein to be sequenced and contained three easily identifiable domains: the N-terminus, the central repeat region and the C-terminus of about 100, 200, and 100 aa, respectively.

The simplicity of the central repeat region composed of about 40 NANP repeats attracted many researchers. A race to develop a vaccine based on this repeat region was very quickly engaged. The group lead by Ruth and Victor Nussenzweig took the synthetic peptide option while the U.S. Army and Navy laboratories opted for a recombinant product (Ballou *et al.*, 1987; Herrington *et al.*, 1987). The synthetic peptide consisted of $(NANP)_3$ segment covalently attached to the tetanus toxoid carrier. The recombinant product contained a segment of 20 NANP repeats attached to an *E. coli* derived protein carrier. This was based on the promising results obtained in *in vitro* studies showing the inhibition of invasion by anti-NANP antibodies (Hollingdale *et al.*, 1984) and protection in mice using the *P. berghei* repeat and the same carrier (Good *et al.*, 1988; Nussenzweig and Nussenzweig, 1989; Zavala *et al.*, 1987).

The great expectations raised by these two trials turned into deep disappointment and frustration since only one out of three and one out of six volunteers, respectively, were protected together with a longer latent period for parasitemia appearance. Our impression and evaluation of that period is that the intense competition and lack of collaboration between the two groups did not favor an in depth and extended evaluation and optimization of the constructs in terms of length of repeats, in one case, and nature of the carrier protein in the other.

The suboptimal results obtained from the first two trials sparked an intense search, on one hand, for other carriers and/or formulations to increase the immunogenicity of the NANP repeat and, on the other hand, for additional domains of the CSP, which would contain T- and B-cell epitopes (Nardin and Nussenzweig, 1993). Particularly interesting was the assembly of helper T- and B-cell epitopes from *P. falciparum* CSP as multiple branched peptides on a lysine scaffold (multiple antigen peptide, MAP). Results obtained in mice with a MAP construct containing a helper T-cell and the *P. berghei* repeat generated indeed an excellent protective response (Tam *et al.*, 1990). Unfortunately, the stepwise assembly of such a construct is not amenable to GMP production due to the difficulty of synthesis reproducibility, homogeneity, and characterization of the final product. This hurdle was surmounted by the chemical conjugation of separately produced and purified scaffolds and linear peptides containing CSP T- and B-cell epitopes (Rose, 1994; Rose *et al.*, 1995). Such a product was tested in a phase one clinical trial (Nardin, 2010; Nardin *et al.*, 2001). Whether the results obtained were not of sufficient interest or the long process of assembling the final product was not suitable for large GMP production, its clinical development was not continued.

Our group in collaboration with groups from ENIRICERCHE and the University of Geneva directed by Antonio Verdini and Paul-Henri Lambert, respectively, established in 1993 a collaboration agreement with the U.S. Army and Navy for the production and clinical development of a MAP antigen containing tt-derived T-cell epitopes colinearly synthesized with $(NANP)_6$. Also this project was terminated due to the problem of GMP compliance as discussed above. Basically, it took about 10years of intense research and dozens of clinical trials before the linear NANP construct alone was abandoned as vaccine candidate (Chulay, 1989; Engers and Godal, 1998; Facer and Tanner, 1997).

One consideration to be made about the MAP and similar multimer products is that antigen immunogenicity may be greatly increased only when weak T-helper epitopes are used. Indeed, when we used strong tt-derived T-cell epitopes colinearly synthesized with $(NANP)_6$ (Valmori *et al.*, 1992), the difference of anti-NANP antibody titers obtained in mice between the MAP construct and the linear one was only marginal (unpublished results). These data were obtained later on when the interest for MAP constructs as malaria vaccines had already diminished. This instance stresses the point that proper controls should have been performed at any moment of vaccine development instead of applying conventional wisdom as often happens.

NANP-based vaccine development was taken up again in the last few years by the groups of Robinson and Pluschke by using conformationally constrained NANP sequences chemically coupled to virosome like particles (VLP) (Bisang *et al.*, 1995, 1998; Moreno *et al.*, 2001; Zurbriggen, 2003). In addition, clinical trials phase 1a and 2a (Genton *et al.*, 2007; Okitsu *et al.*, 2007; Thompson *et al.*, 2008) were conducted in which the NANP construction was used alone or together with a apical membrane antigen 1 (AMA-1) cyclic peptide comprising residues 446–490 of the semiconserved loop I of domain III. The latter product has been shown to induce asexual blood stage parasite growth inhibitory antibodies (Mueller *et al.*, 2003). The phase 2a clinical trial results showed no sterile protection but slower parasite growth was observed (Thompson *et al.*, 2008). On the other hand, the positive results recently obtained in a phase 2a study in

Tanzania in a limited number of children warrant the further exploration of these two combined products or with additional ones in a phase 2b clinical trial (Cech *et al.*, 2011).

As discussed in detail elsewhere (Verdini *et al.*, 2010), although $(NANP)_n$ sequence is simple, its three-dimensional structure is only partially understood. Circular dichroism and Fourier Transform Infrared (FTIR) studies in solution showed that depending on the conditions $(NANP)_n$ polypeptides with $n>20$ assume either a random coil (water) or a β/γ-turns-containing helical conformation (water/trifluoroethanol mixtures and hydrated gels) (Verdini *et al.*, 1991).

The rules for prediction of the disordered state of proteins with repeats (Kajava, 2001) suggest that $(NANP)_n$ sequence is unstructured. On the other hand, the repetitive domain was recently found to have an elongated shape (Plassmeyer *et al.*, 2009) (Fig. 5.4). Molecular modeling predicted that this region can have either regular β-solenoid structures (Brooks

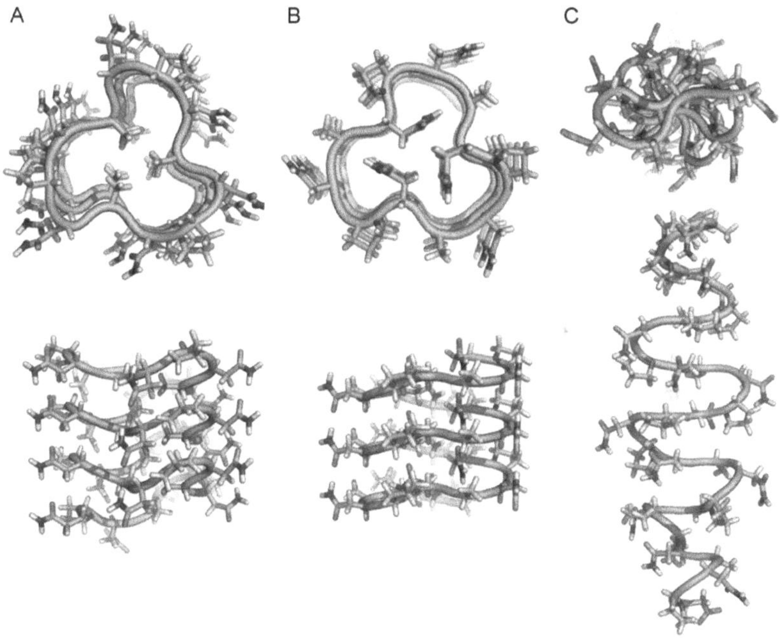

FIGURE 5.4 Structural models for $(NANP)_n$ region of CSP. The backbone of the polypeptide chains is shown as a ribbon and its side-chains have stick representation. Figures are generated using PyMol software (De Lano, 2002). At the top are axial projections and at the bottom are lateral projections of the models A, a β-solenoid model with alanines directed inside of the structure (Kajava and Verdini, unpublished); B, a β-solenoid model with asparagines directed inside of the structure (Brooks *et al.*, 1987) and C, a β-hairpin model (Plassmeyer *et al.*, 2009). (See Color Insert.)

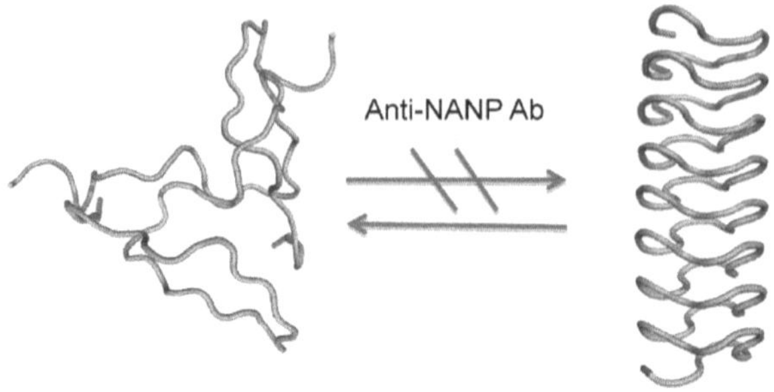

FIGURE 5.5 Hypothetical scheme of inhibition of formation of helical NANP superstructure by antibodies specific for the random coil NANP structure. (See Color Insert.)

et al., 1987; Verdini and Kajava, unpublished data) or made up of tandems of short beta-hairpins (Plassmeyer *et al.*, 2009) (Fig. 5.4). The regular structures are probably assumed for a very short time upon interaction with specific cell membrane components during the sporozoite journey from the skin to the liver (cell traversal or invasion). Thus, it is most likely not accessible to specific B-cells. On the other hand, inhibition of CSP function by antibodies directed against the random coil conformation may be obtained by preventing the formation of the regular beta-turn-containing structures (Fig. 5.5). But this may require the elicitation of high titers of high affinity antibodies, which apparently is very difficult to achieve in humans. Ultimately, the weakest point in developing vaccines based on this sequence may reside in this change of conformation by the NANP repeats.

3.2. CSP C-terminus-based clinical trials

As mentioned above, the disappointing results obtained with the NANP repeat constructs promoted the search of other T- and B-cell epitopes in the N- and C-domains of the *P. falciparum* CSP on which develop other CSP-based vaccine candidates. These studies were performed with synthetic peptides since no recombinant CSP was available. We also tried to express the full-length protein in the *Dictyostelium* expression system developed at the University of Lausanne but the yield was low (Reymond *et al.*, 1995). This forced us to turn to peptide synthesis to construct the N- and C-domains independently. The C-terminus was first synthesized for the 3D7 and 7G8 strains. For our luck, it turned out one of the easiest synthesis we ever performed (Roggero *et al.*, 1995); the N-termini of the two strains followed. All constructs were immunogenic and mouse antibodies against the C-terminal region could inhibit parasite growth (Roggero *et al.*, 1995). The immunological and biological properties of the N- and C-terminus, which comprises helper and cytotoxic T-cells (Table 5.1), and its recognition by antibodies in humans, (Blum-Tirouvanziam *et al.*, 1995; Nardin, 2010; Nardin and Nussenzweig, 1993;

TABLE 5.1 Sequence of synthetic antigens used in clinical trials

Protein	aa	Sequence	References
Pf CSP	282–383	KNNQGNGQGH NMPNDPNRNV DENANANSAV KNNNNEEPSD KHI*KEYLNKI* *QNSLSTEWSP* *CSVTCGNGIQ* *VRIKPGSANK* *PKDELDYAND* *IEKKICKMEK* *CS*	Blum-Tirouvanziam *et al.* (1995), Nardin *et al.* (1989), Reece *et al.* (2004), Sinigaglia *et al.* (1988)
SPf66		CGDELEAETQ NVYAAPNANP YSLFQKEKMV LPNANPPANK KNAGC	Salcedo *et al.* (1991)
Pf MSP3	181–276	RKTKEYAEKA KNAYEKAKNA YQKANQAVLK AKEASSYDYI LGWEFGGGVP EHKKEENMLS HLYVSSKDKE NISKENDDVL DEKEEEAEET EEEELE	Singh *et al.* (2004)
Pf GLURP	85–213	NVPSGLDIDD IPKESIFIQE DQEGQTHSEL NPETSEHSKD LNNNDSKNES SDIISVNNKS NKVQNHFESL SDLELLENSS QDNLDKDTIS TEPFPNQKHK DLQQDLNDEP LEPFPTQIHK DYKEKNLIN	Theisen *et al.* (2000)
Pv CSP N	20–96	THCGHNVDLS KAINLNGVNF NNVDASSLGA *AHVGQSASRG* *RGLGENPDDE* *EGDAKKKKDG* *KKAEPKNPRE* *NKLK*QPG	Arevalo-Herrera *et al.* (1998), Gonzalez *et al.* (2000), Herrera *et al.* (1992a)
Pv CSP C	301–372	NEGANA*PNEK* *SVKE*YLDKVR ATVGTEWTP*C* *SVTCGVGVRV* *RRRVNAANKK* *PEDLTLNDLE* TDVCTMDKCA	
Pv CSP Repeat + p30	96–104	*GDRADGQPAG* *DRADGQPAGD* *RADGQPA* ***FNN*** ***FTVSFWLRVP*** ***KVSASHLE***	Arevalo-Herrera *et al.* (1998); Valmori *et al.* (1992)

CD8+ T cell epitopes in italic.
B and Th epitopes underlined.
In bold, tetanus toxin derived CD4+ T-cell epitope p30.

Nardin *et al.*, 1989; Nussenzweig and Nussenzweig, 1989; Pink and Sinigaglia, 1989; Sinigaglia *et al.*, 1988), the protection studies of the corresponding domain or fragments thereof in *P. berghei* and *Plasmodium yoelii* models (Franke *et al.*, 1997; Migliorini *et al.*, 1993; Renggli *et al.*, 1995; Renia *et al.*, 1991; Roggero *et al.*, 2000; Romero *et al.*, 1990; Weiss *et al.*, 1992), the inhibition of hepatocyte invasion by corresponding mouse antibodies (Roggero *et al.*, 1995) and the biological activity associated with this domain in terms of binding to the hepatocytes (Cerami *et al.*, 1992; Pancake *et al.*, 1992) convinced us to develop this domain into a vaccine candidate.

The C-terminal fragment was assembled by the Fmoc–*t*-butyl protocol and the purified precursor containing two *tert*-butylthiolated cysteine residues was oxidatively folded in solution by the method of Verdini *et al.* (2008). The first trial was a dose and adjuvant finding process (100 vs. 300 μg; alhydrogel vs. Montainde ISA 720) (Lopez *et al.*, 2001). The results obtained in terms of immunogenicity at the T- and B-cell level were promising such that a second larger trial was initiated in which three doses of antigen (10, 30, and 100 μg), together with two adjuvants Montanide ISA 720 and ASO2A, proprietary products of AirLiquid and GlaxoSmith and Kline (GSK), respectively, were injected in groups of six volunteers (Audran *et al.*, 2009). The results showed that the antigen formulation containing ASO2A was superior to that with Montanide in all of the immunological parameters tested. A phase 2a was then planned using the 30-μg dose but only Montanide ISA 720 was used since the use of ASO2A was not granted by GSK. Different reasons were given but none convincing to our opinion. The trial failed to show any sign of protection (Genton *et al.*, 2010). This could be due most likely to the choice of the antigen and adjuvant formulation or, possibly, the experimental challenge used. The challenge was performed in Nijmegen under the supervision of Robert Sauerwein who uses the *P. falciparum* NF54 parasite strain. The other model used by the U.S. Army and Navy is based on the *P. falciparum* 3D7 parasite strain. In spite of calls for global harmonization of protocols in malaria, these straightforward challenge models predictive of protection in the field have never been compared.

4. ERYTROCYTIC SYNTHETIC VACCINES

Erythrocytic stage vaccines are aimed to prevent clinical manifestation and severity of malaria infection. Erythrocytic synthetic vaccine candidates have been modeled on the sequences and structures of *P. falciparum* merozoite specific proteins such as merozoite surface protein 1 (MSP1), MSP2, MSP3, glutamate-rich protein (GLURP), and AMA-1. The SPf 66 was the first such vaccine to be tested in humans (Patarroyo *et al.*, 1988).

4.1. SPf66

SPf66 is a 45-aa long synthetic peptide based on the amino acid sequences of three peptides of relative molecular mass 83, 55, and 35k, supposedly specific for the late schizont and merozoite stages of *P. falciparum* (Patarroyo *et al.*, 1987, 1988) plus 2x-PNANP intercalating sequences: Cys-Gly-Asp-Glu-Leu-Glu-Ala-Glu-Thr-Gln-Asn-Val-Tyr-Ala-Ala-*Pro-Asn-Ala-Asn-Pro*-Tyr-Ser-Leu-Phe-Gln-Lys-Glu-Lys-Met-Val-Leu-*Pro-Asn-Ala-Asn-Pro*-Pro-Ala-Asn-Lys-Lys-Asn-Ala-Gly-Cys. The peptide was assembled using the Merrifield Boc-benzyl synthetic strategy and cysteine residues at both the amino and carboxyl terminal ends were included to induce its polymerization in oxidizing conditions (Rodriguez *et al.*, 1990). A serious limitation of the construct is that two out of three erythrocytic antigens were later not found in the *Plasmodium* genomic sequence. A detailed analysis of the structure and shortcoming of Spf66 is reviewed elsewhere (Verdini *et al.*, 2010).

SPf66 initially showed contradictory results in preclinical trials in non-human primates (Herrera *et al.*, 1992b; Patarroyo *et al.*, 1987; Ruebush *et al.*, 1990), although promising results were observed soon after when it was tested in regions of low endemicity in South America. It was safe and highly immunogenic in adult humans (Amador *et al.*, 1992; Salcedo *et al.*, 1991) and children (Amador *et al.*, 1992; Patarroyo *et al.*, 1992), and showed a protective efficacy against *P. falciparum* of 38–60% in semiimmune Colombian populations subject to natural challenge in a phase 3 clinical trial (Valero *et al.*, 1993). However, the SPf66 did not work as expected outside South America. A lower level of efficacy of SPf66 was observed in a Tanzanian trial (estimated protective efficacy in children aged 1–5 years was 31%) (Alonso *et al.*, 1994). Complete lack of efficacy was later shown in subsequent studies in Gambia (D'Alessandro *et al.*, 1995) and Thailand (Nosten *et al.*, 1996) with an estimated mean protective efficacy of 8–9%, and no significant differences with the control group. These results led to the conclusion that SPf66 does not protect against clinical *P. falciparum* malaria and that further efficacy trials were not justified. On the other hand, the experience gained during these trials served as a basis for future field clinical studies.

4.2. Merozoite surface protein 3

MSP3 is a polymorphic antigen of about 350 aa, which occurs on the surface of merozoites, and has unknown function (Marshall *et al.*, 1992; McColl and Anders, 1997; McColl *et al.*, 1994; Oeuvray *et al.*, 1994). The central and C-terminal regions are predicted to form a helical coiled coil domain (McColl and Anders, 1997) containing two or four strands in register (Burgess *et al.*, 2005; Gondeau *et al.*, 2009). The polymorphic region is mainly N-terminally located while the rest of the protein is conserved.

The *P. falciparum* MSP3 is a malaria vaccine candidate that was identified, characterized, and developed using an ADCI assay (Oeuvray *et al.*, 1994) and correlation of specific antibodies to protection from clinical malaria as surrogates of protection (Roussilhon *et al.*, 2007). Thus, a fully conserved region of MSP3 (amino acids 176–281) was identified (Table 5.1). This region was originally synthesized in our laboratory using the Fmoc–*t*-butyl strategy, and further tested for being a target of human antibodies from malaria–immune adults with ADCI activity. This construct was then tested in a phase 1a clinical trial in which three doses 10, 30, or 100 μg of antigen and two adjuvants (Alhydrogel or Montanide ISA 720) were administered to 36 volunteers (Audran *et al.*, 2005). Both formulations induced cellular and humoral immune responses, and these responses lasted for up to 12 months with the alum-based formulation. The vaccine-induced antibodies showed an inhibition of *P. falciparum* erythrocytic growth *in vitro*, which was, in most cases, as high as or higher than the inhibition induced by natural antibodies from immune African adults (Druilhe *et al.*, 2005). The *in vivo* transfer of sera from the volunteers into *P. falciparum*-infected humanized SCID mice profoundly reduced or abrogated parasitemia. These inhibitory effects were related to the reactivity of the vaccine-induced antibodies with the parasite native protein, which was observed in samples taken 12 months postimmunization in 60% of the volunteers (Druilhe *et al.*, 2005).

Phase 1b clinical trials of the synthetic MSP3 peptide formulated in Alhydrogel in adults and children followed in Burkina Faso and Tanzania, respectively (Lusingu *et al.*, 2009; Sirima *et al.*, 2007). Results obtained in adults indicated that the preparation was safe and no serious adverse reactions were reported in the trial in children. No boosting effect was observed in the adult trial, given that the volunteers had preexisting high antibody titers against the construct. These results supported the testing of the MSP3 formulation in children in a phase 2b trial in Mali. Unfortunately, no conclusion could be drawn since the number of malaria clinical cases was low (P. Druilhe, personal communication). In the meantime, data from a phase 1b trial in children in Burkina Faso indicated that the MSP3 construct gives a protection of about 50% (Sirima *et al.*, 2011). This finding is now being confirmed by a second phase 2b trial in Mali (www.clinicaltrials.gov; P. Druilhe, personal communication).

4.3. Glutamate-rich protein

P. falciparum GLURP is the target of cytophilic antibodies, which are significantly associated with protection against clinical malaria (Meraldi *et al.*, 2004; Oeuvray *et al.*, 2000; Theisen *et al.*, 1998). In this protein of 1271 aa, three major antigenic regions were identified and three long synthetic peptides corresponding to relatively conserved fragments

85–213, 191–287, and 801–920 were produced using the Fmoc–*t*-butyl strategy and tested for their antigenicty and immunogenicity (Meraldi *et al.*, 2004; Theisen *et al.*, 2000) in order to select the best one for development. A phase 1 clinical trial was conducted in healthy adult volunteers with the 85–213 fragment (Table 5.1) combined with either alhydrogel (n=18) or Montanide ISA 720 (n=18) as adjuvants (Hermsen *et al.*, 2007). Subcutaneous immunizations (10, 30, or 100 μg) were administered at days 0, 30, and 120. Adverse events (AE) occurred more frequently with increasing dose of antigen, and were more prevalent in the Montanide ISA 720 group; however, no serious vaccine-related AE were reported. The vaccine-induced dose-dependent cellular and humoral immune responses, with high levels of (mainly cytophilic IgG1) antibodies that recognized parasites in an IFA study and that inhibited parasite growth in an ADCI assay (Hermsen *et al.*, 2007). The GURP vaccine candidate was then developed as a hybrid molecule containing most of the GLURP and MSP3 molecules (Esen *et al.*, 2009; Mordmuller *et al.*, 2010) and it is been tested for protection against malaria in four different sites in Africa (www.clinicaltrials.gov; M. Theisen, personal communication).

5. *P. VIVAX* SYNTHETIC VACCINE

5.1. Epitope mapping and CSP-based preclinical studies

As for *P. falciparum*, the CSP was the first *P. vivax* protein to be sequenced and demonstrated similar structure to that displayed by other malaria parasites (Hoffman, 1996). In this case, the original CSP sequence described by Arnot *et al.* (1985) derived from the *P. vivax* Belem strain, called VK210, contained a central repeat domain composed of 19 repeats of the 9 aa repeat, GDRADGQPA, while the variant type described by Rosenberg *et al.* (1989) designated VK-247 contains repetitive blocks of the sequence ANGAGNQPG. The N- and C-termini where composed of 95 and 92 aa, respectively, and were later shown to contain highly conserved domains (RI: 85–89 aa and RII-Plus: 338–355 aa) involved in parasite binding to host cells (Cerami *et al.*, 1992; Frevert *et al.*, 1993; Rosenberg *et al.*, 1989).

Because of the potential immunological importance of defined epitopes in all three regions of the protein and the disappointing results obtained with the *P. falciparum* NANP repeat constructs, we decided to do an exhaustive search for epitopes with potential value to be included in a vaccine along the entire *P. vivax* sequence. All three regions contained T- and B-cell epitopes, some of which were recognized by a significant number of Colombians (Arevalo-Herrera *et al.*, 1998; Herrera *et al.*, 1992a), as well as by individuals from PNG (George *et al.*, 1990). Great effort was devoted to the identification of epitopes that would stimulate CD8+ T-cells (Arevalo-Herrera *et al.*, 2002).

Using some of these malaria T- and B-cell epitopes (p6, p11, and p25) together with the tetanus toxin universal CD4+ T-cell epitope p30 (Panina-Bordignon *et al.*, 1989) we designed and synthesized a series of eight MAP containing either T- or B-cell epitopes, or combinations of both in different ratios. Immunogenicity of these MAP constructs was tested in *Aotus* monkeys, and as expected, MAP containing T- and B-cell epitopes where the most immunogenic as determined by the production of specific antibodies that recognized the cognate antigen, and the production of *in vitro* IFN-γ production (Herrera *et al.*, 1997). MAP immunogenicity in primates was very encouraging; however, as mentioned above their synthesis was not amenable to GMP production.

Based on the successful synthesis of the *P. falciparum* C- and N-terminal regions, we decided to adopt the same approach with *P. vivax* CSP which in this case included also a peptide based on the repeat region, specifically on the p11 epitope. Long synthetic peptides of 76 and 71 aa denominated N and C comprised the sequence 20–96 and 301–372 of the CSP and a 48-mer peptide denominated R consisted of p11 linearly linked to a 21-mer universal T-cell epitope p30 (Valmori *et al.*, 1992) (Table 5.1). Initially, the N and C peptides as well as p11 were used to determine the prevalence of antibodies to the different regions of the protein in malaria-endemic communities of Colombia. A high percentage of collected sera (n=65) of individuals from Zacarias, a village on the Pacific coast, recognized the different regions of the *P. vivax* CSP. Although the repeat region was the most frequently recognized (88%), about 60% of the sera also recognized epitopes located in the N and C regions, indicating a significant immunogenicity of the three protein regions under natural conditions (Arevalo-Herrera *et al.*, 1998). Similar results were observed in a larger number of subjects (n=80) (Herrera *et al.*, 2004).

Based on these results, we conducted immunogenicity studies both in rodents and primates using the same peptides formulated in two adjuvants, Montanide ISA 720 and Montanide ISA 51, using three immunizations of 50 and 100μg. In rodents, a vigorous antibody response to all peptides was observed although better specific antibody responses were obtained against C and R polypeptides. In contrast, *Aotus* monkeys immunized with the same vaccine formulations displayed a better response to the N polypeptide. In all cases, elicited antibodies not only strongly recognized the three immunogens but all of them also cross-reacted with *P. vivax* sporozoites. Additionally, a comparison of the reactivities of recognized sera from humans naturally exposed to the infection and from peptide-immunized monkeys indicated that the same epitopes were recognized by both species. Peptides also stimulated the *in vitro* production of IFN-γ by *Aotus* peripheral blood mononuclear cells (PBMC). These studies stimulated the initiation of clinical development of these peptides (Arevalo-Herrera *et al.*, 2011b).

Preclinical studies in rodents and primates were simultaneously conducted with a protein fragment corresponding to the *P. vivax* trombosponding-related adhesion protein (TRAP), a protein that appears to participate in sporozoite motility and invasion (Muller *et al.*, 1993a,b; Spaccapelo *et al.*, 1997). A synthetic peptide encompassing the sequence 209–256 of Salvador I strain, located at the N-terminus of the protein, and containing a hepatocyte binding motif CSVTCG in the region II-Plus (Templeton and Kaslow, 1997) was formulated in Freunds and Montanide ISA 729 adjuvants and used to immunized BALB/c mice and *Aotus* monkeys, respectively. Both animal models developed specific antipeptide antibodies that cross-reacted with the parasite in IFAT assays. Partial protection was observed in monkeys after *P. vivax* sporozoite challenge (Herrera *et al.*, 2007).

5.2. CSP-based clinical studies

The high immunogenicity displayed by these three peptides both in terms of antibody and IFN-γ responses, as well as the boosting effect produced in primates by the exposure to *P. vivax* sporozoites, led us to consider the possibility of initiating the clinical development of these vaccine candidates. The N and R constructs were synthesized by the Fmoc–*t*-butyl strategy without any further modification. Instead, the synthesis of the C-terminal fragment required multiple exploratory runs and adaptation of the basic strategy by introducing pseudoproline (oxazolidine) dipeptides at critical points during chain assembly. Such building blocks disrupt on-resin peptide chain aggregation, avoiding collapse of the synthesis (Olugbile *et al.*, 2010). The purified *tert*-butylthiolated precursors were then oxidized and folded in solution via the method of Verdini *et al.* (2008). We therefore conducted a first dose-escalating phase 1 trial in 69 naïve volunteers recruited in Cali, Colombia. We tested the safety, tolerability, and immunogenicity of the three peptides (N, R, and C) formulated in Montanide ISA 720 at 10, 30, and 100 μg/dose for each peptide.

Vaccine formulations were well tolerated and no serious adverse events were observed in any of the vaccines and all three peptides induced rapid antibody production that remained in circulation for about 10 months. As in the studies in primates, these antibodies cross-reacted with sporozoite preparations on IFAT (Herrera *et al.*, 2005) and were able to block *in vitro* parasite invasion of hepatoma cell lines (Arevalo-Herrera *et al.*, 2011a). Moreover, PBMC of most immunized volunteers produced IFN-γ upon peptide *in vitro* stimulation.

In order to optimize the vaccine formulation, a second phase 1 trial was carried out using again Colombian naïve volunteers. A total of 40 young adults, male and female were vaccinated with mixtures of the three peptides formulated in Montanide ISA 720 and in Montanide ISA 51 at doses of 50 and 100 μg. Taking into consideration that the repeat region of the CSP is more immunogenic than the flanking fragments, volunteers were first vaccinated with a mixture of N+C fragments and then the remaining two doses were immunized with a combination of N+R+C. This trial indicated a good reproducibility of safety, tolerability, and immunogenicity of the formulations in both adjuvants, although there was a tendency to greater immunogenicity of all peptides formulated in Montanide ISA 51 (Herrera *et al.*, 2011a). Phase 2a trials are currently being prepared taking advantage of the procedure recently developed to induce *P. vivax* sporozoite infectious challenge in human volunteers (Herrera *et al.*, 2009, 2011b). These studies and those with other *P. vivax* vaccine candidates have been extensively reviewed elsewhere (Arevalo-Herrera *et al.*, 2010; Herrera and Arevalo-Herrera, 2010).

5.3. Studies on the protective efficacy of *P. vivax* vaccines

In contrast to *P. falciparum* which is routinely *in vitro* cultured, *P. vivax* blood forms have been elusive to adapt to *in vitro* growth representing a bottle neck for vaccine and drug discovery and development. Among the constraints imposed by the lack of *in vitro* cultures is the difficulty to continuously produce mature infective gametocytes that could be used to feed laboratory reared *Anopheles* mosquitoes for sporozoite production. *P. vivax* sporozoites are essential for preerythrocytic vaccine testing as well as for assessing the efficacy of new antimalarial drugs with potential effect on parasite liver forms, namely hypnozoites. *P. vivax*-infected patients represent a burdensome substitute to access to parasite blood forms. Therefore, proximity to malaria-endemic areas and access to laboratory bred mosquitos is critical to produce sporozoites. Although inoculation of human volunteers with *P. falciparum* live or attenuated sporozoites has been performed rather routinely for the last few decades, *P. vivax* sporozoites had not been inoculated into humans since 1963. Before then, *P. vivax* parasites were repeatedly used to induce fever in patients suffering neurosyphilis in whom induction of fever was considered a treatment to eliminate *Treponema pallidum* and alleviate patients suffering dementia (Collins *et al.*, 2004). Our access to both patients and mosquitos has allowed us the establishment of a *P. vivax* sporozoite challenge model in which naïve individuals can be exposed to the bite of infected mosquitos and get infected. Infective doses of as low as two mosquito bites reproducibly infected malaria-naïve volunteers. Volunteers exposed to experimental challenge developed patent parasitemia about 11 days post infection and all of them recovered within 1–2 days of a standard antimalarial protocol (Herrera *et al.*, 2009, 2011b).

Sporozoite challenge model represents a valuable tool for vaccine development. First, using this method we are currently planning a *P. vivax* phase 2a efficacy trial in naïve and preimmune volunteers from Colombia vaccinated with CSP long synthetic peptides. Secondly, we are currently setting up the conditions to conduct a phase 2a trial to test the protective efficacy of radiation-attenuated *P. vivax* sporozoites. Although this vaccination method would not be scalable with the current technology, reagents such as cells and sera from vaccinated volunteers would allow the search for correlates of immune protection as well as their use for antigen discovery,

6. FUTURE DEVELOPMENTS

We expect new developments for malaria vaccines in three different complementary areas discussed below.

6.1. Chimeric *P. vivax* CSP-based protein

In contrast to *P. falciparum*, the repeat region of *P. vivax* CSP displays sequence and size polymorphism. Besides the original repeat sequence denominated VK210 (GDRA(D/A)GQPA, a widely distributed and immunodominant variant sequence, denominated VK247, exhibits a completely different sequence (ANGA(G/N/D)QPG) and was found in parasites from different geographic regions of Colombia (Gonzalez *et al.*, 2001). Otherwise, it has been recently shown that the CS protein structure changes during the sporozoite journey leading to adhesive and nonadhesive conformational states (Coppi *et al.*, 2011). Each of these conformations is associated with different functional properties of the protein. The adhesive conformation occurs during sporozoite invasion to hepatocytes when the CS protein is proteolytically processed. It has been found that region I contains the cleavage site (Coppi *et al.*, 2005) and the function of this cleavage is to unmask the cell adhesive TSR in the C-terminus part of the protein. This event could represent an important contribution to the design of vaccines against malaria based on this protein, since antibodies against this region could block the proteolytic processing and therefore the hepatocyte invasion.

Because of the potential role of region I and the repeat region would be similar in both *P. vivax* CSP variant sequences, we have developed a chimeric peptide that includes the N fragment (with special focus in region I), the two repeat variants (VK210 and VK247) and the C fragment. So far, this antigen has been shown to be recognized by sera of individuals from PNG and Colombia and also to be highly immunogenic in mice (unpublished data). We are currently conducting tests to determine the best formulation as well as safety, immunogenicity, and protective efficacy in primates.

6.2. New antigens

Most of the antigens tested in clinical trials were discovered over 20years ago and all present a various degree of polymorphism, which is a serious negative aspect for their development. On the other hand, these proteins present nonpolymorphic, immunogenic, and protective regions that can be exploited for vaccine development as epitomized by the MSP3 and GLURP fragments described above. Three more synthetic antigens of 104, 111, and 145 aa representing nonpolymorphic regions derived from three different proteins are planned to enter phase 1a clinical trials. Two are derived from newly identified proteins, P27A, 223–326 fragment from FF0165c protein (Olugbile *et al.*, 2009) (www.euvaccine.eu), 3290–3420 fragment from Pf3D7_10-2-1519346-1547821 protein (www.plasmodb.org; www.emvda.org; Druilhe, in preparation) and the third one is a segment from LSA3 (P. Druilhe, personal communication).

After the publication of the *P. falciparum* genome (Gardner *et al.*, 2002) it was expected that many new antigens with improved properties than the traditional ones would be identified and developed. To our knowledge, only a few have reached the clinical trial level and are being developed. We thought of identifying and down selecting new potential vaccine antigens via bioinformatics by choosing protein segments with defined secondary structural motifs of size easily achievable by Fmoc–*t*-butyl-based peptide synthesis, which, taken separately, would fold in solution in the native structure (Corradin, 2007; Corradin *et al.*, 2010; Villard *et al.*, 2007). Thus, we first selected α helical coiled coil and unstructured regions which exhibit a clear structural signature. α-Helical coiled coil segments contain at least four repeating heptads, *abcdegf*, where a and d are hydrophobic aa and the remaining aa are usually hydrophilic (Harbury *et al.*, 1993). The intrinsically unstructured regions present a low content of hydrophobic aa and are very common in all genomes (Wright and Dyson, 1999). This strategy is fast and identifies segments, which, by being hydrophilic, are easy to handle (Olugbile *et al.*, 2009; Villard *et al.*, 2007). To the list of α-helical coiled coil and unstructured regions small protein domains can be added (Fig. 5.6) (Corradin *et al.*, 2010). The selected fragments to be explored among these three domains would make an interesting pool of antigens (around 1000) from which select a few most prominent ones through a rigorous selection procedure. These vaccine candidates can then be developed as single molecules as it was the case for the unstructured P27A antigen (Olugbile *et al.*, 2009) or as a string of molecules chemically synthesized (Bernabeu *et al.*, 2011; Olugbile *et al.*, 2011) or produced by DNA recombinant technology. Chemical synthesis through

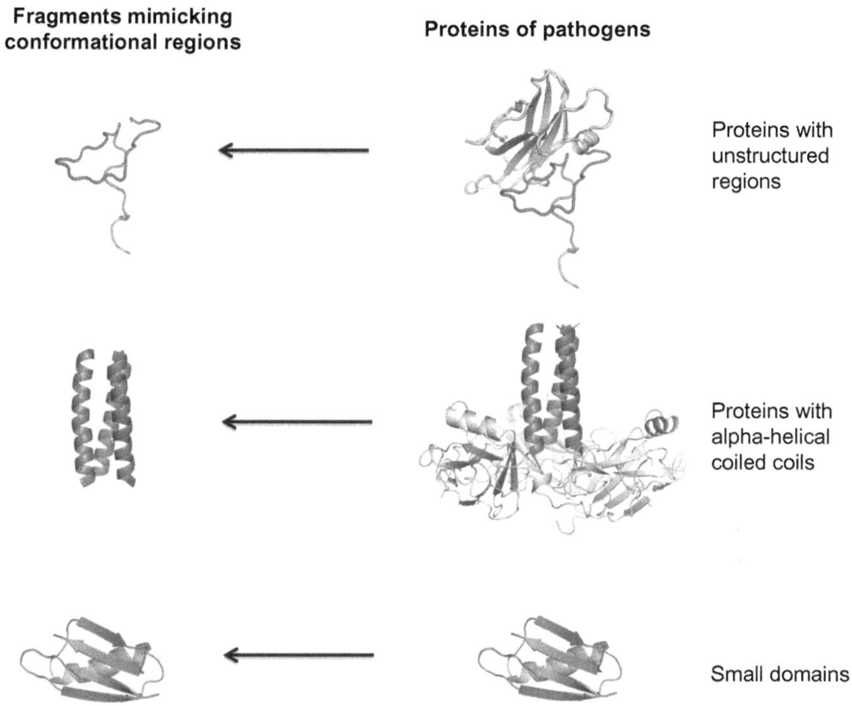

FIGURE 5.6 Examples of protein fragments, which are able to mimic structural epitopes present in native proteins. The predicted number of unstructured, α-helical coiled coil and small domains in *P. falciparum* are 5482, 1392, and 129, respectively (Corradin *et al.*, 2010). (See Color Insert.)

constant improvements in the synthetic strategies and protocols will hopefully allow production of even longer polypeptides to routinely reach 200–250 aa, and positions itself as an attractive route to produce some of these multicomponent antigens.

For the discovery of new liver stage antigens/epitopes, 25,000 properly selected 15 mer were synthesized to activate CD4+ and CD8+ T-cells from immune donors in which IFN-γ production was taken as surrogate of protection (Doolan *et al.*, 2011).

6.3. New tools

Besides the need of testing new antigens, new, predictive tools are necessary to increase the likelihood that the formulations chosen for development in the laboratory are indeed protective in the field. This would reduce the cost and time to bring new candidates for testing in the field. The generation of mice with human immunological properties may indeed help to select the best formulations in terms of immunogenicity and protective properties as recently described (Arnold *et al.*, 2011; Jimenez-Diaz *et al.*, 2009; Morosan *et al.*, 2006). This together with the standardization of *in vitro* assays like growth inhibition assay (GIA) or ADCI and *in vivo* assays of protection with live parasites will reduce the need of multiple and expensive phase 2b clinical trials. It is also of great interest the possibility of developing protection clinical assays using frozen parasites for preerythrocytic and erythrocytic formulations as discussed in a recent workshop (www.euvaccine.eu). This would increase the number of centers in malaria-endemic and nonendemic countries where phase 2a clinical trials can be performed. At this point, as discussed above, sporozoite challenge using the 3D7 and NF54 parasite strains should be compared. In addition, the use of common serum banks to determine the association of protection with a given antigen would offer the possibility of comparing different antigens in a standardized fashion.

Another area of critical importance is the development of human compatible adjuvants which are accessible to everybody without constraints. As seen in the original work of Stoute *et al.* (1997), only one of the three adjuvants used with the RTS, S vaccine candidate, conferred protection in a phase 2a clinical trial with infected mosquitos. These adjuvants are proprietary compounds of GSK and, in general, not available to others. In addition, once their use is granted, it can be revoked anytime. This policy is also followed by all commercial companies. Thus, it was with great expectation that the scientific community welcomed the opening of a center for adjuvant formulations supported by WHO and the Global Adjuvant Development Initiative at the Biochemistry Department, University of Lausanne, Lausanne, Switzerland (Collin and Dubois, 2011). It is hoped that in a few years, new adjuvants will be developed free of intellectual properties and patent issues available to everybody's use (www.transvac.org).

6.4. New networking

All activities illustrated in A and B needs to be coordinated at higher level in such a way to foster collaboration among the different players and avoid unnecessary competition. Search for a malaria vaccine should be a global enterprise where thousands of possible candidates should be produced and compare in a logical, systematic, and collaborative way. Unfortunately, this is not the case due to policies at higher level among foundations and stakeholders, who do not foster true collaboration and coordination to bring forward the best candidates. Some attempts to fill this need have been made by the European Commission, which founded the malaria consortium EMVDA (www.emvda.org) in which different groups were brought together for antigen comparison and development of the best formulations. But it is too little since only a handful of antigens were at disposal while thousands need to be tested. It is our hope that measures to fill this gap will be taken, and an efficacious vaccine will be obtained through a truly global effort.

ACKNOWLEDGMENTS

We like to thank Doctors D. Doolan, P Druilhe, and M. Theisen for sharing unpublished information. Work on *P. falciparum* has been supported by the European Vaccine Initiative and EC LSHP-CT-2007-037506 grants. Work on *P. vivax* has been sponsored by the Colombian Research Fund (Colciencias) as well as by the U.S. National Institute of Allergy and Infectious Diseases (NIAID).

REFERENCES

Alonso, P. L., Tanner, M., Smith, T., Hayes, R. J., Schellenberg, J. A., Lopez, M. C., Bastos de Azevedo, I., Menendez, C., Lyimo, E., Weiss, N., *et al.* (1994). A trial of the synthetic malaria vaccine SPf66 in tanzania: Rationale and design. *Vaccine* **12**(2), 181–186.

Alonso, P. L., Ballou, R., Brown, G., Chitnis, C., Loucq, C., Moorthy, V., Saul, A., and Wirth, D. (2011). A research agenda for malaria eradication: Vaccines. *PLoS Med.* **8**(1), e1000398.

Amador, R., Moreno, A., Murillo, L. A., Sierra, O., Saavedra, D., Rojas, M., Mora, A. L., Rocha, C. L., Alvarado, F., Falla, J. C., *et al.* (1992). Safety and immunogenicity of the synthetic malaria vaccine SPf66 in a large field trial. *J. Infect. Dis.* **166**(1), 139–144.

Aponte, J. J., Menendez, C., Schellenberg, D., Kahigwa, E., Mshinda, H., Vountasou, P., Tanner, M., and Alonso, P. L. (2007). Age interactions in the development of naturally acquired immunity to *Plasmodium falciparum* and its clinical presentation. *PLoS Med.* **4**(7), e242.

Arevalo-Herrera, M., Roggero, M. A., Gonzalez, J. M., Vergara, J., Corradin, G., Lopez, J. A., and Herrera, S. (1998). Mapping and comparison of the B-cell epitopes recognized on the *Plasmodium vivax* circumsporozoite protein by immune Colombians and immunized *Aotus* monkeys. *Ann. Trop. Med. Parasitol.* **92**(5), 539–551.

Arevalo-Herrera, M., Valencia, A. Z., Vergara, J., Bonelo, A., Fleischhauer, K., Gonzalez, J. M., Restrepo, J. C., Lopez, J. A., Valmori, D., Corradin, G., *et al.* (2002). Identification of HLA-A2 restricted CD8(+) T-lymphocyte responses to *Plasmodium vivax* circumsporozoite protein in individuals naturally exposed to malaria. *Parasite Immunol.* **24**(3), 161–169.

Arevalo-Herrera, M., Chitnis, C., and Herrera, S. (2010). Current status of *Plasmodium vivax* vaccine. *Hum. Vaccin.* **6**(1), 124–132.

Arevalo-Herrera, M., Soto, L., Perlaza, B. L., Cespedes, N., Vera, O., Lenis, A. M., Bonelo, A., Corradin, G., and Herrera, S. (2011a). Antibody-mediated and cellular immune responses induced in naive volunteers by vaccination with long synthetic peptides derived from the *Plasmodium vivax* circumsporozoite protein. *Am. J. Trop. Med. Hyg.* **84**(2 Suppl.), 35–42.

Arevalo-Herrera, M., Vera, O., Castellanos, A., Cespedes, N., Soto, L., Corradin, G., and Herrera, S. (2011b). Preclinical vaccine study of *Plasmodium vivax* circumsporozoite protein derived-synthetic polypeptides formulated in montanide ISA 720 and montanide ISA 51 adjuvants. *Am. J. Trop. Med. Hyg.* **84**(2 Suppl.), 21–27.

Arnold, L. A. L., Tyagi, R. K., Meija, P., Swetman, C., Gleeson, J., Perignon, J. L., and Druilhe, P. (2011). Further improvements of the *P. falciparum* humanized mouse model. *PLoS One* **6**(3), 2011.

Arnot, D. E., Barnwell, J. W., Tam, J. P., Nussenzweig, V., Nussenzweig, R. S., and Enea, V. (1985). Circumsporozoite protein of *Plasmodium vivax*: Gene cloning and characterization of the immunodominant epitope. *Science* **230**(4727), 815–818.

Atherton, E., and Sheppard, R. C. (1989). Solid Phase Peptide Synthesis. A Practical Approach. IRL Press, Oxford.

Audran, R., Cachat, M., Lurati, F., Soe, S., Leroy, O., Corradin, G., Druilhe, P., and Spertini, F. (2005). Phase I malaria vaccine trial with a long synthetic peptide derived from the merozoite surface protein 3 antigen. *Infect. Immun.* **73**(12), 8017–8026.

Audran, R., Lurati-Ruiz, F., Genton, B., Blythman, H. E., Ofori-Anyinam, O., Reymond, C., Corradin, G., and Spertini, F. (2009). The synthetic *Plasmodium falciparum* circumsporozoite peptide PfCS102 as a malaria vaccine candidate: A randomized controlled phase I trial. *PLoS One* **4**(10), e7304.

Baird, J. K., Jones, T. R., Danudirgo, E. W., Annis, B. A., Bangs, M. J., Basri, H., Purnomo, H., and Masbar, S. (1991). Age-dependent acquired protection against *Plasmodium falciparum* in people having two years exposure to hyperendemic malaria. *Am. J. Trop. Med. Hyg.* **45** (1), 65–76.

Baird, J. K., Masbar, S., Basri, H., Tirtokusumo, S., Subianto, B., and Hoffman, S. L. (1998). Age-dependent susceptibility to severe disease with primary exposure to *Plasmodium falciparum*. *J. Infect. Dis.* **178**(2), 592–595.

Ballou, W. R., Hoffman, S. L., Sherwood, J. A., Hollingdale, M. R., Neva, F. A., Hockmeyer, W. T., Gordon, D. M., Schneider, I., Wirtz, R. A., Young, J. F., *et al.* (1987). Safety and efficacy of a recombinant DNA *Plasmodium falciparum* sporozoite vaccine. *Lancet* **1**(8545), 1277–1281.

Bergman, M., and Zervas, L. (1932). Über ein allgemeinesVerfahren der peptid-synthese. *Ber. Dtsch. Chem. Ges.* **65,** 1192–1201.

Bernabeu, M., Lopez, F. J., Ferrer, M., Martin-Jaular, L., Razaname, A., Corradin, G., Maier, A. G., del Portillo, H. A., and Fernandez-Becerra, C. (2011). Functional analysis of *Plasmodium vivax* VIR proteins reveals different subcellular localizations and cytoadherence to the ICAM-1 endothelial receptor. *Cell. Microbiol.* doi: 10.1111/j.1462-5822.2011.01726.x. [Epub ahead of print].

Bisang, C., Weber, C., Inglis, J., Schiffer, C. A., Vangunsteren, W. F., Jelesarov, I., Bosshard, H. R., and Robinson, J. A. (1995). Stabilization of type-I beta-turn conformations in peptides containing the npna-repeat motif of the *plasmodium-falciparum* circumsporozoite protein by substituting proline for (S)-alpha-methylproline. *J. Am. Chem. Soc.* **117**(30), 7904–7915.

Bisang, C., Jiang, L. Y., Freund, E., Emery, F., Bauch, C., Matile, H., Pluschke, G., and Robinson, J. A. (1998). Synthesis, conformational properties, and immunogenicity of a cyclic template-bound peptide mimetic containing an NPNA motif from the circumsporozoite protein of *Plasmodium falciparum*. *J. Am. Chem. Soc.* **120**(30), 7439–7449.

Blum-Tirouvanziam, U., Servis, C., Habluetzel, A., Valmori, D., Men, Y., Esposito, F., Del Nero, L., Holmes, N., Fasel, N., and Corradin, G. (1995). Localization of HLA-A2.1-restricted T cell epitopes in the circumsporozoite protein of *Plasmodium falciparum*. *J. Immunol.* **154**(8), 3922–3931.

Bodanszky, M. (1955). Synthesis of peptides by aminolysis of nitrophenyl esters. *Nature* **175** (4459), 685.

Bouharoun-Tayoun, H., Attanath, P., Sabchareon, A., Chongsuphajaisiddhi, T., and Druilhe, P. (1990). Antibodies that protect humans against *Plasmodium falciparum* blood stages do not on their own inhibit parasite growth and invasion *in vitro*, but act in cooperation with monocytes. *J. Exp. Med.* **172**(6), 1633–1641.

Bouharoun-Tayoun, H., Oeuvray, C., Lunel, F., and Druilhe, P. (1995). Mechanisms underlying the monocyte-mediated antibody-dependent killing of *Plasmodium falciparum* asexual blood stages. *J. Exp. Med.* **182**(2), 409–418.

Branch, O., Casapia, W. M., Gamboa, D. V., Hernandez, J. N., Alava, F. F., Roncal, N., Alvarez, E., Perez, E. J., and Gotuzzo, E. (2005). Clustered local transmission and asymptomatic *Plasmodium falciparum* and *Plasmodium vivax* malaria infections in a recently emerged, hypoendemic Peruvian Amazon community. *Malar. J.* **4**, 27.

Brik, A., Keinan, E., and Dawson, P. E. (2000). Protein synthesis by solid-phase chemical ligation using a safety catch linker. *J. Org. Chem.* **65**(12), 3829–3835.

Brooks, B. R., Pastor, R. W., and Carson, F. W. (1987). Theoretically determined three-dimensional structure for the repeating tetrapeptide unit of the circumsporozoite coat protein of the malaria parasite *Plasmodium falciparum*. *Proc. Natl. Acad. Sci. USA* **84**(13), 4470–4474.

Bruce, M. C., Galinski, M. R., Barnwell, J. W., Donnelly, C. A., Walmsley, M., Alpers, M. P., Walliker, D., and Day, K. P. (2000). Genetic diversity and dynamics of *Plasmodium falciparum* and *P. vivax* populations in multiply infected children with asymptomatic malaria infections in Papua New Guinea. *Parasitology* **121**(Pt 3), 257–272.

Burgess, B. R., Schuck, P., and Garboczi, D. N. (2005). Dissection of merozoite surface protein 3, a representative of a family of *Plasmodium falciparum* surface proteins, reveals an oligomeric and highly elongated molecule. *J. Biol. Chem.* **280**(44), 37236–37245.

Canne, L. E., Botti, P., Simon, R. J., Chen, Y. J., Dennis, E. A., and Kent, S. B. H. (1999). Chemical protein synthesis by solid phase ligation of unprotected peptide segments. *J. Am. Chem. Soc.* **121**(38), 8720–8727.

Carpino, L. A. (1957). Oxidative reactions of hydrazines.4. Elimination of nitrogen from 1,1-disubstituted-2-arenesulfonhydrazides. *J. Am. Chem. Soc.* **79**(16), 4427–4431.

Carter, R., and Chen, D. H. (1976). Malaria transmission blocked by immunisation with gametes of the malaria parasite. *Nature* **263**(5572), 57–60.

Carter, R., and Mendis, K. (1992). Transmission immunity in malaria: Reflections on the underlying immune mechanisms during natural infections and following artificial immunization. *Mem. Inst. Oswaldo Cruz* **87**(Suppl. 3), 169–173.

Cech, P. G., Aebi, T., Abdallah, M. S., Mpina, M., Machunda, E. B., Westerfeld, N., Stoffel, S. A., Zurbriggen, R., Pluschke, G., Tanner, M., *et al.* (2011). Virosome-formulated *Plasmodium falciparum* AMA-1 & CSP derived peptides as malaria vaccine: Randomized phase 1b trial in semi-immune adults & children. *PLoS One* **6**(7), e22273.

Cerami, C., Frevert, U., Sinnis, P., Takacs, B., Clavijo, P., Santos, M. J., and Nussenzweig, V. (1992). The basolateral domain of the hepatocyte plasma membrane bears receptors for the circumsporozoite protein of *Plasmodium falciparum* sporozoites. *Cell* **70**(6), 1021–1033.

Chulay, J. D. (1989). Development of sporozoite vaccines for malaria. *Trans. R. Soc. Trop. Med. Hyg.* **83**(Suppl.), 61–66.

Clyde, D. F., McCarthy, V. C., Miller, R. M., and Hornick, R. B. (1973). Specificity of protection of man immunized against sporozoite-induced falciparum malaria. *Am. J. Med. Sci.* **266**(6), 398–403.

Collin, N., and Dubois, P. M. (2011). The vaccine formulation laboratory: A platform for access to adjuvants. *Vaccine* **29**(Suppl. 1), A37–A39.

Collins, W. E., Jeffery, G. M., and Roberts, J. M. (2004). A retrospective examination of reinfection of humans with *Plasmodium vivax*. *Am. J. Trop. Med. Hyg.* **70**(6), 642–644.

Coppi, A., Pinzon-Ortiz, C., Hutter, C., and Sinnis, P. (2005). The plasmodium circumsporozoite protein is proteolytically processed during cell invasion. *J. Exp. Med.* **201**(1), 27–33.

Coppi, A., Natarajan, R., Pradel, G., Bennett, B. L., James, E. R., Roggero, M. A., Corradin, G., Persson, C., Tewari, R., and Sinnis, P. (2011). The malaria circumsporozoite protein has two functional domains, each with distinct roles as sporozoites journey from mosquito to mammalian host. *J. Exp. Med.* **208**(2), 341–356.

Corradin, G. (2007). Peptide based malaria vaccine development: Personal considerations. *Microbes Infect.* **9**(6), 767–771.
Corradin, G., Spertini, F., and Verdini, A. (2004). Medicinal application of long synthetic peptide technology. *Expert Opin. Biol. Ther.* **4**(10), 1629–1639.
Corradin, G., Villard, V., and Kajava, A. V. (2007). Protein structure based strategies for antigen discovery and vaccine development against malaria and other pathogens. *Endocr. Metab. Immune Disord. Drug Targets* **7**(4), 259–265.
Corradin, G., Kajava, A. V., and Verdini, A. (2010). Long synthetic peptides for the production of vaccines and drugs: A technological platform coming of age. *Sci. Transl. Med.* **2**(50), 50rv3.
Curtius, T. (1882). Ueber einige neue hippursäureanalog constituierte synthetisch dargestellte aminosauren. *J. Prakt. Chemie* **26,** 145–208.
Curtius, T. (1902). Synthetische versuche mit hippurazid. *Ber. Dtsch. Chem. Ges.* **35,** 3226–3233.
D'Alessandro, U., Leach, A., Drakeley, C. J., Bennett, S., Olaleye, B. O., Fegan, G. W., Jawara, M., Langerock, P., George, M. O., Targett, G. A., *et al.* (1995). Efficacy trial of malaria vaccine SPf66 in Gambian infants. *Lancet* **346**(8973), 462–467.
Dame, J. B., Williams, J. L., McCutchan, T. F., Weber, J. L., Wirtz, R. A., Hockmeyer, W. T., Maloy, W. L., Haynes, J. D., Schneider, I., Roberts, D., *et al.* (1984). Structure of the gene encoding the immunodominant surface antigen on the sporozoite of the human malaria parasite *Plasmodium falciparum*. *Science* **225**(4662), 593–599.
Denkewalter, R. G., Veber, D. F., Holly, F. W., and Hirschmann, R. (1969). Studies on total synthesis of an enzyme. I. Objective and strategy. *J. Am. Chem. Soc.* **91**(2), 502–503.
De Lano, W. L. (2002). The PyMOL Molecular Graphics System. De Lano Scientific, San Carlos, CA.
Doolan, D. L., Dobano, C., and Baird, J. K. (2009). Acquired immunity to malaria. *Clin. Microbiol. Rev.* **22**(1), 13–36, (Table of Contents).
Doolan, D. L., Douradinha, B., Roddick, J., Robinson, L., Taraika, J., Mark, D., Rarau, P., Mueller, I., Peters, B., Sidney, J., and Sette, A. (2011). Novel Antigen Discovery by Proteome-Wide Screening of CD4 and CD8 T Cell Epitopes Using *P. falciparum* as a Model (A. A. o. I. A. Meeting, Ed.), San Francisco, CA, USA.
Druilhe, P., Spertini, F., Soesoe, D., Corradin, G., Mejia, P., Singh, S., Audran, R., Bouzidi, A., Oeuvray, C., and Roussilhon, C. (2005). A malaria vaccine that elicits in humans antibodies able to kill *Plasmodium falciparum*. *PLoS Med.* **2**(11), e344.
Du Vigneaud, V., Ressler, C., Swan, J. M., Roberts, C. W., and Katsoyannis, P. G. (1954). The synthesis of oxytocin. *J. Am. Chem. Soc.* **76**(12), 3115–3121.
Du, Y. C., Zhang, Y. S., Lu, Z. X., and Tsou, C. L. (1961). Resynthesis of insulin from its glycyl and phenylalanyl chains. *Sci. Sin.* **10**(1), 84–104.
Enea, V., Ellis, J., Zavala, F., Arnot, D. E., Asavanich, A., Masuda, A., Quakyi, I., and Nussenzweig, R. S. (1984). DNA cloning of *Plasmodium falciparum* circumsporozoite gene: Amino acid sequence of repetitive epitope. *Science* **225**(4662), 628–630.
Engers, H. D., and Godal, T. (1998). Malaria vaccine development: Current status. *Parasitol. Today* **14**(2), 56–64.
Esen, M., Kremsner, P. G., Schleucher, R., Gassler, M., Imoukhuede, E. B., Imbault, N., Leroy, O., Jepsen, S., Knudsen, B. W., Schumm, M., *et al.* (2009). Safety and immunogenicity of GMZ2—A MSP3-GLURP fusion protein malaria vaccine candidate. *Vaccine* **27** (49), 6862–6868.
Evans, T. C., Jr., Benner, J., and Xu, M. Q. (1998). Semisynthesis of cytotoxic proteins using a modified protein splicing element. *Protein Sci.* **7**(11), 2256–2264.
Facer, C. A., and Tanner, M. (1997). Clinical trials of malaria vaccines: Progress and prospects. *Adv. Parasitol.* **39,** 1–68.

Feachem, R. G. A., Phillips, A. A., and Targett, G. A. (2009). Shrinking the Malaria Map: A Prospectus on Malaria Elimination. The Global Health Group, San Francisco.
Fischer, E. (1903). Synthese von derivaten der Polypeptid. *Ber. Dtsch. Chem. Ges.* **36,** 2094–2106.
Fischer, E. (1907). Synthese von polypeptiden. XVII. *Ber. Dtsch. Chem. Ges.* **40,** 1754–1767.
Fischer, E., and Fourneau, E. (1901). Ueber einige derivate des glykokolls. *Ber.Dtsch. Chem. Ges.* **34,** 2868–2879.
Franke, E. D., Corradin, G., and Hoffman, S. L. (1997). Induction of protective CTL responses against the *Plasmodium yoelii* circumsporozoite protein by immunization with peptides. *J. Immunol.* **159**(7), 3424–3433.
Frevert, U., Sinnis, P., Cerami, C., Shreffler, W., Takacs, B., and Nussenzweig, V. (1993). Malaria circumsporozoite protein binds to heparan sulfate proteoglycans associated with the surface membrane of hepatocytes. *J. Exp. Med.* **177**(5), 1287–1298.
Gardner, M. J., Hall, N., Fung, E., White, O., Berriman, M., Hyman, R. W., Carlton, J. M., Pain, A., Nelson, K. E., Bowman, S., *et al.* (2002). Genome sequence of the human malaria parasite *Plasmodium falciparum*. *Nature* **419**(6906), 498–511.
Genton, B., Pluschke, G., Degen, L., Kammer, A. R., Westerfeld, N., Okitsu, S. L., Schroller, S., Vounatsou, P., Mueller, M. M., Tanner, M., *et al.* (2007). A randomized placebo-controlled phase Ia malaria vaccine trial of two virosome-formulated synthetic peptides in healthy adult volunteers. *PLoS One* **2**(10), e1018.
Genton, B., D'Acremont, V., Lurati-Ruiz, F., Verhage, D., Audran, R., Hermsen, C., Wolters, L., Reymond, C., Spertini, F., and Sauerwein, R. (2010). Randomized double-blind controlled Phase I/IIa trial to assess the efficacy of malaria vaccine PfCS102 to protect against challenge with *P. falciparum*. *Vaccine* **28**(40), 6573–6580.
George, F. W., 4th, Law, J. L., Rich, K. A., and Martin, W. J. (1990). Identification of a T-cell epitope on the circumsporozoite protein of *Plasmodium vivax*. *Infect. Immun.* **58**(2), 575–578.
Golenser, J., Kamyl, M., Tsafack, A., Marva, E., Cohen, A., Kitrossky, N., and Chevion, M. (1992). Correlation between destruction of malarial parasites by polymorphonuclear leukocytes and oxidative stress. *Free Radic. Res. Commun.* **17**(4), 249–262.
Gondeau, C., Corradin, G., Heitz, F., Le Peuch, C., Balbo, A., Schuck, P., and Kajava, A. V. (2009). The C-terminal domain of *Plasmodium falciparum* merozoite surface protein 3 self-assembles into alpha-helical coiled coil tetramer. *Mol. Biochem. Parasitol.* **165**(2), 153–161.
Gonzalez, J. M., Peter, K., Esposito, F., Nebie, I., Tiercy, J. M., Bonelo, A., Arevalo-Herrera, M., Valmori, D., Romero, P., Herrera, S., *et al.* (2000). HLA-a*0201 restricted CD8+ T-lymphocyte responses to malaria: Identification of new *Plasmodium falciparum* epitopes by IFN-gamma ELISPOT. *Parasite Immunol.* **22**(10), 501–514.
Gonzalez, J. M., Hurtado, S., Arevalo-Herrera, M., and Herrera, S. (2001). Variants of the *Plasmodium vivax* circumsporozoite protein (VK210 and VK247) in Colombian isolates. *Mem. Inst. Oswaldo Cruz* **96**(5), 709–712.
Good, M. F., and Doolan, D. L. (2010). Malaria vaccine design: Immunological considerations. *Immunity* **33**(4), 555–566.
Good, M. F., Berzofsky, J. A., and Miller, L. H. (1988). The T cell response to the malaria circumsporozoite protein: An immunological approach to vaccine development. *Annu. Rev. Immunol.* **6,** 663–688.
Grimaux, E. (1882). Sur des colloides azotes. *Bull. Soc. Chim.* **38,** 64.
Gutte, B., and Merrifield, R. B. (1969). Total synthesis of an enzyme with ribonuclease a activity. *J. Am. Chem. Soc.* **91**(2), 501–502.
Hackeng, T. M., Fernandez, J. A., Dawson, P. E., Kent, S. B., and Griffin, J. H. (2000). Chemical synthesis and spontaneous folding of a multidomain protein: Anticoagulant microprotein S. *Proc. Natl. Acad. Sci. USA* **97**(26), 14074–14078.

Harbury, P. B., Zhang, T., Kim, P. S., and Alber, T. (1993). A switch between two-, three-, and four-stranded coiled coils in GCN4 leucine zipper mutants. *Science* **262**(5138), 1401–1407.

Hay, S. I., Okiro, E. A., Gething, P. W., Patil, A. P., Tatem, A. J., Guerra, C. A., and Snow, R. W. (2010). Estimating the global clinical burden of *Plasmodium falciparum* malaria in 2007. *PLoS Med.* **7**(6), e1000290.

Hermsen, C. C., Verhage, D. F., Telgt, D. S., Teelen, K., Bousema, J. T., Roestenberg, M., Bolad, A., Berzins, K., Corradin, G., Leroy, O., *et al.* (2007). Glutamate-rich protein (GLURP) induces antibodies that inhibit *in vitro* growth of *Plasmodium falciparum* in a phase 1 malaria vaccine trial. *Vaccine* **25**(15), 2930–2940.

Herrera, S., and Arevalo-Herrera, M. (eds.) (2010). Immune Responses to Parasitic Infections Bentham Science Publishers Ltd., CA, (Chapter 4).

Herrera, S., Escobar, P., de Plata, C., Avila, G. I., Corradin, G., and Herrera, M. A. (1992a). Human recognition of T cell epitopes on the *Plasmodium vivax* circumsporozoite protein. *J. Immunol.* **148**(12), 3986–3990.

Herrera, S., Herrera, M. A., Corredor, A., Rosero, F., Clavijo, C., and Guerrero, R. (1992b). Failure of a synthetic vaccine to protect Aotus lemurinus against asexual blood stages of *Plasmodium falciparum. Am. J. Trop. Med. Hyg.* **47**(5), 682–690.

Herrera, S., De Plata, C., Gonzalez, M., Perlaza, B. L., Bettens, F., Corradin, G., and Arevalo-Herrera, M. (1997). Antigenicity and immunogenicity of multiple antigen peptides (MAP) containing *P. vivax* CS epitopes in *Aotus* monkeys. *Parasite Immunol.* **19**(4), 161–170.

Herrera, S., Bonelo, A., Perlaza, B. L., Valencia, A. Z., Cifuentes, C., Hurtado, S., Quintero, G., Lopez, J. A., Corradin, G., and Arevalo-Herrera, M. (2004). Use of long synthetic peptides to study the antigenicity and immunogenicity of the *Plasmodium vivax* circumsporozoite protein. *Int. J. Parasitol.* **34**(13–14), 1535–1546.

Herrera, S., Bonelo, A., Perlaza, B. L., Fernandez, O. L., Victoria, L., Lenis, A. M., Soto, L., Hurtado, H., Acuna, L. M., Velez, J. D., *et al.* (2005). Safety and elicitation of humoral and cellular responses in colombian malaria-naive volunteers by a *Plasmodium vivax* circumsporozoite protein-derived synthetic vaccine. *Am. J. Trop. Med. Hyg.* **73**(5 Suppl.), 3–9.

Herrera, S., Castellanos, A., Arevalo-Herrera, M., Restrepo, N., Gulloso, L., and Corradin, G. (2007). *Plasmodium vivax* thrombospondin related adhesion protein: Immunogenicity and protective efficacy in rodents and *Aotus* monkeys. *Mem. Inst. Oswaldo Cruz* **102**(3), 411–416.

Herrera, S., Fernandez, O., Manzano, M. R., Murrain, B., Vergara, J., Blanco, P., Palacios, R., Velez, J. D., Epstein, J. E., Chen-Mok, M., *et al.* (2009). Successful sporozoite challenge model in human volunteers with *Plasmodium vivax* strain derived from human donors. *Am. J. Trop. Med. Hyg.* **81**(5), 740–746.

Herrera, S., Fernandez, O. L., Vera, O., Cardenas, W., Ramirez, O., Palacios, R., Chen-Mok, M., Corradin, G., and Arevalo-Herrera, M. (2011a). Phase I safety and immunogenicity trial of *Plasmodium vivax* CS derived long synthetic peptides adjuvanted with montanide ISA 720 or montanide ISA 51. *Am. J. Trop. Med. Hyg.* **84**(2 Suppl.), 12–20.

Herrera, S., Solarte, Y., Jordan-Villegas, A., Echavarria, J. F., Rocha, L., Palacios, R., Ramirez, O., Velez, J. D., Epstein, J. E., Richie, T. L., *et al.* (2011b). Consistent safety and infectivity in sporozoite challenge model of *Plasmodium vivax* in malaria-naive human volunteers. *Am. J. Trop. Med. Hyg.* **84**(2 Suppl.), 4–11.

Herrington, D. A., Clyde, D. F., Losonsky, G., Cortesia, M., Murphy, J. R., Davis, J., Baqar, S., Felix, A. M., Heimer, E. P., Gillessen, D., *et al.* (1987). Safety and immunogenicity in man of a synthetic peptide malaria vaccine against *Plasmodium falciparum* sporozoites. *Nature* **328**(6127), 257–259.

Herrington, D., Davis, J., Nardin, E., Beier, M., Cortese, J., Eddy, H., Losonsky, G., Hollingdale, M., Sztein, M., Levine, M., *et al.* (1991). Successful immunization of humans with irradiated malaria sporozoites—humoral and cellular-responses of the protected individuals. *Am. J. Trop. Med. Hyg.* **45**(5), 539–547.

Preventing sporozoite invasion of hepatocytes. Hoffman, S. (ed.) (1996). Malaria Vaccine Development:A Multi-Inmune Responses Approach ASM Press.

Hollingdale, M. R., Nardin, E. H., Tharavanij, S., Schwartz, A. L., and Nussenzweig, R. S. (1984). Inhibition of entry of *Plasmodium falciparum* and *P. vivax* sporozoites into cultured cells; an *in vitro* assay of protective antibodies. *J. Immunol.* **132**(2), 909–913.

Jimenez-Diaz, M. B., Mulet, T., Viera, S., Gomez, V., Garuti, H., Ibanez, J., Alvarez-Doval, A., Shultz, L. D., Martinez, A., Gargallo-Viola, D., *et al.* (2009). Improved murine model of malaria using *Plasmodium falciparum* competent strains and non-myelodepleted NOD-scid IL2Rgammanull mice engrafted with human erythrocytes. *Antimicrob. Agents Chemother.* **53**(10), 4533–4536.

Jones, T. R., Ballou, W. R., and Hoffman, S. L. (1993). Antibodies to the circumsporozoite protein and protective immunity to malaria sporozoites. *Prog. Clin. Parasitol.* **3,** 103–117.

Kajava, A. V. (2001). Review: Proteins with repeated sequence—Structural prediction and modeling. *J. Struct. Biol.* **134**(2–3), 132–144.

Kent, S. B. H. (1980). New aspects of solid phase peptide synthesis. *In* "Biomedical Polymers", (E. P. Goldberg and A. Nakajima, eds.). Academic Press, San Diego.

Kent, S. B. (2009). Total chemical synthesis of proteins. *Chem. Soc. Rev.* **38**(2), 338–351.

Kharazmi, A., Jepsen, S., and Andersen, B. J. (1987). Generation of reactive oxygen radicals by human phagocytic cells activated by *Plasmodium falciparum. Scand. J. Immunol.* **25**(4), 335–341.

Kochar, D. K., Das, A., Kochar, S. K., Saxena, V., Sirohi, P., Garg, S., Kochar, A., Khatri, M. P., and Gupta, V. (2009a). Severe *Plasmodium vivax* malaria: A report on serial cases from Bikaner in northwestern India. *Am. J. Trop. Med. Hyg.* **80**(2), 194–198.

Kochar, S. K., Mahajan, M., Gupta, R. P., Middha, S., Acharya, J., Kochar, A., Das, A., and Kochar, D. K. (2009b). Acute attack of AIP (acute intermittent porphyria) with severe vivax malaria associated with convulsions: A case report. *J. Vector Borne Dis.* **46**(4), 307–309.

Kochendoerfer, G. G., Chen, S. Y., Mao, F., Cressman, S., Traviglia, S., Shao, H., Hunter, C. L., Low, D. W., Cagle, E. N., Carnevali, M., *et al.* (2003). Design and chemical synthesis of a homogeneous polymer-modified erythropoiesis protein. *Science* **299**(5608), 884–887.

Kung, Y. T., Du, Y. C., Huang, W. T., Chen, C. C., Ke, L. T., Hu, S. C., Jiang, R. Q., Chu, S. Q., Niu, C. I., Hsu, J. Z., *et al.* (1965). Malaria Vaccine Development: 20 years of hopes, hypes and limited achievements. Total synthesis of crystalline bovine insulin. *Sci. Sin.* **14**(11), 1710–1716.

Lopez, J. A., Weilenman, C., Audran, R., Roggero, M. A., Bonelo, A., Tiercy, J. M., Spertini, F., and Corradin, G. (2001). A synthetic malaria vaccine elicits a potent CD8(+) and CD4(+) T lymphocyte immune response in humans. Implications for vaccination strategies. *Eur. J. Immunol.* **31**(7), 1989–1998.

Lusingu, J. P., Gesase, S., Msham, S., Francis, F., Lemnge, M., Seth, M., Sembuche, S., Rutta, A., Minja, D., Segeja, M. D., *et al.* (2009). Satisfactory safety and immunogenicity of MSP3 malaria vaccine candidate in Tanzanian children aged 12–24 months. *Malar. J.* **8,** 163.

Lyon, J. A., Thomas, A. W., Hall, T., and Chulay, J. D. (1989). Specificities of antibodies that inhibit merozoite dispersal from malaria-infected erythrocytes. *Mol. Biochem. Parasitol.* **36** (1), 77–85.

Marsh, K., Otoo, L., Hayes, R. J., Carson, D. C., and Greenwood, B. M. (1989). Antibodies to blood stage antigens of *Plasmodium-falciparum* in rural gambians and their relation to protection against infection. *Trans. R. Soc. Trop. Med. Hyg.* **83**(3), 293–303.

Marshall, V. M., Coppel, R. L., Anders, R. F., and Kemp, D. J. (1992). Two novel alleles within subfamilies of the merozoite surface antigen 2 (MSA-2) of *Plasmodium falciparum. Mol. Biochem. Parasitol.* **50**(1), 181–184.

McColl, D. J., and Anders, R. F. (1997). Conservation of structural motifs and antigenic diversity in the *Plasmodium falciparum* merozoite surface protein-3 (MSP-3). *Mol. Biochem. Parasitol.* **90**(1), 21–31.

McColl, D. J., Silva, A., Foley, M., Kun, J. F., Favaloro, J. M., Thompson, J. K., Marshall, V. M., Coppel, R. L., Kemp, D. J., and Anders, R. F. (1994). Molecular variation in a novel polymorphic antigen associated with *Plasmodium falciparum* merozoites. *Mol. Biochem. Parasitol.* **68**(1), 53–67.

McGregor, I. A. (1964). The passive transfer of human malarial immunity. *Am. J. Trop. Med. Hyg.* **13**(Suppl.), 237–239.

McGregor, I. A., Turner, M. W., Williams, K., and Hall, P. (1968). Soluble antigens in the blood of African patients with severe *Plasmodium falciparum* malaria. *Lancet* **1**(7548), 881–884.

Mckay, F. C., and Albertson, N. F. (1957). New amine-masking groups for peptide synthesis. *J. Am. Chem. Soc.* **79**(17), 4686–4690.

Mendis, K. N., Munesinghe, Y. D., de Silva, Y. N., Keragalla, I., and Carter, R. (1987). Malaria transmission-blocking immunity induced by natural infections of *Plasmodium vivax* in humans. *Infect. Immun.* **55**(2), 369–372.

Meraldi, V., Nebie, I., Tiono, A. B., Diallo, D., Sanogo, E., Theisen, M., Druilhe, P., Corradin, G., Moret, R., and Sirima, B. S. (2004). Natural antibody response to Plasmodium falciparum Exp-1, MSP-3 and GLURP long synthetic peptides and association with protection. *Parasite Immunol.* **26**(6–7), 265–272.

Merrifield, R. B. (1962). Peptide synthesis on a solid polymer. *Fed. Proc.* **21**(2), 412.

Merrifield, R. B. (1963). Solid phase peptide synthesis. 1. Synthesis of a tetrapeptide. *J. Am. Chem. Soc.* **85**(14), 2149.

Merrifield, R. B. (1993). Life During a Golden Age of Peptide Chemistry: The Concept and Development of Solid-Phase Peptide Synthesis. American Chemical Society, Washington, DC.

Merrifield, R. B., Stewart, J. M., and Jernberg, N. (1966). Instrument for automated synthesis of peptides. *Anal. Chem.* **38**(13), 1905–1914.

Migliorini, P., Betschart, B., and Corradin, G. (1993). Malaria vaccine: Immunization of mice with a synthetic T cell helper epitope alone leads to protective immunity. *Eur. J. Immunol.* **23**(2), 582–585.

Mojsov, S., and Merrifield, R. B. (1984). An improved synthesis of crystalline mammalian glucagon. *Eur. J. Biochem.* **145**(3), 601–605.

Mordmuller, B., Szywon, K., Greutelaers, B., Esen, M., Mewono, L., Treut, C., Murbeth, R. E., Chilengi, R., Noor, R., Kilama, W. L., *et al.* (2010). Safety and immunogenicity of the malaria vaccine candidate GMZ2 in malaria-exposed, adult individuals from Lambarene, Gabon. *Vaccine* **28**(41), 6698–6703.

Moreno, R., Jiang, L., Moehle, K., Zurbriggen, R., Gluck, R., Robinson, J. A., and Pluschke, G. (2001). Exploiting conformationally constrained peptidomimetics and an efficient human-compatible delivery system in synthetic vaccine design. *Chembiochem* **2**(11), 838–843.

Morosan, S., Hez-Deroubaix, S., Lunel, F., Renia, L., Giannini, C., Van Rooijen, N., Battaglia, S., Blanc, C., Eling, W., Sauerwein, R., *et al.* (2006). Liver-stage development of *Plasmodium falciparum*, in a humanized mouse model. *J. Infect. Dis.* **193**(7), 996–1004.

Mueller, M. S., Renard, A., Boato, F., Vogel, D., Naegeli, M., Zurbriggen, R., Robinson, J. A., and Pluschke, G. (2003). Induction of parasite growth-inhibitory antibodies by a virosomal formulation of a peptidomimetic of loop I from domain III of *Plasmodium falciparum* apical membrane antigen 1. *Infect. Immun.* **71**(8), 4749–4758.

Muir, T. W., Sondhi, D., and Cole, P. A. (1998). Expressed protein ligation: A general method for protein engineering. *Proc. Natl. Acad. Sci. USA* **95**(12), 6705–6710.

Muller, H. M., Reckmann, I., Hollingdale, M. R., Bujard, H., Robson, K. J., and Crisanti, A. (1993a). Thrombospondin related anonymous protein (TRAP) of *Plasmodium falciparum* binds specifically to sulfated glycoconjugates and to HepG2 hepatoma cells suggesting a role for this molecule in sporozoite invasion of hepatocytes. *EMBO J.* **12**(7), 2881–2889.

Muller, H. M., Scarselli, E., and Crisanti, A. (1993b). Thrombospondin related anonymous protein (TRAP) of *Plasmodium falciparum* in parasite-host cell interactions. *Parassitologia* **35** (Suppl.), 69–72.

Nardin, E. (2010). The past decade in malaria synthetic peptide vaccine clinical trials. *Hum. Vaccin.* **6**(1), 27–38.

Nardin, E. H., and Nussenzweig, R. S. (1993). T cell responses to pre-erythrocytic stages of malaria: Role in protection and vaccine development against pre-erythrocytic stages. *Annu. Rev. Immunol.* **11,** 687–727.

Nardin, E. H., Herrington, D. A., Davis, J., Levine, M., Stuber, D., Takacs, B., Caspers, P., Barr, P., Altszuler, R., Clavijo, P., *et al.* (1989). Conserved repetitive epitope recognized by CD4+ clones from a malaria-immunized volunteer. *Science* **246**(4937), 1603–1606.

Nardin, E. H., Calvo-Calle, J. M., Oliveira, G. A., Nussenzweig, R. S., Schneider, M., Tiercy, J. M., Loutan, L., Hochstrasser, D., and Rose, K. (2001). A totally synthetic polyoxime malaria vaccine containing *Plasmodium falciparum* B cell and universal T cell epitopes elicits immune responses in volunteers of diverse HLA types. *J. Immunol.* **166**(1), 481–489.

Nilsson, B. L., Soellner, M. B., and Raines, R. T. (2005). Chemical synthesis of proteins. *Annu. Rev. Biophys. Biomol. Struct.* **34,** 91–118.

Nishiuchi, Y., Inui, T., Nishio, H., Bodi, J., Kimura, T., Tsuji, F. I., and Sakakibara, S. (1998). Chemical synthesis of the precursor molecule of the Aequorea green fluorescent protein, subsequent folding, and development of fluorescence. *Proc. Natl. Acad. Sci. USA* **95**(23), 13549–13554.

Nosten, F., Luxemburger, C., Kyle, D. E., Ballou, W. R., Wittes, J., Wah, E., Chongsuphajaisiddhi, T., Gordon, D. M., White, N. J., Sadoff, J. C., *et al.* (1996). Randomised double-blind placebo-controlled trial of SPf66 malaria vaccine in children in northwestern Thailand. Shoklo SPf66 Malaria Vaccine Trial Group. *Lancet* **348**(9029), 701–707.

Nussenzweig, R. (1980). Use of radiation-attenuated sporozoites in the immunoprophylaxis of malaria. *Int. J. Nucl. Med. Biol.* **7**(2), 89–96.

Nussenzweig, V., and Nussenzweig, R. S. (1989). Circumsporozoite proteins of malaria parasites. *Bull. Mem. Acad. R. Med. Belg.* **144**(11), 493–504.

Nussenzweig, R. S., Vanderberg, J., Most, H., and Orton, C. (1967). Protective immunity produced by the injection of x-irradiated sporozoites of *Plasmodium berghei. Nature* **216** (5111), 160–162.

Oeuvray, C., Bouharoun-Tayoun, H., Gras-Masse, H., Bottius, E., Kaidoh, T., Aikawa, M., Filgueira, M. C., Tartar, A., and Druilhe, P. (1994). Merozoite surface protein-3: A malaria protein inducing antibodies that promote *Plasmodium falciparum* killing by cooperation with blood monocytes. *Blood* **84**(5), 1594–1602.

Oeuvray, C., Theisen, M., Rogier, C., Trape, J. F., Jepsen, S., and Druilhe, P. (2000). Cytophilic immunoglobulin responses to *Plasmodium falciparum* glutamate-rich protein are correlated with protection against clinical malaria in Dielmo, Senegal. *Infect. Immun.* **68**(5), 2617–2620.

Okitsu, S. L., Silvie, O., Westerfeld, N., Curcic, M., Kammer, A. R., Mueller, M. S., Sauerwein, R. W., Robinson, J. A., Genton, B., Mazier, D., *et al.* (2007). A virosomal malaria peptide vaccine elicits a long-lasting sporozoite-inhibitory antibody response in a phase 1a clinical trial. *PLoS One* **2**(12), e1278.

Olugbile, S., Kulangara, C., Bang, G., Bertholet, S., Suzarte, E., Villard, V., Frank, G., Audran, R., Razaname, A., Nebie, I., *et al.* (2009). Vaccine potentials of an intrinsically unstructured fragment derived from the blood stage-associated *Plasmodium falciparum* protein PFF0165c. *Infect. Immun.* **77**(12), 5701–5709.

Olugbile, S., Habel, C., Servis, C., Spertini, F., Verdini, A., and Corradin, G. (2010). Malaria vaccines—The long synthetic peptide approach: Technical and conceptual advancements. *Curr. Opin. Mol. Ther.* **12**(1), 64–76.

Olugbile, S., Villard, V., Bertholet, S., Jafarshad, A., Kulangara, C., Roussilhon, C., Frank, G., Agak, G. W., Felger, I., Nebie, I., *et al.* (2011). Malaria vaccine candidate: Design of a multivalent subunit alpha-helical coiled coil poly-epitope. *Vaccine* **29**(40), 7090–7099.

Overstreet, M. G., Cockburn, I. A., Chen, Y. C., and Zavala, F. (2008). Protective CD8 T cells against *Plasmodium* liver stages: Immunobiology of an 'unnatural' immune response. *Immunol. Rev.* **225,** 272–283.

Pancake, S. J., Holt, G. D., Mellouk, S., and Hoffman, S. L. (1992). Malaria sporozoites and circumsporozoite proteins bind specifically to sulfated glycoconjugates. *J. Cell Biol.* **117** (6), 1351–1357.

Panina-Bordignon, P., Tan, A., Termijtelen, A., Demotz, S., Corradin, G., and Lanzavecchia, A. (1989). Universally immunogenic T cell epitopes: Promiscuous binding to human MHC class II and promiscuous recognition by T cells. *Eur. J. Immunol.* **19**(12), 2237–2242.

Patarroyo, M. E., Romero, P., Torres, M. L., Clavijo, P., Moreno, A., Martinez, A., Rodriguez, R., Guzman, F., and Cabezas, E. (1987). Induction of protective immunity against experimental infection with malaria using synthetic peptides. *Nature* **328**(6131), 629–632.

Patarroyo, M. E., Amador, R., Clavijo, P., Moreno, A., Guzman, F., Romero, P., Tascon, R., Franco, A., Murillo, L. A., Ponton, G., *et al.* (1988). A synthetic vaccine protects humans against challenge with asexual blood stages of *Plasmodium falciparum* malaria. *Nature* **332** (6160), 158–161.

Patarroyo, G., Franco, L., Amador, R., Murillo, L. A., Rocha, C. L., Rojas, M., and Patarroyo, M. E. (1992). Study of the safety and immunogenicity of the synthetic malaria SPf66 vaccine in children aged 1–14 years. *Vaccine* **10**(3), 175–178.

Perignon, J. L., and Druilhe, P. (1994). Immune mechanisms underlying the premunition against *Plasmodium falciparum* malaria. *Mem. Inst. Oswaldo Cruz* **89**(Suppl. 2), 51–53.

Perlaza, B. L., Sauzet, J. P., Balde, A. T., Brahimi, K., Tall, A., Corradin, G., and Druilhe, P. (2001). Long synthetic peptides encompassing the *Plasmodium falciparum* LSA3 are the target of human B and T cells and are potent inducers of B helper, T helper and cytolytic T cell responses in mice. *Eur. J. Immunol.* **31**(7), 2200–2209.

Pink, J. R., and Sinigaglia, F. (1989). Characterizing T-cell epitopes in vaccine candidates. *Immunol. Today* **10**(12), 408–409.

Plassmeyer, M. L., Reiter, K., Shimp, R. L., Jr., Kotova, S., Smith, P. D., Hurt, D. E., House, B., Zou, X., Zhang, Y., Hickman, M., *et al.* (2009). Structure of the *Plasmodium falciparum* circumsporozoite protein, a leading malaria vaccine candidate. *J. Biol. Chem.* **284**(39), 26951–26963.

Poland, J. D., Calisher, C. H., Monath, T. P., Downs, W. G., and Murphy, K. (1981). Persistence of neutralizing antibody 30–35 years after immunization with 17D yellow fever vaccine. *Bull. World Health Organ.* **59**(6), 895–900.

Price, R. N., Douglas, N. M., and Anstey, N. M. (2009). New developments in *Plasmodium vivax* malaria: Severe disease and the rise of chloroquine resistance. *Curr. Opin. Infect. Dis.* **22**(5), 430–435.

Reece, W. H., Pinder, M., Gothard, P. K., Milligan, P., Bojang, K., Doherty, T., Plebanski, M., Akinwunmi, P., Everaere, S., Watkins, K. R., *et al.* (2004). A CD4(+) T-cell immune response to a conserved epitope in the circumsporozoite protein correlates with protection from natural *Plasmodium falciparum* infection and disease. *Nat. Med.* **10**(4), 406–410.

Regnier, F. E. (1983). High-performance liquid chromatography of proteins. *Methods Enzymol.* **91,** 137–190.

Renggli, J., Valmori, D., Romero, J. F., Eberl, G., Romero, P., Betschart, B., and Corradin, G. (1995). CD8+ T-cell protective immunity induced by immunization with *Plasmodium berghei* CS protein-derived synthetic peptides: Evidence that localization of peptide-specific CTLs is crucial for protection against malaria. *Immunol. Lett.* **46**(1–2), 199–205.

Renia, L., Marussig, M. S., Grillot, D., Pied, S., Corradin, G., Miltgen, F., Del Giudice, G., and Mazier, D. (1991). *In vitro* activity of CD4+ and CD8+ T lymphocytes from mice immunized with a synthetic malaria peptide. *Proc. Natl. Acad. Sci. USA* **88**(18), 7963–7967.

Reymond, C. D., Beghdadi-Rais, C., Roggero, M., Duarte, E. A., Desponds, C., Bernard, M., Groux, D., Matile, H., Bron, C., Corradin, G., *et al.* (1995). Anchoring of an immunogenic *Plasmodium falciparum* circumsporozoite protein on the surface of Dictyostelium discoideum. *J. Biol. Chem.* **270**(21), 12941–12947.

Rodriguez, R., Moreno, A., Guzman, F., Calvo, M., and Patarroyo, M. E. (1990). Studies in Owl monkeys leading to the development of a synthetic vaccine against the asexual blood stages of *plasmodium-falciparum*. *Am. J. Trop. Med. Hyg.* **43**(4), 339–354.

Roestenberg, M., McCall, M., Hopman, J., Wiersma, J., Luty, A. J., van Gemert, G. J., van de Vegte-Bolmer, M., van Schaijk, B., Teelen, K., Arens, T., *et al.* (2009). Protection against a malaria challenge by sporozoite inoculation. *N. Engl. J. Med.* **361**(5), 468–477.

Roggero, M. A., Filippi, B., Church, P., Hoffman, S. L., Blum-Tirouvanziam, U., Lopez, J. A., Esposito, F., Matile, H., Reymond, C. D., Fasel, N., *et al.* (1995). Synthesis and immunological characterization of 104-mer and 102-mer peptides corresponding to the N- and C-terminal regions of the *Plasmodium falciparum* CS protein. *Mol. Immunol.* **32**(17–18), 1301–1309.

Roggero, M. A., Meraldi, V., Lopez, J. A., Eberl, G., Romero, J. C., Matile, H., Betschart, B., Corradin, G., and Renggli, J. (2000). The synthetic, oxidized C-terminal fragment of the *Plasmodium berghei* circumsporozoite protein elicits a high protective response. *Eur. J. Immunol.* **30**(9), 2679–2685.

Romero, P., Maryanski, J. L., Cordey, A. S., Corradin, G., Nussenzweig, R. S., and Zavala, F. (1990). Isolation and characterization of protective cytolytic T cells in a rodent malaria model system. *Immunol. Lett.* **25**(1–3), 27–31.

Rose, K. (1994). Facile synthesis of homogeneous artificial proteins. *J. Am. Chem. Soc.* **116**(1), 30–33.

Rose, K., Zeng, W., Brown, L. E., and Jackson, D. C. (1995). A synthetic peptide-based polyoxime vaccine construct of high purity and activity. *Mol. Immunol.* **32**(14–15), 1031–1037.

Rosenberg, R., Wirtz, R. A., Lanar, D. E., Sattabongkot, J., Hall, T., Waters, A. P., and Prasittisuk, C. (1989). Circumsporozoite protein heterogeneity in the human malaria parasite *Plasmodium vivax*. *Science* **245**(4921), 973–976.

Roussilhon, C., Oeuvray, C., Muller-Graf, C., Tall, A., Rogier, C., Trape, J. F., Theisen, M., Balde, A., Perignon, J. L., and Druilhe, P. (2007). Long-term clinical protection from falciparum malaria is strongly associated with IgG3 antibodies to merozoite surface protein 3. *PLoS Med.* **4**(11), e320.

Ruebush, T. K., 2nd., Campbell, G. H., Moreno, A., Patarroyo, M. E., and Collins, W. E. (1990). Immunization of owl monkeys with a combination of Plasmodium falciparum asexual blood-stage synthetic peptide antigens. *Am. J. Trop. Med. Hyg.* **43**(4), 355–366.

Salcedo, M., Barreto, L., Rojas, M., Moya, R., Cote, J., and Patarroyo, M. E. (1991). Studies on the humoral immune response to a synthetic vaccine against *Plasmodium falciparum* malaria. *Clin. Exp. Immunol.* **84**(1), 122–128.

Sauerwein, R. W., Roestenberg, M., and Moorthy, V. S. (2011). Experimental human challenge infections can accelerate clinical malaria vaccine development. *Nat. Rev. Immunol.* **11**(1), 57–64.

Schaal, E. (1871). Ueber einige aus asparagisäure entstchende producte. *Leibig's Annalen der Chemie* **157,** 24–34.

Schneider, J., and Kent, S. B. (1988). Enzymatic activity of a synthetic 99 residue protein corresponding to the putative HIV-1 protease. *Cell* **54**(3), 363–368.

Schnolzer, M., and Kent, S. B. (1992). Constructing proteins by dovetailing unprotected synthetic peptides: Backbone-engineered HIV protease. *Science* **256**(5054), 221–225.

Schofield, L., Villaquiran, J., Ferreira, A., Schellekens, H., Nussenzweig, R., and Nussenzweig, V. (1987). Gamma-interferon, Cd8+ T-cells and antibodies required for immunity to malaria sporozoites. *Nature* **330**(6149), 664–666.

Schwyzer, R. (1953). Coenzym-a—Modellversuche Zur Biologischen Acylierungsreaktion—Uber Die Reaktionsfahigkeit Von Thiolcarbonsauren Und Ihren Estern. *Helvetica Chimica Acta* **36**(2), 414–424.

Schwyzer, R., and Sieber, P. (1963). Total synthesis of adrenocorticotrophic hormone. *Nature* **199**(488), 172.

Sedegah, M., Sim, B. K., Mason, C., Nutman, T., Malik, A., Roberts, C., Johnson, A., Ochola, J., Koech, D., Were, B., *et al.* (1992). Naturally acquired CD8+ cytotoxic T lymphocytes against the *Plasmodium falciparum* circumsporozoite protein. *J. Immunol.* **149**(3), 966–971.

Sheehan, J. C., and Hess, G. P. (1955). A new method of forming peptide bonds. *J. Am. Chem. Soc.* **77**(4), 1067–1068.

Singh, S., Soe, S., Mejia, J. P., Roussilhon, C., Theisen, M., Corradin, G., and Druilhe, P. (2004). Identification of a conserved region of *Plasmodium falciparum* MSP3 targeted by biologically active antibodies to improve vaccine design. *J. Infect. Dis.* **190**(5), 1010–1018.

Sinigaglia, F., Guttinger, M., Kilgus, J., Doran, D. M., Matile, H., Etlinger, H., Trzeciak, A., Gillessen, D., and Pink, J. R. (1988). A malaria T-cell epitope recognized in association with most mouse and human MHC class II molecules. *Nature* **336**(6201), 778–780.

Sinnis, P., and Nussenzweig, V. (1996). *In* "Malaria Vaccine Development: A Multi-Immune Response Approach. Chapter 2. Preventing sporozoite Invasion of Hepatocytes", (S. Hoffman, ed.). American Society for Microbiology, Washington, DC.

Sirima, S. B., Nebie, I., Ouedraogo, A., Tiono, A. B., Konate, A. T., Gansane, A., Derme, A. I., Diarra, A., Soulama, I., Cuzzin-Ouattara, N., *et al.* (2007). Safety and immunogenicity of the *Plasmodium falciparum* merozoite surface protein-3 long synthetic peptide (MSP3-LSP) malaria vaccine in healthy, semi-immune adult males in Burkina Faso, West Africa. *Vaccine* **25**(14), 2723–2732.

Sirima, S., Cousens, S., and Druilhe, P. (2011). Protection against malaria by MSP3 candidate vaccine. *N. Engl. J. Med.* **365**(11), 1062–1064.

Spaccapelo, R., Naitza, S., Robson, K. J., and Crisanti, A. (1997). Thrombospondin-related adhesive protein (TRAP) of *Plasmodium berghei* and parasite motility. *Lancet* **350**(9074), 335.

Stoute, J. A., Slaoui, M., Heppner, D. G., Momin, P., Kester, K. E., Desmons, P., Wellde, B. T., Garcon, N., Krzych, U., Marchand, M., *et al.* (1997). A preliminary evaluation of a recombinant circumsporozoite protein vaccine against *Plasmodium falciparum* malaria. *N. Engl. J. Med.* **336**(2), 86–91.

Sydor, J. R., Mariano, M., Sideris, S., and Nock, S. (2002). Establishment of intein-mediated protein ligation under denaturing conditions: C-terminal labeling of a single-chain antibody for biochip screening. *Bioconjug. Chem.* **13**(4), 707–712.

Tam, J. P., Clavijo, P., Lu, Y. A., Nussenzweig, V., Nussenzweig, R., and Zavala, F. (1990). Incorporation of T and B epitopes of the circumsporozoite protein in a chemically defined synthetic vaccine against malaria. *J. Exp. Med.* **171**(1), 299–306.

Templeton, T. J., and Kaslow, D. C. (1997). Cloning and cross-species comparison of the thrombospondin-related anonymous protein (TRAP) gene from *Plasmodium knowlesi*, *Plasmodium vivax* and *Plasmodium gallinaceum*. *Mol. Biochem. Parasitol.* **84**(1), 13–24.

Theisen, M., Soe, S., Oeuvray, C., Thomas, A. W., Vuust, J., Danielsen, S., Jepsen, S., and Druilhe, P. (1998). The glutamate-rich protein (GLURP) of *Plasmodium falciparum* is a target for antibody-dependent monocyte-mediated inhibition of parasite growth *in vitro*. *Infect. Immun.* **66**(1), 11–17.

Theisen, M., Soe, S., Jessing, S. G., Okkels, L. M., Danielsen, S., Oeuvray, C., Druilhe, P., and Jepsen, S. (2000). Identification of a major B-cell epitope of the *Plasmodium falciparum* glutamate-rich protein (GLURP), targeted by human antibodies mediating parasite killing. *Vaccine* **19**(2–3), 204–212.

Thierry, A. C., Pinaud, S., Bigler, N., Perrenoud, G., Denis, B., Roggero, M. A., Fasel, N., Moulon, C., and Demotz, S. (2001). Long synthetic peptides as biologically active proteins: The example of the chemokines. *Biologicals* **29**(3–4), 259–263.
Thompson, F. M., Porter, D. W., Okitsu, S. L., Westerfeld, N., Vogel, D., Todryk, S., Poulton, I., Correa, S., Hutchings, C., Berthoud, T., *et al.* (2008). Evidence of blood stage efficacy with a virosomal malaria vaccine in a phase IIa clinical trial. *PLoS One* **3**(1), e1493.
Tjitra, E., Anstey, N. M., Sugiarto, P., Warikar, N., Kenangalem, E., Karyana, M., Lampah, D. A., and Price, R. N. (2008). Multidrug-resistant *Plasmodium vivax* associated with severe and fatal malaria: A prospective study in Papua, Indonesia. *PLoS Med.* **5**(6), e128.
Unson, C. G. (2007). Glucagon and the glucagon receptor: Merrifield years at the interface of chemistry and biology. *Int. J. Pept. Res. Ther.* **13**(1–2), 19–27.
Valero, M. V., Amador, L. R., Galindo, C., Figueroa, J., Bello, M. S., Murillo, L. A., Mora, A. L., Patarroyo, G., Rocha, C. L., Rojas, M., *et al.* (1993). Vaccination with SPf66, a chemically synthesised vaccine, against *Plasmodium falciparum* malaria in Colombia. *Lancet* **341**(8847), 705–710.
Valmori, D., Pessi, A., Bianchi, E., and Corradin, G. (1992). Use of human universally antigenic tetanus toxin T cell epitopes as carriers for human vaccination. *J. Immunol.* **149**(2), 717–721.
Verdini, A. S., Chiappinelli, L., and Zanobi, A. (1991). Toward the elucidation of the mechanism of attachment and entry of malaria sporozoites into cells: Synthetic polypeptides from the circumsporozoite protein of *Plasmodium falciparum* bind Ca2+ and interact with model phospholipid membranes. *Biopolymers* **31**(6), 587–594.
Verdini, A., Terenzi, S., Brossard, V., Roggero, M., and Corradin, G. (2008). Oxidative folding of synthetic polypeptides S-protected as tert-butylthio derivatives. *J. Pept. Sci.* **14**(12), 1271–1282.
Verdini, A., Olugbile, S., Corradin, G., and Pink, P. (2010). Malaria Vaccine Development: 20 Years of Hopes, Hypes and Limited Achievements. *In* "Immune Response to Parasitic Infections", (E. Jirillo, ed.), pp. 21–42. Lausanne, Switzerland.
Villard, V., Agak, G. W., Frank, G., Jafarshad, A., Servis, C., Nebie, I., Sirima, S. B., Felger, I., Arevalo-Herrera, M., Herrera, S., *et al.* (2007). Rapid identification of malaria vaccine candidates based on alpha-helical coiled coil protein motif. *PLoS One* **2**(7), e645.
Weiss, W. R., Berzofsky, J. A., Houghten, R. A., Sedegah, M., Hollindale, M., and Hoffman, S. L. (1992). A T cell clone directed at the circumsporozoite protein which protects mice against both *Plasmodium yoelii* and *Plasmodium berghei*. *J. Immunol.* **149**(6), 2103–2109.
World Health Organization (2010). World Malaria Report: 2010. WHO, .
Wright, P. E., and Dyson, H. J. (1999). Intrinsically unstructured proteins: Re-assessing the protein structure-function paradigm. *J. Mol. Biol.* **293**(2), 321–331.
Wünsch, E. (1971). Synthesis of naturally occurring polypeptides, problems of current research. *Angew. Chem. Int. Ed Engl.* **10**(11), 786–795.
Wünsch, E., Jaeger, E., and Scharf, R. (1968). Zur synthese des glucagons. XIX Reindarstellung des synthetischen glucagons. *Chem. Ber.* **101,** 3664–3667.
Yajima, H., and Fujii, N. (1981). Totally synthetic crystalline ribonuclease A. *Biopolymers* **20** (9), 1859–1867.
Zavala, F., Tam, J. P., Barr, P. J., Romero, P. J., Ley, V., Nussenzweig, R. S., and Nussenzweig, V. (1987). Synthetic peptide vaccine confers protection against murine malaria. *J. Exp. Med.* **166**(5), 1591–1596.
Zhang, Y. S. (2010). The first protein ever synthesized *in vitro*—A personal reminiscence of the total synthesis of crystalline insulin. *Sci. China Life Sci.* **53**(1), 16–18.
Zurbriggen, R. (2003). Immunostimulating reconstituted influenza virosomes. *Vaccine* **21** (9–10), 921–924.

CHAPTER 6

Enhancing Cancer Immunotherapy by Intracellular Delivery of Cell-Penetrating Peptides and Stimulation of Pattern-Recognition Receptor Signaling

Helen Y. Wang and **Rong-Fu Wang**

Contents

Department of Pathology and Immunology, Center for Cell and Gene Therapy, Baylor College of Medicine, Houston, Texas, USA
Present address: Center for Inflammation and Epigenetics, The Methodist Hospital Research Institute, Houston, Texas, USA

Advances in Immunology, Volume 114
ISSN 0065-2776, DOI: 10.1016/B978-0-12-396548-6.00006-8

Abstract The importance of T-cell-mediated antitumor immunity has been demonstrated in both animal models and human cancer immunotherapy. In the past 30 years, T-cell-based immunotherapy has been improved with an objective clinical response rate of up to 72%. Identification of MHC class I- and II-restricted tumor antigens recognized by tumor-reactive T cells has generated a resurgence of interest in cancer vaccines. Although clinical trials with cancer peptide/protein vaccines have only met a limited success, several phase II/III clinical trials are either completed or ongoing with encouraging results. Recent advances in immunotherapy have led to the approval of two anticancer drugs (sipuleucel-T vaccine and anti-CTLA-4 antibody) by the US FDA for the treatment of metastatic castration-resistant prostate cancer and melanoma, respectively. Intracellular delivery of antigenic peptides into dendritic cells (DCs) prolongs antigen presentation of antigen-presenting cells to T cells, thus further improving clinical efficacy of peptide/protein cancer vaccines. Because innate immune responses are critically important to provide sensing and initiating of adaptive immunity, combined use of cell-penetrating peptide vaccines with stimulation of innate immune signaling may produce potent antitumor immune responses. We will discuss the recent progress and novel strategies in cancer immunotherapy.

1. INTRODUCTION

The host immune system consisting of innate and adaptive immunity plays an essential role in immunosurveillance, recognition, and destruction of cancer cells (Schreiber *et al.*, 2011; Vesely *et al.*, 2011). T cell-mediated antitumor immunity has been demonstrated in murine tumor models 30 years ago by adoptive transfer experiments (Greenberg, 1991; Rosenberg, 1990; Rosenberg *et al.*, 2008). Recently, adoptive T-cell therapy has been successfully used to treat many human cancers such as melanoma, renal cell carcinoma, and lymphoma with varying degrees of tumor regression (Lesterhuis *et al.*, 2011; Rosenberg, 2011; Rosenberg *et al.*, 2008; Tey *et al.*, 2006). Although $CD4^+$ and $CD8^+$ T cells are the major components of T-cell-mediated antitumor immunity, natural killer (NK), NK1.1 T (NKT), and $\gamma\delta$ T cells may also play a role in immunosurveillance against cancer

(Diefenbach and Raulet, 2001; Vesely *et al.*, 2011; Wang, 2001). Using tumor-reactive T cells, many immunogenic tumor antigens have been identified (Boon *et al.*, 1994; Wang and Rosenberg, 1999). Clinical studies using molecularly defined MHC class I-restricted tumor antigens show that peptide vaccines can induce antigen-specific immune responses in the patients who received peptide vaccines, but overall immune responses elicited by the use of $CD8^+$ T-cell peptides are weak in several early clinical studies. However, several tumor antigens, including gp100 and MAGE-3, have been used in phase II and III clinical trials with encouraging results. Recently, antigen-presenting cells (APCs) loaded with tumor antigens have been approved by US Federal Food Administration (FDA) for the treatment of prostate cancer. This is an important milestone in the field of cancer immunology. However, blood APC-based vaccines require autologous cells from the patients and are expensive ($93,000 for a course of three treatments) with an average extension of survival of 4.1 months. To further improve broad application and clinical efficacy of cancer vaccines, we need to develop peptide/protein-based vaccines as a more broadly applicable and less expensive anticancer drugs. Further, recent studies have identified several checkpoints or roadblocks for T-cell activation and function (Callahan *et al.*, 2010; Chambers *et al.*, 2001; Zhu *et al.*, 2011). These include coinhibitory molecules and other negative regulators in T cells and dendritic cells (DCs), as well as immune suppression mediated by regulatory T cells (Zhu *et al.*, 2011). To enhance antitumor immunity, it is necessary to remove these roadblocks so that T cells can be fully activated and to mediate the eradication of cancer cells through modulating innate immune signaling. Importantly, anti-CTLA-4 (cytotoxic T-lymphocyte-associated protein 4) antibody therapy has a proven therapeutic effect on metastatic melanoma and has recently been approved by US FDA for the treatment of metastatic melanoma (Hodi *et al.*, 2010; Royal *et al.*, 2010). With encouraging results of clinical trials and FDA approval of two anticancer immunotherapy drugs, development of synthetic peptide/protein-based cancer vaccines will be the next frontline in the field of cancer immunotherapy and vaccines. In this chapter, we discuss a novel strategy for enhancing antitumor immune responses by intracellular delivery of peptides into DCs and stimulation of innate immune signaling to overcome immune suppression.

2. ADOPTIVE CELL THERAPY: HISTORY AND RECENT PROGRESSES

2.1. LAK and cytokine-induced killer cell therapy

In the early 1980s, lymphocyte-activated killer (LAK) cells were first used in mouse models and human cancer patients (Grimm *et al.*, 1982; Muul *et al.*, 1987). LAK cells are generated from the peripheral blood mononuclear cells (PBMCs) following *ex vivo* expansion in the presence of interleukin (IL)-2 and are capable of killing fresh tumor cells without requirement of MHC restriction. Clinical studies show modest efficacy against melanoma and renal carcinoma cancer (Rosenberg *et al.*, 1987; Takayama *et al.*, 2000). In the early 1990s, cytokine-induced killer (CIK) cells are generated from PBMCs in the presence of interferon (IFN)-γ on day 0, followed by adding anti-CD3 and IL-2 on day 1, with continued addition of IL-2 during 21–28 days of culture (Schmidt-Wolf *et al.*, 1991). These $CD3^+$ $CD56^+$ CIK cells are converted from $CD3^+$ $CD56^-$ cells and expanded up to 1000-fold after 21–28 days with mixed cell populations (2% NK cells, and >90% CD3 and $CD56^+$ T cells) and show strong cytotoxicity against many tumor cell targets without MHC restriction (Linn *et al.*, 2002). Thus, these cells may function similar to NK-like T cells. It is not clear how they recognize tumor targets and what antigens they recognize on tumor cells. Although CIK cells have been tested in a clinical setting for a variety of cancers, data on the efficacy of CIK therapy are limited. The first report of the international registry on CIK treatment of 426 patients shows that a large-scale expansion of CIK cells *ex vivo* is possible and cell infusion is safe (Hontscha *et al.*, 2011). The clinical response rate of CIK is 51/384 (13%) with complete and partial responses, 40/384 (10%) with minor response, and 161/384 (42%) with a stable disease (Hontscha *et al.*, 2011). Several groups report that combination of CIK or tumor-infiltrating lymphocyte (TIL) with chemotherapy produces better clinical response rates and reduces the percentage of relapse compared with chemotherapy alone (Dudley *et al.*, 2002; Jiang *et al.*, 2005). With encouraging clinical evidence of CIK therapy, it is important to conduct randomized clinical trials to determine the clinical benefit of cancer patients who receive CIK alone, chemotherapy alone, and CIK plus chemotherapy in the near future.

2.2. Adoptive T-cell therapy with TILs

Adoptive cell therapy (ACT) with TILs has emerged as the most effective treatment for patients with metastatic melanoma. TIL-based therapy was first reported in 1988, and clinical studies with TIL plus IL-2 showed 34% objective response rate compared with 16% clinical response with IL-2 alone (Rosenberg, 2000; Rosenberg *et al.*, 1988, 1994). Importantly, ACT with TILs has been dramatically improved for clinical efficacy by introducing treatment with a nonmyeloablative preparative immunodepleting regimen consisting of cyclophosphamide and fludarabine before T-cell infusion (Dudley *et al.*, 2002). Objective clinical response rates have been observed in 49–72% of patients with metastatic melanoma refractory to all other treatments (Rosenberg, 2011; Rosenberg *et al.*, 2008). This regimen depletes circulating lymphocytes as well as those at tumor sites for a week before host hematopoietic cell recovery, thus likely removing suppressive Treg cells and allowing antitumor T cells to survive and expand in patients after adoptive transfer. The unique features of ACT are that clinical responses can be durable (>5 years) and low percentages of relapse (Rosenberg *et al.*, 2011). More recently, whole body irradiation was added to the cyclophosphamide and fludarabine lymphodepleting preparative regimen before adoptive T-cell transfer. These further modifications result in the highest objective clinical responses in all patients receiving treatment (Wrzesinski *et al.*, 2010). However, because the difficulties associated with generation and expansion of TILs derived from tumor tissues and variable availability of such tumor tissues in cancer patients, ACT with autologous TILs is not suitable for many cancer patients, in particular, those with cancer other than melanoma. The success rate for generating TILs from other types of cancer is much lower than that seen in melanoma. Thus, use of T cells transduced with retroviruses or lentiviruses encoding T-cell receptors (TCRs) that recognized tumor antigens or with genes encoding cytokines or costimulatory molecules has made ACT available for patients with different types of cancer. Alternatively, these peripheral T cells will be stimulated with antigenic peptides to generate antigen-specific T cells. This approach has been successfully used to treat lymphoma and melanoma with antigen-specific T cells (Hunder *et al.*, 2008; Leen *et al.*, 2006; Wolf *et al.*, 2003; Yee *et al.*, 2000, 2002). Despite impressive clinical response rates of ACT in cancer therapy in phase I/II clinical studies, so far no ACT treatment has been approved as an anticancer drug. This may be due to difficulties in patentability of many immunotherapeutic strategies or technologies, individualized treatment associated with high costs, and lack of funding and interests by the pharmaceutical companies. However, with recent successes and promising clinical results, ACT or other immune cell transfer therapies are likely to move into phase III trials and obtain FDA approval as anticancer drugs.

3. APC-BASED VACCINES: THE FIRST FDA APPROVED DRUG FOR PROSTATE CANCER

Professional APCs such as DCs can potently induce antigen-specific T cells. DC loaded with cancer antigens or tumor lysates has been used to vaccinate cancer patients with limited success. However, the US FDA recently approved the first therapeutic cancer vaccine drug (Provenge, Dendreon) for the treatment of metastatic castration-resistant prostate cancer. The sipuleucel-T vaccines consist of blood APCs, including monocytes and DCs, loaded with a fusion protein (PA2024) of the prostate antigen prostatic acid phosphatase linked to an immunostimulatory granulocyte–macrophage colony-stimulating factor. Although tumor regressions, radiographic, and prostate-specific antigen responses occurred very rarely, an overall survival benefit of 4.1 months was observed for the sipuleucel-T group versus the placebo group. This constitutes an important milestone in the field of cancer immunotherapy. However, because of the individual patient-specific nature and the high cost of this treatment ($93,000 for three infusions), it is very challenging to implement this treatment in the large eligible patient population. Direct *in vivo* targeting and activation of DC with broadly injectable immunogens for cancer treatment are desirable. Moreover, the clinical efficacy of cancer vaccines remains to be improved. To achieve this purpose, the most appropriate tumor antigens and/or immune targets for immunotherapy of distinct cancer types need to be identified.

4. TUMOR ANTIGENS RECOGNIZED BY TUMOR-REACTIVE T CELLS

4.1. Tumor antigens recognized by CD8$^+$ T cells

In 1991, the first human tumor antigen was identified by screening cDNA expression library with tumor-reactive CD8$^+$ T cells (Van der Bruggen *et al.*, 1991). Since then, many tumor antigens have been identified using T cells with antitumor activity (Table 6.1). These tumor antigens can be classified into several types: (1) tissue-specific tumor antigens with higher expression in cancer cells compared with normal cells; (2) tumor-specific and shared antigens that are expressed in cancer and testis, but not in other normal tissues; (3) tumor-specific and unique antigens. Some of them, including gp100, MAGE-3, and NY-ESO-1, have been testing in phase II/III clinical trials with encouraging results. It should be noted that chronic infection or chronic inflammation has caused about 20% of human cancers (Coussens and Werb, 2002; De Marzo *et al.*, 2007). Epstein–Barr virus (EBV), a human gamma herpesvirus with tropism for B cells, has been implicated in the pathogenesis of a variety of human tumors, including immunoblastic lymphoma, Burkitt lymphoma, nasopharyngeal carcinoma, and Hodgkin disease (Leen *et al.*, 2007; Young and Rickinson, 2004). Infection with oncogenic human papilloma virus (HPV) is causally linked to the development of cervical cancer (Melief and van der Burg, 2008). Hepatitis B virus (HBV) and HCV infection of liver cells is a primary factor in the development of liver cancer (Coussens and Werb, 2002; Karin *et al.*, 2006; Peto, 2001). Viral antigens derived from EBV, HPV, and HBV are not the subject of this review but have been extensively used to develop prophylactic and therapeutic vaccines against viral infection and cancer (Huang *et al.*, 2011; Kwak *et al.*, 2011; Long *et al.*, 2011; van der Burg and Melief, 2011).

TABLE 6.1 Tumor antigens recognized by $CD8^+$ T cells

Antigens	MHC class I restrictions	Peptide epitopes	References
Tissue-specific antigens			
gp100	A2	KTWGQYWQV	Bakker *et al.* (1994)
	A2	AMLGTHTMEV	Tsai *et al.* (1997)
	A2	MLGTHTMEV	Tsai *et al.* (1997)
	A2	SLADTNSLAV	Tsai *et al.* (1997)
	A2	ITDQVPFSV	Kawakami *et al.* (1995)
	A2	LLDGTATLRL	Kawakami *et al.* (1994a)
	A2	YLEPGPVTA	Cox *et al.* (1994)
	A2	VLYRYGSFSV	Kawakami *et al.* (1995)
	A2	RLMKQDFSV	Kawakami *et al.* (1998)
	A2	RLPRIFCSC	Kawakami *et al.* (1998)
	A3	LIYRRRLMK	Kawakami *et al.* (1998)
	A3	ALNFPGSQK	Kawashima *et al.* (1998)
	A3	SLIYRRRLMK	Kawashima *et al.* (1998)
	A3	ALLAVGATK	Skipper *et al.* (1996)
	A24	VYFFLPDHL	Robbins *et al.* (1997)
	A*6801	HTMEVTVYHR	Sensi *et al.* (2002)
	B*3501	VPLDCVLYRY	Benlalam *et al.* (2003)
	Cw8	SNDGPTLI	Castelli *et al.* (1999)
MART-1/ Melan-A	A2	AAGIGILTV	Coulie *et al.* (1994), Kawakami *et al.* (1994b)
	A2	ILTVILGVL	Castelli *et al.* (1995)
	A2	EAAGIGILTV	Schneider *et al.* (1998)
	B45	AEEAAGIGIL	Schneider *et al.* (1998)
gp75/TRP-1	A31	MSLQRQFLR	Wang *et al.* (1996b)
TRP-2	A2	SVYDFFVWL	Parkhurst *et al.* (1998)
	A2	TLDSQVMSL	Noppen *et al.* (2000)
	A31	LLGPGRPYR	Wang *et al.* (1996a)
	A33	LLGPGRPYR	Wang *et al.* (1998a)
	A68	EVISCKLIKR	Lupetti *et al.* (1998)
	Cw8	ANDPIFVVL	Castelli *et al.* (1999)
Tyrosinase	A1	KCDICTDEY	Kittlesen *et al.* (1998)
	A1	SSDYVIPIGTY	Kawakami *et al.* (1998)
	A2	YMDGTMSQV	Wolfel *et al.* (1994)
	A2	MLLAVLYCL	Wolfel *et al.* (1994)
	A24	AFLPWHRLF	Kang *et al.* (1995)
	B44	SEIWRDIDF	Brichard *et al.* (1996)
	B*3501	TPRLPSSADVEF	Benlalam *et al.* (2003)

(*continued*)

TABLE 6.1 *(continued)*

Antigens	MHC class I restrictions	Peptide epitopes	References
Tumor-specific shared antigens			
BAGE	Cw16	AARAVFLAL	Boel *et al.* (1995)
CAMEL	A2	MLMAQEALAFL	Aarnoudse *et al.* (1999)
MAGE-A1	A1	EADPTGHSY	Traversari *et al.* (1992)
	A3	SLFRAVITK	Chaux *et al.* (1999a)
	A24	NYKHCFPEI	Fujie *et al.* (1999)
	A28	EVYDGREHSA	Chaux *et al.* (1999a)
	B37	REPVTKAEML	Tanzarella *et al.* (1999)
	B53	DPARYEFLW	Chaux *et al.* (1999a)
	Cw2	SAFPTTINF	Chaux *et al.* (1999a)
	Cw3	SAYGEPRKL	Chaux *et al.* (1999a)
	Cw16	SAYGEPRKL	Van der Bruggen *et al.* (1994b)
MAGE-A2	A2	KMVELVHFL	Visseren *et al.* (1997)
	A2	YLQLVFGIEV	Visseren *et al.* (1997)
	A24	EYLQLVFGI	Tahara *et al.* (1999)
	B37	REPVTKAEML	Tanzarella *et al.* (1999)
MAGE-A3	A1	EADPIGHLY	Gaugler *et al.* (1994)
	A2	FLWGPRALV	Van der Bruggen *et al.* (1994a)
	A24	TFPDLESEF	Oiso *et al.* (1999)
	A24	IMPKAGLLI	Tanaka *et al.* (1997)
	B44	MEVDPIGHLY	Fleischhauer *et al.* (1995), Herman *et al.* (1996)
	B52	WQYFFPVIF	Russo *et al.* (2000)
	B37	REPVTKAEML	Tanzarella *et al.* (1999)
	B*3501	EVDPIGHLY	Benlalam *et al.* (2003)
MAGE-A4	A2	GVYDGREHTV	Duffour *et al.* (1999)
MAGE-A6	A34	MVKISGGPR	Zorn and Hercend (1999)
	B37	REPVTKAEML	Tanzarella *et al.* (1999)
	B*3501	EVDPIGHVY	Benlalam *et al.* (2003)
MAGE-A10	A2	GLYDGMEHL	Huang *et al.* (1999)
MAGE-A12	Cw7	VRIGHLYIL	Heidecker *et al.* (2000), Panelli *et al.* (2000)
NY-ESO-1	A2	SLLMWITQCFL	Jager *et al.* (1998)
	A2	SLLMWITQC	Jager *et al.* (1998)
	A2	QLSLLMWIT	Jager *et al.* (1998)
	A31	ASGPGGGAPR	Wang *et al.* (1998b)
	B*3501	MPFATPMEA	Benlalam *et al.* (2003)

TABLE 6.1 *(continued)*

Antigens	MHC class I restrictions	Peptide epitopes	References
SSX-2	A2	KASEKIFYV	Ayyoub *et al.* (2002)
Tumor-specific unique antigens			
β-Catenin	A24 S	YLDSGIHF	Robbins *et al.* (1996)
Caspase-8	B35	FPSDSWCYF	Mandruzzato *et al.* (1997)
CDK-4	A2	ACDPHSGHFV	Wolfel *et al.* (1995)

4.2. Tumor antigens recognized by CD4$^+$ Th and Treg cells

Given the importance of CD4$^+$ T cells in antitumor immunity, it is critical to identify MHC class II-restricted tumor antigens capable of stimulating CD4$^+$ Th cells. There are several strategies to identify MHC class II antigens recognized by CD4$^+$ T cells: (1) genetic targeting expression (GTE) system using tumor-reactive human T cells isolated from patients with cancer or other immune-related diseases, (2) use of HLA-DR transgenic (Tg) mice for identification of MHC class II-restricted antigens *in vivo*, (3) peptide stimulation *in vitro* using candidate antigens overexpressed in cancer cells. Many tumor antigens capable of stimulating CD4$^+$ T cells have been identified (Table 6.2).

4.2.1. GTE system

We have developed GTE system for identification of antigens recognized by CD4$^+$ T cells (Wang and Rosenberg, 1999; Wang *et al.*, 1999a,b). The GTE system comprises two essential components: (A) generation of a highly transfectable HEK293IMDR cell line and (B) the creation of an Ii fusion library from tumor cells such that the Ii fusion proteins are targeted to the endosomal/lysosomal compartment for efficient antigen processing and presentation for T-cell recognition (Wang and Rosenberg, 1999; Wang *et al.*, 1999b). Using this system, many tumor antigens have successfully been identified. For example, we identified a mutated fibronectin as a tumor antigen recognized by HLA-DR2-restricted CD4$^+$ T cells. A mutation in this gene results in the substitution of lysine for glutamic acid and gives rise to a new T-cell epitope recognized by CD4$^+$ T cells (Wang *et al.*, 2002b). Analysis of cytokine profiles and suppressive activity of these T cells reveal that they are CD4$^+$ Th1 cells, secreting IFN-γ and IL-2, but no suppressive function. Because elevated percentage of CD4$^+$ Treg cells are present in tumor tissues, we have recently generated many such tumor/antigen-specific CD4$^+$ Treg cell clones from TILs in surgically removed tumor samples. Using the same strategy for Th1 cells, we identified LAGE1 and ARTC1 as antigenic ligands for CD4$^+$ Treg

TABLE 6.2 MHC class II-restricted melanoma antigens recognized by $CD4^+$ T cells

Tumor antigens	HLA restrictions	Peptides	References
Mutated/fusion antigens			
TPI	HLA-DR1	GELIG**I**LNAAKVPAD	Wang *et al.* (1999a), Pieper *et al.* (1999)
LDFP	HLA-DR1	PVIWRRAPA	Wang *et al.* (1999b)
	HLA-DR1	WRRAPAPGA	Wang *et al.* (1999b)
CDC27	HLA-DR4	FSWAMDLDPKGA	Wang *et al.* (1999a)
	Fibronectin	HLA-DR2	
		PSVGQQMIFE**K**HGFR RTTPP	Wang *et al.* (2002b)
Neo-PAP	HLA-DR7	RVIKNSIRLTL	Topalian *et al.* (2002)
ARTC1	HLA-DR1	YSVYFNLPADTIYTN	Wang *et al.* (2005)
Nonmutated antigens			
Tyrosinase	HLA-DR4	QNILLSNAPLGPQFP	Topalian *et al.* (1996)
	HLA-DR4	SYLQDSDPDSFQD	Topalian *et al.* (1996)
	HLA-DR15	FLLHHAFVDSIFEQWL QRHRP	Kobayashi *et al.* (1998)
gp100	HLA-DR4	WNRQ**LYPEWTEAQ**RLD	Touloukian *et al.* (2000)
	HLA-DR7	GPT**LIGANASFS**IALN	Kobayashi *et al.* (2001a)
	HLA-DR7/ DR53	TGRA**MLGTHTMEV**TVYH	Lapointe *et al.* (2001), Kobayashi *et al.* (2001a)
	HLA-DR7	SLAV**VSTQLIMPG**QE	Kobayashi *et al.* (2001a)
MART-1	HLA-DR4	RNGYRALMDKSLHVGT QCALTRR	Zarour *et al.* (2000)
MAGE-A1	HLA-DR13	LLKYRAREPVTKAE	Chaux *et al.* (1999a)
MAGE-A2	HAL-DR1	LLKYRAREPVTKAE	Chaux *et al.* (1999a)
MAGE-3	HLA-DR11	TSYVKVLHHMVKISG	Manici *et al.* (1999)
	HLA-DR13	AELVHFLLLKYRAR	Chaux *et al.* (1999b)
	HLA-DR13	FLLLKYRAREPVTKAE	Chaux *et al.* (1999b)
	HLA-DP4	TQHFVQENYLEY	Schultz *et al.* (2000)
	HLA-DR1, 4, 7, 11	FFPVIFSKASSSLQL	Kobayashi *et al.* (2001b)
	HLA-DR1, 4, 11	RKVAELVHFLLLKYR	Consogno *et al.* (2003)
MAGE-A6	HLA-DR13	LLKYRAREPVTKAE	Chaux *et al.* (1999a)
LAGE1	HLA-DR13	RL**LQLHITMPF**SS	Wang *et al.* (2004)
CAMEL	HLA-DR11/12	PWKRSWSA	Slager *et al.* (2003)
NY-ESO-1	HLA-DR4	LPVPGV**LLKEFTVSG**NILTI	Zeng *et al.* (2000)
	HLA-DP4	**WITQCFLPV**FLAQP PSGQRR	Zeng *et al.* (2001)
hTRT	HLA-DR7	RPGLLGASVLGLDDI	Schroers *et al.* (2002)
Eph	HLA-DR11	DVTFNIACKKCG	Chiari *et al.* (2000)

Note: Amino acid sequence in bold stands for mutated or core sequence for recognition.

cells, providing direct evidence that antigen-specific $CD4^+$ Treg cells are present at tumor sites and mediate antigen-specific and local immune suppression of antitumor immunity (Wang *et al.*, 2004, 2005).

4.2.2. Use of HLA-DR Tg mice and *in vitro* peptide stimulation

MHC class II-restricted epitopes can be identified by using HLA-DR Tg mice in combination peptide stimulation *in vitro*. HLA-DR4 Tg mice were used to identify $CD4^+$ T-cell epitopes from candidate antigens (Touloukian *et al.*, 2000; Zeng *et al.*, 2000). HLA-DR Tg mice might have advantages for identifying putative peptides, as they should have a high precursor frequency of antigen-specific T cells after immunization. Once candidate peptides are known, one can generate antigen-specific $CD4^+$ T cells from human PBMCs stimulated with synthetic candidate peptides. Therefore, the combined use of immunization of DR Tg mice with the intact protein antigens and stimulated with the peptides predicted by a computer-assisted algorithm may avoid the need to stimulate human PBMCs with a large number of peptides. NY-ESO-1 is a potent immunogen recognized by both antibody and T cells (Chen *et al.*, 1997; Jager *et al.*, 1998; Wang *et al.*, 1998b). Of particular interest is that 10–13% of patients with advanced cancer developed a high titer of antibody (Stockert *et al.*, 1998; Zeng *et al.*, 2000). We identified a T-cell epitope presented by HLA-DP4, a predominant allele expressed in 40–70% of the population (Zeng *et al.*, 2001). Identification of DP4-restricted T-cell peptides from MAGE-3 and NY-ESO-1 could be of great benefit for more than 50% of patients with cancer. These studies suggest that, unlike LAGE-1, NY-ESO-1 may preferentially activate $CD4^+$ Th cells. However, a recent study shows that NY-ESO-1 can also induce Treg cells (Vence *et al.*, 2007). Interestingly, several MHC class II peptides recognized by $CD4^+$ T cells have been identified from EBNA1 as well as other viral antigens (Bickham *et al.*, 2001; Leen *et al.*, 2001; Munz *et al.*, 2000; Paludan and Munz, 2003; Voo *et al.*, 2002). T-cell peptides derived from EBV viral antigens are capable of stimulating $CD4^+$ Th1 and Treg cells (Marshall *et al.*, 2003; Voo *et al.*, 2005). It appears that the same T-cell epitope from EBNA1 can stimulate both Th1 and Treg cells (Voo *et al.*, 2005). Thus, it is likely that both tumor and viral antigens can activate effector and Treg cells, depending on particular epitope affinity and cytokine milieu. Although IL-17-producing T (Th17) cells are present in many human cancer tissues, very little is known about their antigen specificity. In particular, the role of Th17 cells in cancer immunity and tumor progression is not clear and requires further study.

5. CURRENT PROGRESSES OF SYNTHETIC PEPTIDE VACCINES

Identification of these MHC class I-restricted antigens has set the stage for developing peptide-based cancer vaccines, although some evidence for a therapeutic effect on tumor growth inhibition and regression was observed in patients who received peptide vaccines (Marchand *et al.*, 1999; Rosenberg *et al.*, 1998). However, objective complete clinical responses were sporadic, even though CTL reactivity was clearly evident after one round of stimulation *in vitro* of PBMC from the majority of vaccinated patients (Rosenberg *et al.*, 2004). Analysis of the infiltrating lymphocytes in skin and tumor biopsies using T-cell-specific peptide–major histocompatibility complex tetramers showed generation of antigen-specific $CD8^+$ T cells (Yee *et al.*, 2000). Recently, a multicenter phase II clinical trial of melanoma patients with gp100 peptide with or without IL-2 shows that the gp100 peptide vaccine plus IL-2-treated group had a significant improvement in overall clinical response compared with the IL-2-only group (16% vs. 6%) as well as longer progression-free survival (Schwartzentruber *et al.*, 2011). The median overall survival was also improved in the gp100 peptide vaccine plus IL-2 group compared to the IL-2-only group (17.8 vs. 11.1 months). Similarly, MAGE-3 peptide/protein vaccines are ongoing in phase III clinical trials (Bilusic and Madan, 2011; Cecco *et al.*, 2011). The clinical efficacy of peptide vaccines may be further improved by the use of DCs loaded with cancer peptides or by the use of synthetic long peptides harboring both CD4 and CD8 T-cell epitopes (Melief and van der Burg, 2008; Chapters 3 and 4). A major challenge in cancer vaccine development is how to generate strong and long-lasting antitumor immunity through optimal delivery of well-chosen tumor-associated antigens.

6. ENHANCING ANTITUMOR IMMUNITY BY INTRACELLULAR DELIVERY OF PEPTIDES INTO DCs

Although mature DCs are more potent than immature DCs in priming and eliciting T-cell responses (Apetoh *et al.*, 2011; Delamarre and Mellman, 2011; Tacken and Figdor, 2011), they lose the ability to efficiently take up exogenous antigens, particularly for MHC class II-restricted antigens (Banchereau and Steinman, 1998). As a result, peptide-pulsed DCs as vaccines have several limitations. For example, peptide degradation, rapid MHC class I turnover, and the disassociation of peptide from MHC class I molecules during the preparation and injection of DC/peptides may result in short half-lives of MHC class I/peptide complexes on the DC surface, leading to weak T-cell responses. We developed a novel strategy to overcome these problems by the use of cell-penetrating peptides (CPPs) for intracellular delivery of cancer peptides into DCs (Wang and Wang, 2002; Wang *et al.*, 2002a). Intracellular delivery of peptides into DCs could allow DCs to continuously process and present the internalized peptides to T cells for an extended period of time. Several potent CPPs have been identified from proteins, including the Tat protein of human immunodeficiency virus, the VP22 protein of herpes simplex virus, and fibroblast growth factor (Berry, 2008; Deshayes *et al.*, 2005; Edenhofer, 2008; Gupta *et al.*, 2005; Torchilin, 2006), although some long synthetic peptides can also penetrate selectively into DCs (Melief and van der Burg, 2008). Among them, the 11-mer TAT peptide (YGRKKRRQRRR) and other CPPs have been well studied for the transduction of biologically active proteins into cells both *in vitro* and *in vivo* (Gupta *et al.*, 2005). We found that both CPP1-TRP2 or TAT-TRP2 peptides can translocate intracellularly into mature DCs and prolong DCs to process the internalized peptides and to present MHC–peptide complexes to antigen-specific T cells (Wang and Wang, 2002; Wang *et al.*, 2002a). Immunization of mice with DCs transduced with CPP1-TRP-2 or TAT-TRP2 resulted in complete protection against B16 tumor as well as significant inhibition of the preestablished B16 tumor (Wang and Wang, 2002; Wang *et al.*, 2002a). Although both DC/TRP2 and DC/TAT-TRP2 immunization increased the number of TRP2-specific $CD8^+$ T cells detected by K^b/TRP2 tetramers, T-cell activity elicited by DC/TAT-TRP2 was 3- to 10-fold higher than that induced by DC/TRP2 (Wang *et al.*, 2002a). Consistent with previous studies showing that $CD4^+$ T cells are required for an antitumor effect, our studies show a similar requirement for DC/TAT-TRP-2-induced antitumor immunity, suggesting that both CPP1- and TAT-mediated antigen delivery of a self-peptide may have general applications for enhancing T-cell-based cancer therapy, and $CD4^+$ T-cell response is required for generating optimal antitumor immunity. More recently, we initiated a phase I clinical trial for prostate cancer using TAT-NY-ESO-1 peptides. Clinical studies show that TAT-NY-ESO-1 peptide vaccines are safe and induced antigen-specific T-cell responses (R.-F.W. Guru Sonpavde and Teresa G. Hayes, unpublished data).

7. ENHANCING IMMUNE RESPONSES AND BLOCKING IMMUNE SUPPRESSION BY STIMULATION OF INNATE IMMUNE RECEPTORS

7.1. Innate immune receptors and signaling

Toll-like receptors (TLRs), NOD-like receptors (NLRs), RIG-I-like receptors (RLRs), and AIM-2-like receptors have emerged as innate pattern recognition receptors (PRRs) that can detect a variety of invading pathogens and intracellular ligands, thus serving as a first line of defense against infectious pathogens and cancer. These germline-encoded PRRs are expressed in DCs and other immune cells, and can recognize structure-conserved molecules, such as pathogen-associated molecular patterns (PAMPs) and damage-associated molecular patterns (DAMPs). Recognition of PAMPs or DAMPs by PRRs triggers the activation of several key signaling pathways, including NF-κB, type I IFN, and inflammasome, leading to the production of inflammatory cytokines, which, in turn, promote DC maturation programs for the induction of adaptive immune responses (Iwasaki and Medzhitov, 2004; Takeda and Akira, 2005). TLRs are expressed on the cell surface (TLR1, TLR2, TLR4, and TLR5) or in the endosome (TLR3, TLR7, TLR8, and TLR9). By contrast, several intracellular PRRs such as RIG-I and MDA5 are in the cytoplasm and responsible for the recognition of invading viruses (Akira *et al.*, 2006; Kato *et al.*, 2005; Yoneyama *et al.*, 2004). NLRs represent a large family of protein receptors/regulators harboring an initiating signal domain, such as the caspase recruitment domain (CARD), pyrin domain (PYRIN) or baculovirus inhibitor-of-apoptosis repeat (BIR) domain, a nucleotide-binding oligomerization domain (NOD), and an LRR domain. Activation of such cytoplasmic receptors by invading pathogens including bacteria and viruses activates inflammasome consisting of caspase-1 and ASC and leads to the production of proinflammatory cytokines such as IL-1b and IL-18. Thus, TLRs, NLRs, and RLRs are critical in bridging innate and adaptive immune responses by activating several key signaling pathways and in producing many important cytokines as mediators. Thus, they represent a potent means of modulating immune responses in cancer immunotherapy. Both natural and synthetic ligands for TLRs and RLRs have been identified and characterized for their recognition, but only a limited number of ligands have been identified for NLRs. These ligands of PRRs, in particular TLRs, have been used as potent vaccine adjuvants to enhance immune responses. The most significant development of cancer vaccine studies is to include various TLR agonists to vaccine formulations, including TLR-3 (poly I:C), TLR-4 (monophosphoryl lipid A; MPL), TLR-5 (flagellin), TLR-7 (imiquimod), and TLR-9 (CpG) (Duthie *et al.*, 2011). The types of signaling and cytokines by immune cells after TLR stimulation control $CD4^+$ T-cell differentiation into Th1, Th2, Th17, and Treg cells. However, stimulation of immune cells such as DCs and T cells by most TLR-based adjuvants produces proinflammatory cytokines and promotes Th1 and $CD8^+$ T responses (Manicassamy and Pulendran, 2009).

7.2. Blocking negative regulators of innate immune signaling

Although innate immune responses are critically important as sensors to induce adaptive immunity, tight regulation of innate signaling pathways is essential for both innate and adaptive immunities; otherwise, aberrant immune responses may occur, leading to severe or even fatal consequences. Similarly, DC maturation and activation are controlled by both positive and negative regulators, thus leading to immunity or tolerance induction. To generate potent antitumor immunity, we need to block negative regulators in immune cells such as DCs and T cells. For example,

A20-silenced DCs produce potent antitumor immunity (Song *et al.*, 2008). We recently identified several negative regulators (NLRC5 and NLRX1) that inhibit NF-κB and type I IFN signaling (Cui *et al.*, 2010; Xia *et al.*, 2011). Similarly, several key negative regulators such as CTLA-4 and programmed cell death 1 (PD-1) play a critical role in the inhibition of T-cell activation. Blockade of CTLA-4 and/or PD-1 results in T-cell activation and enhances nonspecific immune responses (Chambers *et al.*, 2001; Zhu *et al.*, 2011). These antibody-based immunotherapies are currently under active clinical trials (Callahan *et al.*, 2010), and anti-CTLA-4 antibody therapy has been approved by US FDA for the treatment of metastatic melanoma (Hodi *et al.*, 2010).

7.3. Overcoming Treg cell-mediated immune suppression by TLR signaling

As Treg cells have accumulated in the tumor microenvironment, it is necessary to develop novel strategies to overcome this type of immune suppression; otherwise, the immune response induced by cancer vaccines will be weak and transient. To block immune suppression mediated by Treg cells, we found that TLR8 ligands (ssRNA40 and Poly-G10 oligonucleotides) can directly reverse the suppressive function of human (but not murine) Treg cells in the absence of DCs. Using RNA interference technology, we identified the TLR8–MyD88 signaling pathway that is required for the reversal of Treg cell function by Poly-G oligonucleotides (Peng *et al.*, 2005). More importantly, we demonstrated that the suppressive function of $CD8^+$ Treg cells and γδ-TCR Treg cells can also be reversed after Poly-G oligonucleotide treatment (Kiniwa *et al.*, 2007; Peng *et al.*, 2007), suggesting that these cells share a common TLR8 signaling-mediated mechanism. Recent studies show that TLR2 ligands can reverse the suppressive function of human Treg cells (Nyirenda *et al.*, 2011; Oberg *et al.*, 2010). However, murine TLR2-deficient mice reduce the number of $CD4^+$ $CD25^+$ Treg cells (Netea *et al.*, 2004). Activation of TLR2 with its ligand (Pam3Cys) directly increases the proliferation of murine Treg cells and transiently reverses their suppressive function (Liu *et al.*, 2006; Sutmuller *et al.*, 2006). However, engagement of TLR2 with polysaccharide A of *Bacteroides fragilis* enhances the suppressive function of Treg cells (Round *et al.*, 2011). These studies demonstrated that TLR signaling is critically important in modulating immune responses.

8. CONCLUSIONS

In the past 30 years, significant progress has been made in the field of cancer immunotherapy. While clinical validation and development has been slow, recent approval of two immunotherapy drugs (sipuleucel-T and anti-CTLA-4 antibody) has boosted the development of immunotherapy as important and promising treatment of patients with cancer. As ACT is the most powerful treatment of cancer with up to 72% objective clinical response rate, it is important to move forward with phase III clinical trials with tumor-specific T cells and CIK effector cells. Like APC-based therapy, the limitation of ACT is individualized medicine, and it is very challenging to broaden its application with retroviruses or lentiviruses expressing antigen-specific TCR. For these reasons, development of peptide/protein cancer vaccines has great potential. With encouraging results from recent multicenter clinical trials with gp100 and MAGE-A3, many therapeutic companies will step in the field and develop therapeutic peptide cancer vaccines for many types of cancer. The key issues will be how to further improve immune responses and clinical efficacy of peptide cancer vaccines. To achieve this goal, (1) we need to develop *in vivo* targeted delivery of peptides into APCs such as DCs with CPPs-linked cancer peptides (long peptide)/proteins, or nanoparticles; (2) we need to overcome immune suppression mediated by Treg cells and other immune cells; (3) importantly, peptide vaccines should be combined with strategies that block negative regulators or immune suppression to achieve maximal antitumor immunity and clinical responses. However, because immune responses measured in the blood do not necessarily correlate with clinical efficacy or survival, it is important to probe the reasons for these clinical observations. Because pretreatment of patients with chemodepleting regimens improves the clinical benefit of ACT, it is reasonable to believe that combined use of immunotherapy with chemotherapy can enhance immune responses and clinical outcomes. Recent advances and rapid progress in the field of cancer immunotherapy represent an unprecedented opportunity for the development of therapeutic cancer vaccines in the next few years.

ACKNOWLEDGMENTS

This work was supported in part by grants from National Cancer Institute, National Institutes of Health, and Cancer Research Institute.

REFERENCES

Aarnoudse, C. A., van den Doel, P. B., Heemskerk, B., and Schrier, P. I. (1999). Interleukin-2-induced, melanoma-specific T cells recognize CAMEL, an unexpected translation product of LAGE-1. *Int. J. Cancer* **82,** 442–448.

Akira, S., Uematsu, S., and Takeuchi, O. (2006). Pathogen recognition and innate immunity. *Cell* **124,** 783–801.

Apetoh, L., Locher, C., Ghiringhelli, F., Kroemer, G., and Zitvogel, L. (2011). Harnessing dendritic cells in cancer. *Semin. Immunol.* **23,** 42–49.

Ayyoub, M., Stevanovic, S., Sahin, U., Guillaume, P., Servis, C., Rimoldi, D., Valmori, D., Romero, P., Cerottini, J. C., Rammensee, H. G., *et al.* (2002). Proteasome-assisted identification of a SSX-2-derived epitope recognized by tumor-reactive CTL infiltrating metastatic melanoma. *J. Immunol.* **168,** 1717–1722.

Bakker, A. B. H., Schreurs, M. W. J., de Boer, A. J., Kawakami, Y., Rosenberg, S. A., Adema, G. J., and Figdor, C. G. (1994). Melanocyte lineage-specific antigen gp100 is recognized by melanocyte-derived tumor-infiltrating lymphocytes. *J. Exp. Med.* **179,** 1005–1009.

Banchereau, J., and Steinman, R. M. (1998). Dendritic cells and the control of immunity. *Nature* **392,** 245–252.

Benlalam, H., Linard, B., Guilloux, Y., Moreau-Aubry, A., Derre, L., Diez, E., Dreno, B., Jotereau, F., and Labarriere, N. (2003). Identification of five new HLA-B*3501-restricted epitopes derived from common melanoma-associated antigens, spontaneously recognized by tumor-infiltrating lymphocytes. *J. Immunol.* **171,** 6283–6289.

Berry, C. C. (2008). Intracellular delivery of nanoparticles via the HIV-1 tat peptide. *Nanomedicine* **3,** 357–365.

Bickham, K., Munz, C., Tsang, M. L., Larsson, M., Fonteneau, J. F., Bhardwaj, N., and Steinman, R. (2001). EBNA1-specific CD4+ T cells in healthy carriers of Epstein-Barr virus are primarily Th1 in function. *J. Clin. Invest.* **107,** 121–130.

Bilusic, M., and Madan, R. A. (2011). Therapeutic cancer vaccines: The latest advancement in targeted therapy. *Am. J. Ther.* In Press (Epublication Feb. 2011).

Boel, P., Wildmann, C., Sensi, M. L., Brasseur, R., Renauld, J. C., Coulie, P., Boon, T., and Van der Bruggen, P. (1995). BAGE: A new gene encoding an antigen recognized on human melanomas by cytolytic T lymphocytes. *Immunity* **2,** 167–175.

Boon, T., Cerottini, J.-C., Van Den Eynde, B., Van der Bruggen, P., and Van Pel, A. (1994). Tumor antigens recognized by T lymphocytes. *Annu. Rev. Immunol.* **12,** 337–365.

Brichard, V. G., Herman, J., Van Pel, A., Wildmann, C., Gaugler, B., Wolfel, T., Boon, T., and Lethe, B. (1996). A tyrosinase nonpeptide presented by HLA-B44 is recognized on a human melanoma by autologous cytolytic T lymphocytes. *Eur. J. Immunol.* **26,** 224–230.

Callahan, M. K., Wolchok, J. D., and Allison, J. P. (2010). Anti-CTLA-4 antibody therapy: Immune monitoring during clinical development of a novel immunotherapy. *Semin. Oncol.* **37,** 473–484.

Castelli, C., Storkus, W. J., Maeurer, M. J., Martin, D. M., Huang, E. C., Pramanik, B. N., Nagabhushan, T. L., Parmiani, G., and Lotze, M. T. (1995). Mass spectrometric identification of a naturally processed melanoma peptide recognized by CD8+ cytotoxic T lymphocytes. *J. Exp. Med.* **181,** 363–368.

Castelli, C., Tarsini, P., Mazzocchi, A., Rini, F., Rivoltini, L., Ravagnani, F., Gallino, F., Belli, F., and Parmiani, G. (1999). Novel HLA-Cw8-restricted T cell epitopes derived from tyrosinase-related protein-2 and gp100 melanoma antigens. *J. Immunol.* **162,** 1739–1748.

Cecco, S., Muraro, E., Giacomin, E., Martorelli, D., Lazzarini, R., Baldo, P., and Dolcetti, R. (2011). Cancer vaccines in phase II/III clinical trials: State of the art and future perspectives. *Curr. Cancer Drug Targets* **11,** 85–102.

Chambers, C. A., Kuhns, M. S., Egen, J. G., and Allison, J. P. (2001). CTLA-4-mediated inhibition in regulation of T cell responses: Mechanisms and manipulation in tumor immunotherapy. *Annu. Rev. Immunol.* **19,** 565–594.

Chaux, P., Luiten, R., Demotte, N., Vantomme, V., Stroobant, V., Traversari, C., Russo, V., Schultz, E., Cornelis, G. R., Boon, T., *et al.* (1999a). Identification of five MAGE-A1 epitopes recognized by cytolytic T lymphocytes obtained by in vitro stimulation with dendritic cells transduced with MAGE-A1. *J. Immunol.* **163,** 2928–2936.

Chaux, P., Vantomme, V., Stroobant, V., Thielemans, K., Corthals, J., Luiten, R., Eggermont, A. M., Boon, T., and van der Bruggen, P. (1999b). Identification of MAGE-3 epitopes presented by HLA-DR molecules to CD4(+) T lymphocytes. *J. Exp. Med.* **189,** 767–778.

Chen, Y. T., Scanlan, M. J., Sahin, U., Tureci, O., Gure, A. O., Tsang, S., Williamson, B., Stockert, E., Pfreundschuh, M., and Old, L. J. (1997). A testicular antigen aberrantly expressed in human cancers detected by autologous antibody screening. *Proc. Natl. Acad. Sci. USA* **94,** 1914–1918.

Chiari, R., Hames, G., Stroobant, V., Texier, C., Maillere, B., Boon, T., and Coulie, P. G. (2000). Identification of a tumor-specific shared antigen derived from an Eph receptor and presented to CD4 T cells on HLA class II molecules. *Cancer Res.* **60,** 4855–4863.

Consogno, G., Manici, S., Facchinetti, V., Bachi, A., Hammer, J., Conti-Fine, B. M., Rugarli, C., Traversari, C., and Protti, M. P. (2003). Identification of immunodominant regions among promiscuous HLA-DR-restricted CD4+ T-cell epitopes on the tumor antigen MAGE-3. *Blood* **101,** 1038–1044.

Coulie, P. G., Brichard, V., Van Pel, A., Wolfel, T., Schneider, J., Traversari, C., Mattei, S., De Plaen, E. D., Lurquin, C., Szikora, J.-P., *et al.* (1994). A new gene coding for a differentiation antigen recognized by autologous cytolytic T lymphocytes on HLA-A2 melanomas. *J. Exp. Med.* **180,** 35–42.

Coussens, L. M., and Werb, Z. (2002). Inflammation and cancer. *Nature* **420,** 860–867.

Cox, A. L., Skipper, J., Cehn, Y., Henderson, R. A., Darrow, T. L., Shabanowitz, J., Engelhard, V. H., Hunt, D. F., and Slingluff, C. L. (1994). Identification of a peptide recognized by five melanoma-specific human cytotoxic T cell lines. *Science* **264,** 716–719.

Cui, J., Zhu, L., Xia, X., Wang, H. Y., Legras, X., Hong, J., Ji, J., Shen, P., Zheng, S., Chen, Z. J., *et al.* (2010). NLRC5 negatively regulates the NF-kappaB and type I interferon signaling pathways. *Cell* **141,** 483–496.

De Marzo, A. M., Platz, E. A., Sutcliffe, S., Xu, J., Gronberg, H., Drake, C. G., Nakai, Y., Isaacs, W. B., and Nelson, W. G. (2007). Inflammation in prostate carcinogenesis. *Nat. Rev. Cancer* **7,** 256–269.

Delamarre, L., and Mellman, I. (2011). Harnessing dendritic cells for immunotherapy. *Semin. Immunol.* **23,** 2–11.

Deshayes, S., Morris, M. C., Divita, G., and Heitz, F. (2005). Cell-penetrating peptides: Tools for intracellular delivery of therapeutics. *Cell. Mol. Life Sci.* **62,** 1839–1849.

Diefenbach, A., and Raulet, D. H. (2001). Strategies for target cell recognition by natural killer cells. *Immunol. Rev.* **181,** 170–184.

Dudley, M. E., Wunderlich, J. R., Robbins, P. F., Yang, J. C., Hwu, P., Schwartzentruber, D. J., Topalian, S. L., Sherry, R., Restifo, N. P., Hubicki, A. M., *et al.* (2002). Cancer regression and autoimmunity in patients after clonal repopulation with antitumor lymphocytes. *Science* **19,** 19.

Duffour, M. T., Chaux, P., Lurquin, C., Cornelis, G., Boon, T., and van der Bruggen, P. (1999). A MAGE-A4 peptide presented by HLA-A2 is recognized by cytolytic T lymphocytes. *Eur. J. Immunol.* **29,** 3329–3337.

Duthie, M. S., Windish, H. P., Fox, C. B., and Reed, S. G. (2011). Use of defined TLR ligands as adjuvants within human vaccines. *Immunol. Rev.* **239,** 178–196.

Edenhofer, F. (2008). Protein transduction revisited: Novel insights into the mechanism underlying intracellular delivery of proteins. *Curr. Pharm. Des.* **14,** 3628–3636.

Fleischhauer, K., Avila, D., Vilbois, F., Traversari, C., Bordignon, C., and Wallny, H. J. (1995). Characterization of natural peptide ligands for HLA-B*4402 and -B*4403: Implications for peptide involvement in allorecognition of a single amino acid change in the HLA-B44 heavy chain. *Tissue Antigens* **44,** 311–317.

Fujie, T., Tahara, K., Tanaka, F., Mori, M., Takesako, K., and Akiyoshi, T. (1999). A MAGE-1-encoded HLA-A24-binding synthetic peptide induces specific anti-tumor cytotoxic T lymphocytes. *Int. J. Cancer* **80,** 169–172.

Gaugler, B., Van Den Eynde, B., Van der Bruggen, P., Romero, P., Gaforio, J. J., De Plaen, E., Lethe, B., Brasseur, F., and Boon, T. (1994). Human gene MAGE-3 codes for an antigen recognized on a melanoma by autologous cytolytic T lymphocytes. *J. Exp. Med.* **179,** 921–930.

Greenberg, P. D. (1991). Adoptive T cell therapy of tumors: Mechanisms operative in the recognition and elimination of tumor cells. *Adv. Immunol.* **49,** 281–355.

Grimm, E. A., Mazumder, A., Zhang, H. Z., and Rosenberg, S. A. (1982). Lymphokine-activated killer cell phenomenon. Lysis of natural killer-resistant fresh solid tumor cells by interleukin 2-activated autologous human peripheral blood lymphocytes. *J. Exp. Med.* **155,** 1823–1841.

Gupta, B., Levchenko, T. S., and Torchilin, V. P. (2005). Intracellular delivery of large molecules and small particles by cell-penetrating proteins and peptides. *Adv. Drug Deliv. Rev.* **57,** 637–651.

Heidecker, L., Brasseur, F., Probst-Kepper, M., Gueguen, M., Boon, T., and Van den Eynde, B. J. (2000). Cytolytic T lymphocytes raised against a human bladder carcinoma recognize an antigen encoded by gene MAGE-A12. *J. Immunol.* **164,** 6041–6045.

Herman, J., van der Bruggen, P., Luescher, I. F., Mandruzzato, S., Romero, P., Thonnard, J., Fleischhauer, K., Boon, T., and Coulie, P. G. (1996). A peptide encoded by the human MAGE3 gene and presented by HLA-B44 induces cytolytic T lymphocytes that recognize tumor cells expressing MAGE3. *Immunogenetics* **43,** 377–383.

Hodi, F. S., O'Day, S. J., McDermott, D. F., Weber, R. W., Sosman, J. A., Haanen, J. B., Gonzalez, R., Robert, C., Schadendorf, D., Hassel, J. C., *et al.* (2010). Improved survival with ipilimumab in patients with metastatic melanoma. *N. Engl. J. Med.* **363,** 711–723.

Hontscha, C., Borck, Y., Zhou, H., Messmer, D., and Schmidt-Wolf, I. G. (2011). Clinical trials on CIK cells: First report of the international registry on CIK cells (IRCC). *J. Cancer Res. Clin. Oncol.* **137,** 305–310.

Huang, L. Q., Brasseur, F., Serrano, A., De Plaen, E., van der Bruggen, P., Boon, T., and Van Pel, A. (1999). Cytolytic T lymphocytes recognize an antigen encoded by MAGE-A10 on a human melanoma. *J. Immunol.* **162,** 6849–6854.

Huang, L. M., Lu, C. Y., and Chen, D. S. (2011). Hepatitis B virus infection, its sequelae, and prevention by vaccination. *Curr. Opin. Immunol.* **23,** 237–243.

Hunder, N. N., Wallen, H., Cao, J., Hendricks, D. W., Reilly, J. Z., Rodmyre, R., Jungbluth, A., Gnjatic, S., Thompson, J. A., and Yee, C. (2008). Treatment of metastatic melanoma with autologous CD4+ T cells against NY-ESO-1. *N. Engl. J. Med.* **358,** 2698–2703.

Iwasaki, A., and Medzhitov, R. (2004). Toll-like receptor control of the adaptive immune responses. *Nat. Immunol.* **5,** 987–995.

Jager, E., Chen, Y. T., Drijfhout, J. W., Karbach, J., Ringhoffer, M., Jager, D., Arand, M., Wada, H., Noguchi, Y., Stockert, E., *et al.* (1998). Simultaneous humoral and cellular immune response against cancer-testis antigen NY-ESO-1: Definition of human histocompatibility leukocyte antigen (HLA)-A2-binding peptide epitopes. *J. Exp. Med.* **187,** 265–270.

Jiang, H., Liu, K. Y., Tong, C. R., Jiang, B., and Lu, D. P. (2005). The efficacy of chemotherapy in combination with auto-cytokine-induced killer cells in acute leukemia. *Zhonghua Nei Ke Za Zhi* **44,** 198–201.

Kang, X.-Q., Kawakami, Y., Sakaguchi, K., El-Gamil, M., Wang, R.-F., Yannelli, J. R., Appella, E., Rosenberg, S. A., and Robbins, P. F. (1995). Identification of a tyrosinase epitope reocognized by HLA-A24 restricted tumor-infiltrating lymphocytes. *J. Immunol.* **155,** 1343–1348.

Karin, M., Lawrence, T., and Nizet, V. (2006). Innate immunity gone awry: Linking microbial infections to chronic inflammation and cancer. *Cell* **124,** 823–835.

Kato, H., Sato, S., Yoneyama, M., Yamamoto, M., Uematsu, S., Matsui, K., Tsujimura, T., Takeda, K., Fujita, T., Takeuchi, O., *et al.* (2005). Cell type-specific involvement of RIG-I in antiviral response. *Immunity* **23,** 19–28.

Kawakami, Y., Eliyahu, S., Delgaldo, C. H., Robbins, P. F., Rivoltini, L., Topalian, S. L., Miki, T., and Rosenberg, S. A. (1994a). Cloning of the gene coding for a shared human melanoma antigen recognized by autologous T cells infiltrating into tumor. *Proc. Natl. Acad. Sci. USA* **91,** 3515–3519.

Kawakami, Y., Eliyahu, S., Sakaguchi, K., Robbins, P. F., Rivoltini, L., Yannelli, J. B., Appella, E., and Rosenberg, S. A. (1994b). Identification of the immunodominant peptides of the MART-1 human melanoma antigen recognized by the majority of HLA-A2 restricted tumor infiltrating lymphocytes. *J. Exp. Med.* **180,** 347–352.

Kawakami, Y., Eliyahu, S., Jennings, C., Sakaguchi, K., Kang, X., Southwood, S., Robbins, P. F., Sette, A., Appella, E., and Rosenberg, S. A. (1995). Recognition of multiple epitopes in the human melanoma antigen gp100 by tumor-infiltrating T lymphocytes associated with in vivo tumor regression. *J. Immunol.* **154,** 3961–3968.

Kawakami, Y., Robbins, P. F., Wang, X., Tupesis, J. P., Parkhurst, M. R., Kang, X., Sakaguchi, K., Appella, E., and Rosenberg, S. A. (1998). Identification of new melanoma epitopes on melanosomal proteins recognized by tumor infiltrating T lymphocytes restricted by HLA-A1, - A2, and -A3 alleles. *J. Immunol.* **161,** 6985–6992.

Kawashima, I., Tsai, V., Southwood, S., Takesako, K., Celis, E., and Sette, A. (1998). Identification of gp100-derived, melanoma-specific cytotoxic T- lymphocyte epitopes restricted by HLA-A3 supertype molecules by primary in vitro immunization with peptide-pulsed dendritic cells. *Int. J. Cancer* **78,** 518–524.

Kiniwa, Y., Miyahara, Y., Wang, H. Y., Peng, W., Peng, G., Wheeler, T. M., Thompson, T., Old, L. J., and Wang, R. F. (2007). CD8+ Foxp3+ regulatory T cells mediate immunosuppression in prostate cancer. *Clin. Cancer Res.* **13,** 6947–6958.

Kittlesen, D. J., Thompson, L. W., Gulden, P. H., Skipper, J. C., Colella, T. A., Shabanowitz, J., Hunt, D. F., Engelhard, V. H., Slingluff, C. L., Jr., and Shabanowitz, J. A. (1998). Human melanoma patients recognize an HLA-A1-restricted CTL epitope from tyrosinase containing two cysteine residues: Implications for tumor vaccine development. *J. Immunol.* **160,** 2099–2106.

Kobayashi, H., Kokubo, T., Takahashi, M., Sato, K., Miyokawa, N., Kimura, S., Kinouchi, R., and Katagiri, M. (1998). Tyrosinase epitope recognized by an HLA-DR-restricted T-cell line from a Vogt-Koyanagi-Harada disease patient. *Immunogenetics* **47,** 398–403.

Kobayashi, H., Lu, J., and Celis, E. (2001a). Identification of helper T-cell epitopes that encompass or lie proximal to cytotoxic T-cell epitopes in the gp100 melanoma tumor antigen. *Cancer Res.* **61,** 7577–7584.

Kobayashi, H., Song, Y., Hoon, D. S., Appella, E., and Celis, E. (2001b). Tumor-reactive T helper lymphocytes recognize a promiscuous MAGE-A3 epitope presented by various major histocompatibility complex class II alleles. *Cancer Res.* **61,** 4773–4778.

Kwak, K., Yemelyanova, A., and Roden, R. B. (2011). Prevention of cancer by prophylactic human papillomavirus vaccines. *Curr. Opin. Immunol.* **23,** 244–251.

Lapointe, R., Royal, R. E., Reeves, M. E., Altomare, I., Robbins, P. F., and Hwu, P. (2001). Retrovirally transduced human dendritic cells can generate T cells recognizing multiple MHC class I and class II epitopes from the melanoma antigen glycoprotein 100. *J. Immunol.* **167,** 4758–4764.

Leen, A., Meij, P., Redchenko, I., Middeldorp, J., Bloemena, E., Rickinson, A., and Blake, N. (2001). Differential immunogenicity of Epstein-Barr virus latent-cycle proteins for human CD4(+) T-helper 1 responses. *J. Virol.* **75,** 8649–8659.

Leen, A. M., Myers, G. D., Sili, U., Huls, M. H., Weiss, H., Leung, K. S., Carrum, G., Krance, R. A., Chang, C. C., Molldrem, J. J., *et al.* (2006). Monoculture-derived T lymphocytes specific for multiple viruses expand and produce clinically relevant effects in immunocompromised individuals. *Nat. Med.* **12,** 1160–1166.

Leen, A. M., Rooney, C. M., and Foster, A. E. (2007). Improving T cell therapy for cancer. *Annu. Rev. Immunol.* **25,** 243–265.

Lesterhuis, W. J., Haanen, J. B., and Punt, C. J. (2011). Cancer immunotherapy—Revisited. *Nat. Rev. Drug Discov.* **10,** 591–600.

Linn, Y. C., Lau, L. C., and Hui, K. M. (2002). Generation of cytokine-induced killer cells from leukaemic samples with in vitro cytotoxicity against autologous and allogeneic leukaemic blasts. *Br. J. Haematol.* **116,** 78–86.

Liu, H., Komai-Koma, M., Xu, D., and Liew, F. Y. (2006). Toll-like receptor 2 signaling modulates the functions of CD4+CD25+ regulatory T cells. *Proc. Natl. Acad. Sci. USA* **103,** 7048–7053.

Long, H. M., Taylor, G. S., and Rickinson, A. B. (2011). Immune defence against EBV and EBV-associated disease. *Curr. Opin. Immunol.* **23,** 258–264.

Lupetti, R., Pisarra, P., Verrecchia, A., Farina, C., Nicolini, G., Anichini, A., Bordignon, C., Sensi, M., Parmiani, G., and Traversari, C. (1998). Translation of a retained intron in tyrosinase-related protein (TRP) 2 mRNA generates a new cytotoxic T lymphocyte (CTL)-defined and shared human melanoma antigen not expressed in normal cells of the melanocytic lineage. *J. Exp. Med.* **188,** 1005–1016.

Mandruzzato, S., Brasseur, F., Andry, G., Boon, T., and van der Bruggen, P. (1997). A CASP-8 mutation recognized by cytolytic T lymphocytes on a human head and neck carcinoma. *J. Exp. Med.* **186,** 785–793.

Manicassamy, S., and Pulendran, B. (2009). Modulation of adaptive immunity with Toll-like receptors. *Semin. Immunol.* **21,** 185–193.

Manici, S., Sturniolo, T., Imro, M. A., Hammer, J., Sinigaglia, F., Noppen, C., Spagnoli, G., Mazzi, B., Bellone, M., Dellabona, P., *et al.* (1999). Melanoma cells present a MAGE-3 epitope to CD4(+) cytotoxic T cells in association with histocompatibility leukocyte antigen DR11. *J. Exp. Med.* **189,** 871–876.

Marchand, M., van Baren, N., Weynants, P., Brichard, V., Dreno, B., Tessier, M. H., Rankin, E., Parmiani, G., Arienti, F., Humblet, Y., *et al.* (1999). Tumor regressions observed in patients with metastatic melanoma treated with an antigenic peptide encoded by gene MAGE-3 and presented by HLA- A1. *Int. J. Cancer* **80,** 219–230.

Marshall, N. A., Vickers, M. A., and Barker, R. N. (2003). Regulatory T cells secreting IL-10 dominate the immune response to EBV latent membrane protein 1. *J. Immunol.* **170,** 6183–6189.

Melief, C. J., and van der Burg, S. H. (2008). Immunotherapy of established (pre)malignant disease by synthetic long peptide vaccines. *Nat. Rev. Cancer* **8,** 351–360.

Munz, C., Bickham, K. L., Subklewe, M., Tsang, M. L., Chahroudi, A., Kurilla, M. G., Zhang, D., O'Donnell, M., and Steinman, R. M. (2000). Human CD4(+) T lymphocytes consistently respond to the latent Epstein-Barr virus nuclear antigen EBNA1. *J. Exp. Med.* **191,** 1649–1660.

Muul, L. M., Nason-Burchenal, K., Carter, C. S., Cullis, H., Slavin, D., Hyatt, C., Director, E. P., Leitman, S. F., Klein, H. G., and Rosenberg, S. A. (1987). Development of an automated closed system for generation of human lymphokine-activated killer (LAK) cells for use in adoptive immunotherapy. *J. Immunol. Methods* **101,** 171–181.

Netea, M. G., Sutmuller, R., Hermann, C., Van der Graaf, C. A., Van der Meer, J. W., van Krieken, J. H., Hartung, T., Adema, G., and Kullberg, B. J. (2004). Toll-like receptor 2 suppresses immunity against Candida albicans through induction of IL-10 and regulatory T cells. *J. Immunol.* **172,** 3712–3718.

Noppen, C., Levy, F., Burri, L., Zajac, P., Remmel, E., Schaefer, C., Luscher, U., Heberer, M., and Spagnoli, G. C. (2000). Naturally processed and concealed HLA-A2.1-restricted epitopes from tumor-associated antigen tyrosinase-related protein-2. *Int. J. Cancer* **87,** 241–246.

Nyirenda, M. H., Sanvito, L., Darlington, P. J., O'Brien, K., Zhang, G. X., Constantinescu, C. S., Bar-Or, A., and Gran, B. (2011). TLR2 Stimulation drives human naive and effector regulatory T cells into a Th17-like phenotype with reduced suppressive function. *J. Immunol.* **187,** 2278–2290.

Oberg, H. H., Ly, T. T., Ussat, S., Meyer, T., Kabelitz, D., and Wesch, D. (2010). Differential but direct abolishment of human regulatory T cell suppressive capacity by various TLR2 ligands. *J. Immunol.* **184,** 4733–4740.

Oiso, M., Eura, M., Katsura, F., Takiguchi, M., Sobao, Y., Masuyama, K., Nakashima, M., Itoh, K., and Ishikawa, T. (1999). A newly identified MAGE-3-derived epitope recognized by HLA-A24-restricted cytotoxic T lymphocytes. *Int. J. Cancer* **81,** 387–394.

Paludan, C., and Munz, C. (2003). CD4+ T cell responses in the immune control against latent infection by Epstein-Barr virus. *Curr. Mol. Med.* **3,** 341–347.

Panelli, M. C., Bettinotti, M. P., Lally, K., Ohnmacht, G. A., Li, Y., Robbins, P., Riker, A., Rosenberg, S. A., and Marincola, F. M. (2000). A tumor-infiltrating lymphocyte from a melanoma metastasis with decreased expression of melanoma differentiation antigens recognizes MAGE-12. *J. Immunol.* **164,** 4382–4392.

Parkhurst, M. R., Fitzgerald, E. B., Southwood, S., Sette, A., Rosenberg, S. A., and Kawakami, Y. (1998). Identification of a shared HLA-A*0201-restricted T-cell epitope from the melanoma antigen tyrosinase-related protein 2 (TRP2). *Cancer Res.* **58,** 4895–4901.

Peng, G., Guo, Z., Kiniwa, Y., Voo, K. S., Peng, W., Fu, T., Wang, D. Y., Li, Y., Wang, H. Y., and Wang, R.-F. (2005). Toll-like receptor 8 mediated-reversal of CD4+ regulatory T cell function. *Science* **309,** 1380–1384.

Peng, G., Wang, H. Y., Peng, W., Kiniwa, Y., Seo, K., and Wang, R.-F. (2007). Tumor-infiltrating gamma-delta T cells suppress T and dendritic cell function via mechanisms controlled by a unique Toll-like receptor signaling pathway. *Immunity* **27,** 334–348.

Peto, J. (2001). Cancer epidemiology in the last century and the next decade. *Nature* **411,** 390–395.

Pieper, R., Christian, R. E., Gonzales, M. I., Nishimura, M. I., Gupta, G., Settlage, R. E., Shabanowitz, J., Rosenberg, S. A., Hunt, D. F., and Topalian, S. L. (1999). Biochemical identification of a mutated human melanoma antigen recognized by CD4(+) T cells. *J. Exp. Med.* **189,** 757–766.

Robbins, P. F., El-Gamil, M., Li, Y. F., Kawakami, Y., Loftus, D., Appella, E., and Rosenberg, S. A. (1996). A mutated beta-catenin gene encodes a melanoma-specific antigen recognized by tumor infiltrating lymphocytes. *J. Exp. Med.* **183,** 1185–1192.

Robbins, P., El-Gamil, M., Li, Y. F., Fitzgerald, E., Kawakami, Y., and Rosenberg, S. A. (1997). The intronic region of an incompletely spliced gp100 gene transcript encodes an epitope recognized by melanoma-reactive tumor-infiltrating lymphocytes. *J. Immunol.* **159,** 303–308.

Rosenberg, S. A. (1990). Adoptive immunotherapy for cancer. *Sci. Am.* **262,** 62–69.

Rosenberg, S. A. (2000). Interleukin-2 and the development of immunotherapy for the treatment of patients with cancer. *Cancer J. Sci. Am.* **6** (Suppl. 1), S2–S7.

Rosenberg, S. A. (2011). Cell transfer immunotherapy for metastatic solid cancer—what clinicians need to know. *Nat. Rev. Clin. Oncol.* **8,** 577–585.

Rosenberg, S. A., Lotze, M. T., Muul, L. M., Chang, A. E., Avis, F. P., Leitman, S., Linehan, W. M., Robertson, C. N., Lee, R. E., Rubin, J. T., *et al.* (1987). A progress report on the treatment of 157 patients with advanced cancer using lymphokine-activated killer cells and interleukin-2 or high-dose interleukin-2 alone. *N. Engl. J. Med.* **316,** 889–897.

Rosenberg, S. A., Packard, B. S., Aebersold, P. M., Solomon, D., Topalian, S. L., Toy, S. T., Simon, P., Lotze, M. T., Yang, J. C., Seipp, C. A., *et al.* (1988). Use of tumor infiltrating lymphocytes and interleukin-2 in the immunotherapy of patients with metastatic melanoma. A Preliminary report. *N. Engl. J. Med.* **319,** 1676–1680.

Rosenberg, S. A., Yannelli, J. R., Yang, J. C., Topalian, S. L., Schwartzentruber, D. J., Weber, J. S., Parkinson, D. R., Seipp, C. A., Einhorn, J. H., and White, D. E. (1994). Treatment of patients with metastatic melanoma with autologous tumor-infiltrating lymphocytes and interleukin 2. *J. Natl. Cancer Inst.* **86,** 1159–1166.

Rosenberg, S. A., Yang, J. C., Schwartzentruber, D. J., Hwu, P., Marincola, F. M., Topalian, S. L., Restifo, N. P., Dudley, M. E., Schwarz, S. L., Spiess, P. J., *et al.* (1998). Immunologic and therapeutic evaluation of a synthetic tumor-associated peptide vaccine for the treatment of patients with metastatic melanoma. *Nat. Med.* **4,** 321–327.

Rosenberg, S. A., Yang, J. C., and Restifo, N. P. (2004). Cancer immunotherapy: Moving beyond current vaccines. *Nat. Med.* **10,** 909–915.

Rosenberg, S. A., Restifo, N. P., Yang, J. C., Morgan, R. A., and Dudley, M. E. (2008). Adoptive cell transfer: A clinical path to effective cancer immunotherapy. *Nat. Rev. Cancer* **8,** 299–308.

Rosenberg, S. A., Yang, J. C., Sherry, R. M., Kammula, U. S., Hughes, M. S., Phan, G. Q., Citrin, D. E., Restifo, N. P., Robbins, P. F., Wunderlich, J. R., *et al.* (2011). Durable complete responses in heavily pretreated patients with metastatic melanoma using T-cell transfer immunotherapy. *Clin. Cancer Res.* **17,** 4550–4557.

Round, J. L., Lee, S. M., Li, J., Tran, G., Jabri, B., Chatila, T. A., and Mazmanian, S. K. (2011). The Toll-like receptor 2 pathway establishes colonization by a commensal of the human microbiota. *Science* **332,** 974–977.

Royal, R. E., Levy, C., Turner, K., Mathur, A., Hughes, M., Kammula, U. S., Sherry, R. M., Topalian, S. L., Yang, J. C., Lowy, I., *et al.* (2010). Phase 2 trial of single agent ipilimumab (anti-CTLA-4) for locally advanced or metastatic pancreatic adenocarcinoma. *J. Immunother.* **33,** 828–833.

Russo, V., Tanzarella, S., Dalerba, P., Rigatti, D., Rovere, P., Villa, A., Bordignon, C., and Traversari, C. (2000). Dendritic cells acquire the MAGE-3 human tumor antigen from apoptotic cells and induce a class I-restricted T cell response. *Proc. Natl. Acad. Sci. USA* **97,** 2185–2190.

Schmidt-Wolf, I. G., Negrin, R. S., Kiem, H. P., Blume, K. G., and Weissman, I. L. (1991). Use of a SCID mouse/human lymphoma model to evaluate cytokine-induced killer cells with potent antitumor cell activity. *J. Exp. Med.* **174,** 139–149.

Schneider, J., Brichard, V., Boon, T., Meyer zum Buschenfelde, K. H., and Wolfel, T. (1998). Overlapping peptides of melanocyte differentiation antigen Melan-A/MART-1 recognized by autologous cytolytic T lymphocytes in association with HLA-B45.1 and HLA-A2.1. *Int. J. Cancer* **75,** 451–458.

Schreiber, R. D., Old, L. J., and Smyth, M. J. (2011). Cancer immunoediting: Integrating immunity's roles in cancer suppression and promotion. *Science* **331,** 1565–1570.

Schroers, R., Huang, X. F., Hammer, J., Zhang, J., and Chen, S. Y. (2002). Identification of HLA DR7-restricted epitopes from human telomerase reverse transcriptase recognized by CD4+ T-helper cells. *Cancer Res.* **62,** 2600–2605.

Schultz, E. S., Lethe, B., Cambiaso, C. L., Van Snick, J., Chaux, P., Corthals, J., Heirman, C., Thielemans, K., Boon, T., and van der Bruggen, P. (2000). A MAGE-A3 peptide presented by HLA-DP4 is recognized on tumor cells by CD4+ cytolytic T lymphocytes. *Cancer Res.* **60,** 6272–6275.

Schwartzentruber, D. J., Lawson, D. H., Richards, J. M., Conry, R. M., Miller, D. M., Treisman, J., Gailani, F., Riley, L., Conlon, K., Pockaj, B., *et al.* (2011). gp100 peptide vaccine and interleukin-2 in patients with advanced melanoma. *N. Engl. J. Med.* **364,** 2119–2127.

Sensi, M., Pellegatta, S., Vegetti, C., Nicolini, G., Parmiani, G., and Anichini, A. (2002). Identification of a novel gp100/pMel17 peptide presented by HLA-A*6801 and recognized on human melanoma by cytolytic T cell clones. *Tissue Antigens* **59,** 273–279.

Skipper, J. C., Kittlesen, D. J., Hendrickson, R. C., Deacon, D. D., Harthun, N. L., Wagner, S. N., Hunt, D. F., Engelhard, V. H., and Slingluff, C. L., Jr. (1996). Shared epitopes for HLA-A3-restricted melanoma-reactive human CTL include a naturally processed epitope from Pmel-17/gp100. *J. Immunol.* **157,** 5027–5033.

Slager, E. H., Borghi, M., van der Minne, C. E., Aarnoudse, C. A., Havenga, M. J., Schrier, P. I., Osanto, S., and Griffioen, M. (2003). CD4+ Th2 cell recognition of HLA-DR-restricted epitopes derived from CAMEL: A tumor antigen translated in an alternative open reading frame. *J. Immunol.* **170,** 1490–1497.

Song, X. T., Evel-Kabler, K., Shen, L., Rollins, L., Huang, X. F., and Chen, S. Y. (2008). A20 is an antigen presentation attenuator, and its inhibition overcomes regulatory T cell-mediated suppression. *Nat. Med.* **14,** 258–265.

Stockert, E., Jager, E., Chen, Y. T., Scanlan, M. J., Gout, I., Karbach, J., Arand, M., Knuth, A., and Old, L. J. (1998). A survey of the humoral immune response of cancer patients to a panel of human tumor antigens. *J. Exp. Med.* **187,** 1349–1354.

Sutmuller, R. P., den Brok, M. H., Kramer, M., Bennink, E. J., Toonen, L. W., Kullberg, B. J., Joosten, L. A., Akira, S., Netea, M. G., and Adema, G. J. (2006). Toll-like receptor 2 controls expansion and function of regulatory T cells. *J. Clin. Invest.* **116,** 485–494.

Tacken, P. J., and Figdor, C. G. (2011). Targeted antigen delivery and activation of dendritic cells in vivo: Steps towards cost effective vaccines. *Semin. Immunol.* **23,** 12–20.

Tahara, K., Takesako, K., Sette, A., Celis, E., Kitano, S., and Akiyoshi, T. (1999). Identification of a MAGE-2-encoded human leukocyte antigen-A24-binding synthetic peptide that induces specific antitumor cytotoxic T lymphocytes. *Clin. Cancer Res.* **5,** 2236–2241.

Takayama, T., Sekine, T., Makuuchi, M., Yamasaki, S., Kosuge, T., Yamamoto, J., Shimada, K., Sakamoto, M., Hirohashi, S., Ohashi, Y., *et al.* (2000). Adoptive immunotherapy to lower postsurgical recurrence rates of hepatocellular carcinoma: A randomised trial. *Lancet* **356,** 802–807.

Takeda, K., and Akira, S. (2005). Toll-like receptors in innate immunity. *Int. Immunol.* **17,** 1–14.

Tanaka, F., Fujie, T., Tahara, K., Mori, M., Takesako, K., Sette, A., Celis, E., and Akiyoshi, T. (1997). Induction of antitumor cytotoxic T lymphocytes with a MAGE-3-encoded synthetic peptide presented by human leukocytes antigen-A24. *Cancer Res.* **57,** 4465–4468.

Tanzarella, S., Russo, V., Lionello, I., Dalerba, P., Rigatti, D., Bordignon, C., and Traversari, C. (1999). Identification of a promiscuous T-cell epitope encoded by multiple members of the MAGE family. *Cancer Res.* **59,** 2668–2674.

Tey, S. K., Bollard, C. M., and Heslop, H. E. (2006). Adoptive T-cell transfer in cancer immunotherapy. *Immunol. Cell Biol.* **84,** 281–289.

Topalian, S. L., Gonzales, M. I., Parkhurst, M., Li, Y. F., Southwood, S., Sette, A., Rosenberg, S. A., and Robbins, P. F. (1996). Melanoma-specific CD4+ T cells recognize nonmutated HLA-DR-restricted tyrosinase epitopes. *J. Exp. Med.* **183,** 1965–1971.

Topalian, S. L., Gonzales, M. I., Ward, Y., Wang, X., and Wang, R. F. (2002). Revelation of a cryptic major histocompatibility complex class II- restricted tumor epitope in a novel RNA-processing enzyme. *Cancer Res.* **62,** 5505–5509.

Torchilin, V. P. (2006). Recent approaches to intracellular delivery of drugs and DNA and organelle targeting. *Annu. Rev. Biomed. Eng.* **8,** 343–375.

Touloukian, C. E., Leitner, W. W., Topalian, S. L., Li, Y. F., Robbins, P. F., Rosenberg, S. A., and Restifo, N. P. (2000). Identification of a MHC class II-restricted human gp100 epitope using DR4-IE transgenic mice. *J. Immunol.* **164,** 3535–3542.

Traversari, C., Van der Bruggen, P., Luescher, I. F., Lurquin, C., Chomez, P., Van Pel, A., De Plaen, E., Amar-Costesec, A., and Boon, T. (1992). A nonapeptide encoded by human gene MAGE-1 is recognized on HLA-A1 by cytolytic T lymphocytes directed against tumor antigen MZ2-E. *J. Exp. Med.* **176,** 1453–1457.

Tsai, V., Southwood, S., Sidney, J., Sakaguchi, K., Kawakami, Y., Appella, E., Sette, A., and Celis, E. (1997). Identification of subdominant CTL epitopes of the GP100 melanoma-associated tumor antigen by primary in vitro immunization with peptide-pulsed dendritic cells. *J. Immunol.* **158,** 1796–1802.

Van der Bruggen, P., Traversari, C., Chomez, P., Lurquin, C., DePlaen, E., Van Den Eynde, B., Knuth, A., and Boon, T. (1991). A gene encoding an antigen recognized by cytolytic T lymphocytes on a human melanoma. *Science* **254,** 1643–1647.

Van der Bruggen, P., Bastin, J., Gajewski, T., Coulie, P. G., Boel, P., de Smet, C., Traversari, C., Townsend, A., and Boon, T. (1994a). A peptide encoded by human gene MAGE-3 and presented by HLA-A2 induces cytolytic T lymphocytes that recognize tumor cells expressing MAGE-3. *Eur. J. Immunol.* **24,** 3038–3043.

Van der Bruggen, P., Szikora, J.-P., Boel, P., Wildmann, C., Somville, M., Sensi, M., and Boon, T. (1994b). Autologous cytolytic T lymphocytes recognize a MAGE-1 nonapeptide on melanomas expressing Cw1601. *Eur. J. Immunol.* **24,** 2134–2140.

van der Burg, S. H., and Melief, C. J. (2011). Therapeutic vaccination against human papilloma virus induced malignancies. *Curr. Opin. Immunol.* **23,** 252–257.

Vence, L., Palucka, A. K., Fay, J. W., Ito, T., Liu, Y. J., Banchereau, J., and Ueno, H. (2007). Circulating tumor antigen-specific regulatory T cells in patients with metastatic melanoma. *Proc. Natl. Acad. Sci. USA* **104,** 20884–20889.

Vesely, M. D., Kershaw, M. H., Schreiber, R. D., and Smyth, M. J. (2011). Natural innate and adaptive immunity to cancer. *Annu. Rev. Immunol.* **29,** 235–271.

Visseren, M. J., van der Burg, S. H., van der Voort, E. I., Brandt, R. M., Schrier, P. I., van der Bruggen, P., Boon, T., Melief, C. J., and Kast, W. M. (1997). Identification of HLA-A*0201-restricted CTL epitopes encoded by the tumor-specific MAGE-2 gene product. *Int. J. Cancer* **73,** 125–130.

Voo, K. S., Fu, T., Heslop, H. E., Brenner, M. K., Rooney, C. M., and Wang, R. F. (2002). Identification of HLA-DP3-restricted peptides from EBNA1 recognized by CD4(+) T cells. *Cancer Res.* **62,** 7195–7199.

Voo, K. S., Peng, G., Guo, Z., Fu, T., Li, Y., Frappier, L., and Wang, R. F. (2005). Functional characterization of EBV-encoded nuclear antigen 1-specific CD4+ helper and regulatory T cells elicited by in vitro peptide stimulation. *Cancer Res.* **65,** 1577–1586.

Wang, R.-F. (2001). The role of MHC class II-restricted tumor antigens and CD4+ T cells in antitumor immunity. *Trends Immunol.* **22,** 269–276.

Wang, R. F., and Rosenberg, S. A. (1999). Human tumor antigens for cancer vaccine development. *Immunol. Rev.* **170,** 85–100.

Wang, R.-F., and Wang, H. Y. (2002). Enhancement of antitumor immunity by prolonging antigen presentation on dendritic cells. *Nat. Biotechnol.* **20,** 149–156.

Wang, R.-F., Appella, E., Kawakami, Y., Kang, X., and Rosenberg, S. A. (1996a). Identification of TRP-2 as a human tumor antigen recognized by cytotoxic T lymphocytes. *J. Exp. Med.* **184,** 2207–2216.

Wang, R.-F., Parkhurst, M. R., Kawakami, Y., Robbins, P. F., and Rosenberg, S. A. (1996b). Utilization of an alternative open reading frame of a normal gene in generating a novel human cancer antigen. *J. Exp. Med.* **183,** 1131–1140.

Wang, R.-F., Johnston, S., Southwood, S., Sette, A., and Rosenberg, S. A. (1998a). Recognition of an antigenic peptide derived from TRP-2 by cytotoxic T lymphocytes in the context of HLA-A31 and -A33. *J. Immunol.* **160,** 890–897.

Wang, R.-F., Johnston, S. L., Zeng, G., Schwartzentruber, D. J., and Rosenberg, S. A. (1998b). A breast and melanoma-shared tumor antigen: T cell responses to antigenic peptides translated from different open reading frames. *J. Immunol.* **161,** 3596–3606.

Wang, R.-F., Wang, X., Atwood, A. C., Topalian, S. L., and Rosenberg, S. A. (1999a). Cloning genes encoding MHC class II-restricted antigens: Mutated CDC27 as a tumor antigen. *Science* **284,** 1351–1354.

Wang, R.-F., Wang, X., and Rosenberg, S. A. (1999b). Identification of a novel MHC class II-restricted tumor antigen resulting from a chromosomal rearrangement recognized by CD4+ T cells. *J. Exp. Med.* **189,** 1659–1667.

Wang, H. Y., Fu, T., Wang, G., Gang, Z., Donna, M. P.-L., Yang, J. C., Restifo, N. P., Hwu, P., and Wang, R.-F. (2002a). Induction of CD4+ T cell-dependent antitumor immunity by TAT-mediated tumor antigen delivery into dendritic cells. *J. Clin. Invest.* **109,** 1463–1470.

Wang, H. Y., Zhou, J., Zhu, K., Riker, A. I., Marincola, F. M., and Wang, R.-F. (2002b). Identification of a mutated fibronectin as a tumor antigen recognized by CD4+ T cells: Its role in extracellular matrix formation and tumor metastasis. *J. Exp. Med.* **195,** 1397–1406.

Wang, H. Y., Lee, D. A., Peng, G., Guo, Z., Li, Y., Kiniwa, Y., Shevach, E. M., and Wang, R.-F. (2004). Tumor-specific human CD4+ regulatory T cells and their ligands: Implication for immunotherapy. *Immunity* **20,** 107–118.

Wang, H. Y., Peng, G., Guo, Z., Shevach, E. M., and Wang, R.-F. (2005). Recognition of a new ARTC1 peptide ligand uniquely expressed in tumor cells by antigen-specific CD4+ regulatory T cells. *J. Immunol.* **174,** 2661–2670.

Wolf, A. M., Wolf, D., Steurer, M., Gastl, G., Gunsilius, E., and Grubeck-Loebenstein, B. (2003). Increase of regulatory T cells in the peripheral blood of cancer patients. *Clin. Cancer Res.* **9,** 606–612.

Wolfel, T., Van Pel, A., Brichard, V., Schneider, J., Seliger, B., Meyer Zum Buschenfelde, K.-H., and Boon, T. (1994). Two tyrosinase nonapeptides recognized on HLA-A2 melanomas by autologous cytolytic T lymphocytes. *Eur. J. Immunol.* **24,** 759–764.

Wolfel, T., Hauer, M., Schneider, J., Serrano, M., Wolfel, C., Klehmann-Hieb, E., De Plaen, E., Hankeln, T., Meyer Zum Buschenfelde, K.-H., and Beach, D. (1995). A p16INK4a-insensitive CDK4 mutant targeted by cytolytic T lymphocytes in a human melanoma. *Science* **269,** 1281–1284.

Wrzesinski, C., Paulos, C. M., Kaiser, A., Muranski, P., Palmer, D. C., Gattinoni, L., Yu, Z., Rosenberg, S. A., and Restifo, N. P. (2010). Increased intensity lymphodepletion enhances tumor treatment efficacy of adoptively transferred tumor-specific T cells. *J. Immunother.* **33,** 1–7.

Xia, X., Cui, J., Wang, H. Y., Zhu, L., Matsueda, S., Wang, Q., Yang, X., Hong, J., Songyang, Z., Chen, Z., *et al.* (2011). NLRX1 negatively regulates TLR-induced NF-κB signaling by targeting TRAF6 and IKK. *Immunity* **34,** 843–853.

Yee, C., Thompson, J. A., Roche, P., Byrd, D. R., Lee, P. P., Piepkorn, M., Kenyon, K., Davis, M. M., Riddell, S. R., and Greenberg, P. D. (2000). Melanocyte destruction after antigen-specific immunotherapy of melanoma. Direct evidence of T cell-mediated vitiligo. *J. Exp. Med.* **192,** 1637–1644.

Yee, C., Thompson, J. A., Byrd, D., Riddell, S. R., Roche, P., Celis, E., and Greenberg, P. D. (2002). Adoptive T cell therapy using antigen-specific CD8+ T cell clones for the treatment of patients with metastatic melanoma: In vivo persistence, migration, and antitumor effect of transferred T cells. *Proc. Natl. Acad. Sci. USA* **99,** 16168–16173.

Yoneyama, M., Kikuchi, M., Natsukawa, T., Shinobu, N., Imaizumi, T., Miyagishi, M., Taira, K., Akira, S., and Fujita, T. (2004). The RNA helicase RIG-I has an essential function in double-stranded RNA-induced innate antiviral responses. *Nat. Immunol.* **5,** 730–737.

Young, L. S., and Rickinson, A. B. (2004). Epstein-Barr virus: 40 years on. *Nat. Rev. Cancer* **4,** 757–768.

Zarour, H. M., Kirkwood, J. M., Kierstead, L. S., Herr, W., Brusic, V., Slingluff, C. L., Jr., Sidney, J., Sette, A., and Storkus, W. J. (2000). Melan-A/MART-1(51-73) represents an immunogenic HLA-DR4-restricted epitope recognized by melanoma-reactive CD4(+) T cells. *Proc. Natl. Acad. Sci. USA* **97,** 400–405.

Zeng, G., Touloukian, C. E., Wang, X., Restifo, N. P., Rosenberg, S. A., and Wang, R.-F. (2000). Identification of CD4+ T cell epitopes from NY-ESO-1 presented by HLA-DR molecules. *J. Immunol.* **165,** 1153–1159.

Zeng, G., Wang, X., Robbins, P. F., Rosenberg, S. A., and Wang, R.-F. (2001). CD4+ T cell recognition of MHC class II-restricted epitopes from NY-ESO-1 presented by a prevalent HLA-DP4 allele: Association with NY-ESO-1 antibody production. *Proc. Natl. Acad. Sci. USA* **98,** 3964–3969.

Zhu, Y., Yao, S., and Chen, L. (2011). Cell surface signaling molecules in the control of immune responses: A tide model. *Immunity* **34,** 466–478.

Zorn, E., and Hercend, T. (1999). A MAGE-6-encoded peptide is recognized by expanded lymphocytes infiltrating a spontaneously regressing human primary melanoma lesion. *Eur. J. Immunol.* **29,** 602–607.

CHAPTER 7

TLR Ligand–Peptide Conjugate Vaccines: Toward Clinical Application

Gijs G.P. Zom,* Selina Khan,* Dmitri V. Filippov,† and Ferry Ossendorp*

Contents

Abstract

Approaches to treat cancer with therapeutic vaccination have made significant progress. In order to induce efficient antitumor immunity, a vaccine should target and activate antigen-presenting cells, such as the dendritic cell, while delivering the tumor-derived

* Department of Immunohematology and Blood Transfusion, Leiden University Medical Centre, Leiden, The Netherlands
† Leiden Institute of Chemistry, Leiden University, Leiden, The Netherlands

Advances in Immunology, Volume 114
ISSN 0065-2776, DOI: 10.1016/B978-0-12-396548-6.00007-X

antigen of choice. Conjugates of synthetic peptides and ligands of pattern-recognition receptors (PRRs) combine these features and, given their synthetic nature, can be produced under GMP conditions. Therefore, conjugation of antigenic peptides to potent PRR ligands is a promising vaccination approach for the treatment of cancer. This review focuses on the different PRR families that can be exploited for the design of conjugates and explores the results obtained so far with PRR ligands conjugated to antigen. The uptake and processing of Toll-like receptor ligand–peptide conjugates are discussed in more detail, as well as future directions that may further enhance the immunogenicity of conjugates.

1. INTRODUCTION

Cancer is routinely treated by surgery, chemotherapy, and radiation. Although refinement of these therapies has resulted in considerably lower incidences of side effects with maintenance of efficacy, the call for better targeted therapies has become stronger. In recent years, considerable progress was achieved in the field of immunotherapy.

Several immunotherapeutic antibodies against cancer are on the market, while also tumor antigen-based specific vaccine formulations are currently being developed (Buonerba *et al.*, 2011; Pedicord *et al.*, 2011; Zarour and Ferrone, 2011).

Cancer patients often show detectable tumor-antigen specific T-cell immunity, but a process of tolerance seems to overpower the eradication of tumor cells. Several approaches to overcome or to modulate the tolerant or suppressed state of tumor-specific T-cells are in clinical studies now, like CTLA-4 and PD-1 blockade (Pedicord *et al.*, 2011; Rosenblatt *et al.*, 2011). Besides, there is much progress in optimizing vaccine formulations to more effectively prime or (re)activate tumor-specific T-cells. This review focuses on optimal vaccine formulations, in more detail on synthetically defined structures that harbor the right properties for specific T-cell activation.

To achieve a state of effective antitumor immunity, a triad of immune-related hallmarks can be defined. First, a therapy should be targeted against the central antigen-presenting cell (APC), the dendritic cell (DC). This goal can be met by making use of the broad array of receptors that DCs express. At the same time, a DC should be matured in such a way that a process is set into action that will ultimately lead to presentation of tumor antigens in their MHC class I or II molecules, combined with the upregulation of costimulatory molecules. Third, the antigen that is delivered to the DC should be highly tumor specific in order to achieve antitumor immunity and evade tolerance induction.

These three hallmarks can also potentially be combined in one molecule. Conjugating antigen to a targeting molecule, such as a Toll-like receptor ligand (TLR ligand), enables the efficient delivery of tumor-derived antigen to DCs while maturing these DCs to induce (cross-) presentation to tumor-specific T-helper cells (Th cells) and cytotoxic T-cells (CTLs) (Segura and Villadangos, 2009). It is well established that besides specific CTLs, also tumor-specific Th cells are essential for proper antitumor cellular immunity. This was already demonstrated in our group over a decade ago by immunizing mice with a peptide containing either a specific or an irrelevant Th epitope and subsequently inoculating these mice with a MHC class II negative tumor. Only mice that received the tumor-specific Th epitope-containing peptide were protected from tumor outgrowth. $CD8^+$ T-cells were identified as the effector cells responsible for tumor eradication, while it was shown that $CD4^+$ T-cells were not able to directly recognize the tumor cells but rather cross-presented tumor antigen by local MHC class II expressing APCs (Ossendorp *et al.*, 1998). In the same period, it was firmly established in our and other groups that T help cells for CTL priming was mainly mediated by Th–DC cell–cell contact via the CD40–CD40L interaction (Bennett *et al.*, 1998; Ridge *et al.*, 1998; Schoenberger *et al.*, 1998). Therefore, effective tumor-specific vaccines should include tumor antigen-specific Th and CTL epitope sequences.

2. TARGETING AND DC MATURATION

2.1. Central role of DCs in vaccine development

DCs play a crucial role in the initiation and control of T-cell-mediated immune responses. In the peripheral tissues, DCs reside in an immature state where they sample antigens and pathogens from their surroundings. After antigen capture in the presence of a danger signal, such as bacterial unmethylated CpG DNA or LPS, DCs undergo a complex maturation process and *in vivo* the DCs home to the T-cell-rich areas of the lymphoid organs, where they present antigenic peptides to specific T-cells and direct the T-cell differentiation into effector or memory T-cells. DCs have been shown to be very potent in antigen ingestion and in presenting exogenously derived peptides into their MHC class I route, a process known as cross-presentation. This feature, together with their capacity to express an array of sensing receptors which can activate these specialized cells to initiate and regulate specific T-cell immunity underlines that DC is the central cell type to target vaccines for infectious diseases and cancer to. Our studies with *in vivo* transferred DCs as a cellular vaccine showed that maturation signals with TLR ligands could effectively substitute the required Th signals via CD40–CD40L interaction for optimal CTL induction in mice (Schuurhuis *et al.*, 2000). The maturation signals provided by CD40 and TLRs not only give rise to elevated expression of costimulatory molecules like CD80 and CD86 and production of cytokines like IL-12, but also the MHC class I processing machinery is strongly enhanced especially by the upregulation of the proteasome activator PA28β (Ossendorp *et al.*, 2005). Together, the entire maturation process allows DCs to optimally prime naive T lymphocytes. In addition, different DC subsets can induce development of both Th1 and Th2 effector cells, depending on a combination of antigen dose and the type of ligand with which the DCs are activated (Flinsenberg *et al.*, 2011; Steinman, 2008). This implicates that the choice for an optimal vaccine formulation including the type of adjuvant depends on the type of pathogen and the immunological character of the disease.

2.2. Pattern-recognition receptor families and their ligands

The first line of defense against pathogens is represented by the pattern-recognition receptors (PRRs; Akira *et al.*, 2006). These sensing receptors of the innate immune system detect pathogen-associated molecular patterns (PAMPs), molecules that specifically occur in microbes but not in mammalian cells. Recognition of PAMPs by PRRs triggers specific signaling pathways that induce immune responses against microbes. Detection of PAMPs by the PRRs of DCs induces signals leading to the ability of DCs to efficiently prime specific cellular T-cell responses (Banchereau *et al.*, 2000; Mellman and Steinman, 2001). This stimulatory effect on these innate immune receptors is therefore essential for the action of successful vaccines. In fact, molecularly well-defined PAMPs can be regarded as a new generation of adjuvants to be included in improved vaccine formulations. TLRs (Gay and Gangloff, 2007), the nucleotide-binding oligomerization domain-like or Nod-like receptors (NLRs; Franchi *et al.*, 2009), the retinoic acid-inducible gene-I-like or RIG-like receptors (RLRs; Takeuchi and Akira, 2008), and the C-type lectin receptors (CLRs; Osorio and Reis e Sousa, 2011) are the four known families of PRRs.

The C-type lectin family of proteins, which is not in the scope of this review, consists of over a thousand members, which all share the property of possessing a C-type carbohydrate recognition domain, localized in a unique structural fold. Functions of this family of proteins are very diverse, though many CLR proteins are able to recognize carbohydrate structures, such as glucans, fucose, and high-mannose structures. These structures are important constituents of viruses, fungi, (myco)bacteria, and parasites. The few CLRs that have been shown to self-sufficiently induce myeloid cell activation and, further downstream, adaptive immune responses signal through the spleen tyrosine kinase (Syk) adaptor protein. CLRs either bind Syk *in trans* via ITAM-bearing adaptors or, more rarely, directly bind Syk through a cytoplasmic single tyrosine-based motif (Mocsai *et al.*, 2010; Osorio and Reis e Sousa, 2011). Most of the CLRs signaling through Syk have the ability to activate NFκB, a process for which the adaptor protein CARD9 is required. Upon phagocytosis, CARD9 was seen to be rapidly recruited to the phagosomes (Goodridge *et al.*, 2009). Therefore, specific CLR targeting, either by itself or in combination with other PRRs, is also a promising approach for effective vaccine formulations but will not be further discussed here.

2.2.1. The TLR family

The founding member of the TLR family, the protein Toll, was originally identified in 1985 as a developmental protein in *Drosophila* (Anderson *et al.*, 1985). More than a decade later, Toll was found to have a role in the detection of fungal pathogens (Lemaitre *et al.*, 1996). Mammalian analogues were identified shortly thereafter, together making up the TLR family (Kawai and Akira, 2010; Poltorak *et al.*, 1998). Thus far, 13 TLRs have been identified in mammals, of which TLR1–10 are expressed in humans. Although mice lack expression of TLR10, they do express TLR11–13 (Chaturvedi and Pierce, 2009).

TLRs are transmembrane proteins that are characterized by extracellular, transmembrane, and cytosolic domains (Gay and Gangloff, 2007). The extracellular domains containing leucine-rich repeats (LRRs) with horseshoe-like shapes are involved in recognition of common molecular patterns derived from diverse microbes (Jin and Lee, 2008). TLRs are expressed either on the cell surface (TLR1, 2, 4, 5, 6, and 10) or on membranes of intracellular organelles, such as endosomes (TLR3, 7, 8, and 9). The natural ligands for the endosomal receptors turned out to be nucleic acid-based molecules. Bacterial DNA having unmethylated CpG motifs are ligands for TLR9 and viral single-stranded RNAs are ligands for TLR7 and 8, while the ligands of TLR3 are double-stranded viral RNAs (Gay and Gangloff, 2007). The cell surface-expressed TLR1, 2, 4, 5, 6, and 10 recognize molecular patterns of extracellular microbes (Monie *et al.*, 2009).

TLR2 can detect a wide variety of ligands derived from bacteria, viruses, parasites, and fungi. The ligand specificity is often determined by the interaction of TLR2 with other TLRs, such as TLR1, 6, or 10, or non-TLR molecules, such as dectin-1, CD14, or CD36. The formation of a heterodimer with TLR1 enables TLR2 to identify triacyl lipoproteins or lipopeptides from (myco)bacterial origin, such as Pam_3CSK_4 and peptidoglycan (PGA; Gay and Gangloff, 2007; Spohn *et al.*, 2004). Heterodimerization of TLR2 and 6 enables the detection of diacyl lipopeptides and zymosan. Lipopolysaccharide (LPS) is a ligand for TLR4 and flagellin for TLR5 (Bryant *et al.*, 2010).

Upon binding their cognate ligand, most TLRs activate the adaptor protein MyD88 via their cytoplasmic tail (also Toll/IL-1 receptor domain; TIR), although some, like TLR3 and -4, make use of the TRIF/IRF3 pathway as well. This interaction leads to the triggering of IL-1 receptor-associated kinases, tumor necrosis factor (TNF) receptor-associated factor 6, and TGFβ-activated kinase 1 (TAK1). Triggering of TLRs ultimately leads to the activation of nuclear factor κB (NFκB), activating protein-1, and/or IRF3. Depending on the trigger, the activation of these transcription factors leads to transcription of type 1 interferons and/or proinflammatory cytokines such as IL-1β, IL-12, and TNFα (Kawai and Akira, 2010). TLRs are expressed on several cell types but virtually all TLRs are expressed on DCs allowing these specialized cells to sense all possible pathogens and danger signals. Since most of the TLR ligands are known, and as they are generally small molecules of well-defined composition, these molecules can be synthetically produced and included in defined vaccine formulations.

2.2.2. Internalization of TLR ligands

As described above, TLRs interact, either at the cell surface or intracellularly, with their corresponding TLR ligands. Given the restricted number of germline-encoded TLRs available to detect a broad variety of structurally different ligands, it is reasonable to expect that additional proteins participate in a modulatory and combinatorial manner to ensure recognition of the different ligands.

For obvious reasons, ligands targeting the intracellular receptors, TLR3, TLR7, TLR8, and TLR9, must be internalized independent of their respective TLRs. Multiple mechanisms have indeed been shown to facilitate uptake of nucleic acid ligands; the mode of uptake depends not only on the nature of the ligand but also on the cell type involved. For instance, CpG-ODN type B is internalized by mouse DCs in a caveolin-dependent but clathrin-independent route (Khan *et al.*, 2007), whereas monocyte-derived DCs internalize poly(I:C) dsRNA in a clathrin-dependent manner (Itoh *et al.*, 2008).

It has been shown that both CpG as well as GpC motifs containing oligodeoxynucleotide (ODN) are internalized to equal extent (Heit *et al.*, 2003). This has led to the suggestion that scavenger receptors might be involved in aiding the uptake of nucleic acids in a sequence-specific independent manner. However, recently CXCL16, a membrane-bound scavenger receptor type expressed on plasmacytoid DCs (pDCs), was found to support uptake of CpG–ODN type A but not internalization of CpG–ODN type B, arguing that some specificity does exist in terms of sequence recognition (Gursel *et al.*, 2006).

In contrast, CD14, a glycosylphosphatidylinositol-anchored membrane-associated protein, which is a well-established component of the cell surface expressed TLR4 ligand binding complex, was reported to mediate uptake of Poly(I:C) into TLR3-containing endosomes, thereby promoting TLR3 activation (Lee *et al.*, 2006) as well as to promote uptake of nucleic acids such as ssRNA and CpG–ODN type B (Baumann *et al.*, 2010). These data further suggest that some ancillary proteins involved in internalization possess sequence preference, whereas others are less restricted.

Interestingly, several studies show that a variety of ligands targeting the extracellular TLRs, like TLR2, are also internalized independently of their TLRs. This seems puzzling but most likely reflects the fact that the TLRs are sensing receptors rather than uptake receptors. In this respect, the diacylated lipopeptide FSL-1, a TLR2 ligand, was shown to be internalized by macrophages in a TLR2-independent process but requiring the expression of CD14 as well as CD36 proteins (a B-class scavenger receptor; Shamsul *et al.*, 2010).

Similarly, Mantovani and coworkers found that the outer membrane protein A (OmpA), a component of the outer membrane of *Enterobacteriaceae*, activates DCs and macrophages in a TLR2-dependent manner, but that internalization of OmpA was mediated by two members of the SR-1 scavenger receptor family, LOX-1 and SREC-I (Jeannin *et al.*, 2005). Recently, we found that the two stereoisomers (R- and S-stereochemistry at C-2 of the glycerol moiety) of the TLR2 ligand Pam_3CSK_4 derivatives are internalized independently of TLR2 expression, but in a clathrin- and caveolin-dependent manner (Khan *et al.*, 2007, 2009), suggesting that the receptor complex involved is less selective.

Identification and characterization of the receptors involved in uptake of the individual TLR ligands will be of high importance in the light of rational adjuvant design for defined vaccine formulations.

2.2.3. Cytoplasmic PRR families

The recognition of PAMPs can also take place in the cytosol. Here, the NLR family is able to detect components of the bacterial PGA layer. The Nod1 and Nod2 proteins recognize D-Glu-meso-diaminopimelic acid dipeptide and GlcNAc-MurNAc-L-alanine-D-glutamate (muramyl dipeptide, MDP), respectively. The expression of several antibacterial compounds, such as defensins, cryptidin, and peptidoglycan-recognition proteins (PGRPs), is dependent on Nod1 and Nod2, underlining their importance in antibacterial immunity.

Upon activation of Nod1 and Nod2, the receptor-interacting protein 2 (RIP2) can bind the caspase recruitment domain (CARD) of Nod1 and Nod2. RIP2 ultimately activates NFκB by enabling ubiquitination of NFκB essential modulator.

Nod1 was shown to induce expression of IL-1β. Expression of the proinflammatory IL-1β is dependent on cleavage of the pro-IL-1β precursor by caspase-1, which is activated by the inflammasome (Kufer and Sansonetti, 2007). Additionally, the Nod2-ligand MDP was shown to induce the release of stored pro-IL-1β in a caspase-1-dependent fashion. The released IL-1β is subsequently involved in Nod2-associated MAPK activation which ultimately leads to proinflammatory cytokine production (Hedl and Abraham, 2011). As the triggering of NLR signaling cascades leads to maturation of DCs and promotes proinflammatory cytokine production, the question is raised whether this proinflammatory state of a DC is also accompanied by enhanced cross-presentation. Indeed, as shown by Asano *et al.* (2010), NLR enhances DC cross-presentation when Nod ligands were injected together with an antigenic protein. This was shown using $CD8^+$ DCs, the DC subset which is known to be a highly efficient cross-presenting DC (Shortman and Heath, 2010).

The cytosol also contains another family of PRRs, RLRs. All three family members known to date, RIG-I, MDA5, and LGP2, are DExD/H box RNA helicases that are able to detect PAMPs in viral RNA or processed self-RNA. Upon recognition of their ligands, signaling by RLRs typically occurs through activation of the adaptor protein IPS-1, via CARD–CARD interactions. Upon binding IPS-1, the RLRs are relocated to IPS-1-associated intracellular membranes, where an IPS-1 signalosome is formed. Ultimately, the formation of the signalosome leads to activation of a transcription program, resulting in IFN production (Loo and Gale, 2011). Importantly, RLR signaling shares many components of signaling cascades triggered by TNF receptor 1 and TLRs (Kawai and Akira, 2009).

3. SYNTHETIC PEPTIDE VACCINATION

From a historic vaccine development perspective, whole tumor cell lysates came to the attention of researchers as a putative novel treatment of cancer. Although enhanced T-cell responses and (temporary) remission of tumors were observed using tumor lysates or DCs pulsed with these lysates (Geiger *et al.*, 2001; Ribas *et al.*, 2010), the popularity of this technique has diminished as it lacks adequate specificity, and the obtained results have not led to a breakthrough. Also, vaccination with tumor-specific protein alone is not strong enough to induce antitumor immunity. Therefore, current research has been focusing more and more on the use of synthetically well-defined adjuvants and tumor-specific peptides.

3.1. Human papillomavirus as a tumor antigen

In order to explore the potency of a novel vaccine formulation, the best choice for a malignant tumor model is one of which the tumor antigens are well defined. Human papillomavirus (HPV)-induced tumors fit this requirement as the viral antigens presented by all tumor cells are by definition nonself. Besides being a cause of approximately 30% of head-and-neck cancer, vulvar cancer, and penile cancer, HPV is mainly known to be the causative agent of nearly all cases of cervical cancer. Of the high-risk HPV serotypes identified thus far, the HPV16 serotype is the predominant serotype, accounting for approximately 50% of all cervical cancers (zur Hausen, 2002). The clearance of HPV infections and frequent spontaneous regression of low-grade cervical intraepithelial lesions indicate that immunity succeeds in controlling HPV before malignancies develop (de Jong *et al.*, 2004; Frazer, 2004; Koutsky, 1997; Sasadeusz *et al.*, 2001). A large body of evidence shows the important role of HPV-specific T-cells in protection against disease. Failure of immune control allows HPV infections to flare up to establish HPV persistence and HPV-induced cancer (de Jong *et al.*, 2004; de Vos van Steenwijk *et al.*, 2010; Palefsky, 2000; Palefsky and Holly, 2003; Sasadeusz *et al.*, 2001).

3.2. Short versus long peptide vaccination

It is well established that T-cells play an important role in the elimination of malignant cells. Since CTLs recognize small protein fragments presented by MHC class I molecules, it proved to be possible to achieve protective T-cell immunity by vaccination with synthetic peptides, representing 9–11-amino acid-long sequences, against viruses (Kast *et al.*, 1991; Schultz *et al.*, 2004) and also against HPV16-induced tumors (Feltkamp *et al.*, 1993). However, further research indicated major flaws in the concept of vaccination with the exact MHC class I binding peptides. First of all, peptide-specific tolerance can be induced, associated with enhanced tumor outgrowth instead of protection (Toes *et al.*, 1996a,b). Secondly, the lack of induction of specific T-cell help lead to suboptimal and short-lived $CD8^+$ T-cell responses, which is caused by the lack of proper Th cell-mediated signaling through DCs (Melief *et al.*, 2000; van den Broeke *et al.*, 2003; van Poelgeest *et al.*, 2005).

To compare the therapeutic potency of an exact MHC class I binding peptide with that of a long peptide incorporating the same HPV16 E7 CTL epitope but in addition an HPV16 Th epitope, we tested short and long peptide vaccines in a therapeutic setting in mice (Zwaveling *et al.*, 2002). Vaccinations with the HPV16-derived 35-amino acid-long E7 peptide resulted in the induction of far more robust E7-specific CTL responses than vaccinations with the short peptide containing the minimal CTL epitope correlating with effective tumor clearance.

4. CONJUGATION OF ANTIGEN TO TLR LIGANDS

In a survey of the status of melanoma vaccines, the overall objective response rate in a series of 440 patients treated with various melanoma-specific vaccines was only 2.6% (Rosenberg *et al.*, 2004). It was concluded that the immunotherapeutic approaches need drastic improvement. Since most peptide vaccination trials to date were carried out by injecting exact MHC class I binding peptides, often without TLR ligand, this evaluation is certainly justified. Measures for improved clinical results with cancer peptide-based vaccines include use of long peptides incorporating both MHC class I and class II tumor-associated epitopes. Linking class I and II epitopes is more effective than mixing class I and II epitopes (Zwaveling *et al.*, 2002). Additionally, the choice of TLR ligands for obtaining optimal efficacy of human DC activation therapy may differ from that in the mouse. Notably, the CpG receptor TLR9 in human beings is only expressed on pDCs and not, like in the mouse, on myeloid DC. Nonetheless, rapid and robust CTL responses were induced by combining MART1/Melan-A HLA-A2 peptide vaccination with CpG ODN 7909 (Speiser *et al.*, 2005), in line with our results in mice. Therefore, conjugation of TLR ligands to peptides for vaccination may be a promising strategy to induce effective antitumor immunity. However, in vaccine design studies, it should be noted that the polarity and quality of an immune response may differ depending on the chosen adjuvant ligand. A Th2-skewed response is obviously highly unwanted when aiming at inducing antitumor cellular immunity.

The potency of CpG DNA to induce efficient activation of DCs and production of cytokines and chemokines has led several laboratories to chemically conjugate whole protein antigens to CpG for induction of the development of adaptive antigen-specific immune response (Klinman *et al.*, 2004). Cho *et al.* were the first to show that conjugation of CpG to ovalbumin (OVA) protein induced specific $CD8^+$ T-cells in a Th cell-independent manner (Cho *et al.*, 2000). In line with this study, several other groups have demonstrated a robust immunostimulatory capacity of CpG-conjugated proteins in different model systems (Heit *et al.*, 2005; Klinman *et al.*, 2004; Maurer *et al.*, 2002; Shirota *et al.*, 2001; Tighe *et al.*, 2000).

It was also reported that CpG linked to FITC-labeled OVA was taken up more efficiently than nonconjugated OVA, and that within 30–45min, the CpG–OVA was translocated to LAMP1 positive endosomal–lysosomal compartments (Heit *et al.*, 2005). Heit *et al.* (2003) showed that cross-presentation of OVA-linked CpG occurred independently from TLR9 expression, but that TLR9 expression was essential for activation of the DCs. This makes sense, considering that the TLR9 is mainly expressed in the ER and is recruited to the endosomes upon DC maturation (Ahmad-Nejad *et al.*, 2002; Latz *et al.*, 2004). It also suggests that a still unknown scavenger receptor recognizing nonspecific DNA sequence is likely to be involved in the internalization of CpG.

Aside from CpG DNA, other TLR ligands have also been explored as potent adjuvants for vaccines. Nonhuman primates (NHPs) were immunized with a vaccine containing a commercial TLR7 ligand conjugated to HIV Gag protein. As compared to immunization with HIV Gag alone, or a mixture of Gag and either CpG or the TLR7 ligand, NHPs immunized with the conjugate showed an enhanced magnitude and altered quality of the Th1 type immune responses and induction of specific $CD8^+$ T-cells (Wille-Reece *et al.*, 2005). The same group also used the TLR7/8 ligand R848 in combination with HIV Gag vaccination and observed that it was a rather weak inducer of primary Th1 and $CD8^+$ T-cell responses. However, when a structurally and functionally similar TLR7/8 ligand was conjugated to HIV Gag, Th1 and $CD8^+$ T-cell responses were enhanced, accompanied by a relatively high expression of CD127, a marker of memory formation (Wille-Reece *et al.*, 2005). Well-defined conjugates containing a different TLR7 ligand, based on an 8-oxoadenine core (Fig. 7.1, construct **2***), attached to peptides containing the OVA-derived CTL epitope (SIINFEKL) have been reported by us (Weterings *et al.*, 2006). These compounds did not show any DC-activating capacity while the presentation of the model epitope by the DCs could still be observed. This lack of the DC activation capacity could be explained by the poor binding of the conjugate to TLR7 due to steric bulk of the peptide moiety. Interestingly, slightly different 8-oxoadenine derivative attached to mouse serum albumin via a hydrazone-based

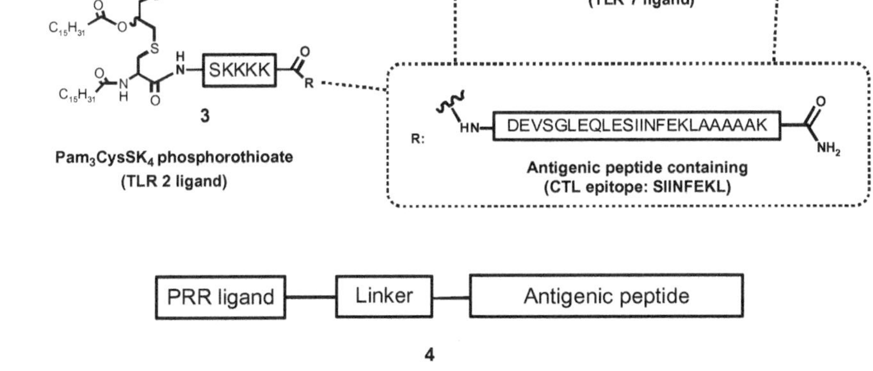

FIGURE 7.1 Structures of the conjugates consisting of a TLR ligand and an antigenic peptide (**1**, **2**, **3**), for the references see text. Schematic representation of the design of such conjugates (**4**).

linker did lead to the release of proinflammatory cytokines *in vitro* (Wu *et al.*, 2007). The fact that the immunomodulatory activity was preserved in this latter case could be explained by a different mode of attachment of the TLR ligand to the antigen or by the release of the free ligand by intracellular hydrolytic degradation of the hydrazone.

Bacterial lipoproteins and their synthetic analogues have been shown to be strong immune modulators during the early phase after induction (Hohlich *et al.*, 2003). Moreover, a robust priming of virus-specific CTLs was seen when mice were injected with an MHC class I epitope conjugated to the TLR2 ligand Pam_3CSK_4 (Deres *et al.*, 1989). Similar TLR2 targeting Pam_2Cys conjugates have been used to promote immune responses against viral, bacterial, and protein antigens (Jackson *et al.*, 2004). Th, antibody, and CTL responses were improved upon conjugation. Importantly, protective as well as therapeutic responses against OVA-expressing tumors were induced in mice upon vaccination with a Pam_2Cys conjugate. Protective immunity was also induced using a Pam_3CSK_4 conjugate containing a SV40-derived peptide (Obert *et al.*, 1998).

4.1. TLR ligands conjugated to peptide

In comparison to conjugation of TLR ligands to tumor-derived proteins, relatively less effort was made in the field of conjugation of TLR ligands to antigenic peptides. A study by Daftarian *et al.* (2005) reported potent activity against vaccinia virus expressing full-length HIV antigen, induced in a model with CpG conjugated to peptides containing the minimal CTL and Th epitopes from HIV Gag or pol proteins. Another study applied synthetic HSV2-derived peptides conjugated to a palmitic acid moiety, a ligand for TLR2. The authors observed the induction of HSV2-specific CTL responses, and these immunized mice were protected from HSV2 challenge (Zhang *et al.*, 2009).

4.1.1. Downstream trafficking and processing of TLR ligand–peptide conjugates

In our group, it was shown that a synthetic long peptide conjugated to either CpG or Pam_3CSK_4 (Fig. 7.1, constructs **1** and **3**) induces DC maturation to the same extent as the free TLR ligand, proving that the maturating potential of the TLR ligand is not affected by conjugation to a peptide. Subsequently, peptide was taken up more rapidly in DCs when conjugated to a TLR ligand, both *in vitro* and *in vivo*. Besides, conjugation of peptide to the TLR ligands greatly enhanced *in vitro* antigen presentation as compared to a mixture of free TLR ligand and peptide. Moreover, both conjugates enhanced T-cell priming *in vivo*. Investigation of antigen-processing routes showed that MHC class I presentation was dependent on endosomal acidification, proteasomal cleavage, and TAP translocation. The uptake of peptide conjugated to either CpG or Pam_3CSK_4 was independent of expression of their respective TLR, an observation that was already reported for the endosomally expressed TLR9, but was now also surprisingly observed for the surface-expressed TLR2. However, TLR expression and downstream TLR signaling were shown to be essential for DC maturation and $CD8^+$ T-cell priming. A difference between the CpG- and Pam_3CSK_4-conjugate is found in the uptake route: while uptake of the Pam_3CSK_4-conjugate was dependent on clathrin-coated pits and caveolae formation, uptake of the CpG conjugate was shown to be independent of clathrin-coated pits, but partly dependent on caveolae formation (Khan *et al.*, 2007).

The question remains what happens with the endocytosed conjugates in processing routes. Most probably, the peptide is enzymatically cleaved in the endosomes, removing the peptide from the TLR ligand. The peptide is then available for MHC class 2 loading in the endosomal pathway or ends up in the cytosol where proteasomal degradation, TAP translocation, and MHC class I loading are taking place. The role of the free TLR ligand inside a DC may vary. As efficient T-cell priming is also observed by CpG-conjugates, it seems plausible that, after endosomal cleavage, the free CpG can interact with its cognate receptor, the endosomally expressed TLR9, as opposed to the TLR2 ligand Pam_3CSK_4 which exerts its DC maturing effect at the cell surface. In future research, this issue could be addressed by introducing a universal linker between the TLR ligand and peptide. In this manner, the potency of conjugates consisting of divergent antigenic peptides can be standardized.

Targeting DCs with a TLR ligand–peptide conjugate was shown to lead to the formation of an intracellular antigen depot. This depot enables prolonged antigen presentation and subsequent T-cell priming, which was not observed when DCs were pulsed with the short OVA-derived SIINFEKL peptide (van Montfoort *et al.*, 2009). Moreover, sustained antigen presentation from an internal depot was also observed when DCs were pulsed with IgG-OVA, the uptake of which is Fc-receptor dependent and also induces a DC maturation signal (Schuurhuis *et al.*, 2002). This specific antigen storage function of DCs, in contrast to macrophages which rapidly degrade antigen, is a crucial quality of DCs to sustain antigen presentation in MHC class I to optimally raise CTL immunity. It was speculated that DCs require an antigen depot function for MHC class I cross-presentation because of the unstable nature of MHC class I–peptide complexes in contrast to MHC class II (van Montfoort *et al.*, 2009). The depot will serve as a reservoir to constantly replenish new peptide fragments for MHC class I presentation. One of the reasons for DCs to require sustained peptide presentation for several days is the time needed to migrate from the infection site to draining lymphoid organs. Indeed, 2weeks after s.c. vaccination of TLR ligand–peptide conjugates, very effective CTL priming was observed, induced with one to two log lower doses of conjugate than with mixtures of peptide with TLR ligand (Khan *et al.*, 2012, submitted for publication). Therefore, next to DC maturation signals, proper antigen targeting and handling by DC are essential for optimal vaccine formulations.

4.1.2. Influence of ligand chirality on TLR2-mediated activity

A chiral center at C-2 of the glycerol moiety in Pam_3CSK_4 gives way to the existence of two diastereomers of the TLR2 ligand, namely Pam-R and Pam-S. Previously, it was shown that the Pam-R-epimer is the more potent variant, based on IL-6 and IL-8 production or antibody response in mice injected with whole protein together with Pam-R (Asai *et al.*, 2007; Makimura *et al.*, 2006; Metzger *et al.*, 1991). When using the natural racemic mixture of Pam-R and Pam-S as a vaccine adjuvant, it should be excluded that the Pam-S-epimer has an inhibitory effect on the potency of Pam-R or vice versa. In our group, we showed that the racemic mixture of Pam-R and Pam-S is just as potent as Pam-R alone in DC maturation, antigen presentation, and T-cell priming (Khan *et al.*, 2009).

4.1.3. Induction of antitumor immunity by use of TLR ligand–peptide conjugates

Pam_2Cys-conjugated peptides containing a synthetically linked CTL and Th epitope sequence were effective in tumor control in two mouse models as shown by Jackson *et al.* (2004). To determine whether Pam_3CSK_4 conjugated to natural long peptides have the potency to induce antitumor immunity, we immunized mice with a combination of two conjugates, one containing a CTL epitope and one containing a Th epitope of OVA. Other groups included mice immunized with just one of both conjugates or a mixture of free Pam_3CSK_4 and the two peptides. Mice were subsequently challenged with the aggressive B16-OVA melanoma tumor. Significantly more mice of the group that received both conjugates survived the tumor challenge on a long-term basis, as compared to the group that received a mixture of free Pam_3CSK_4 and the CTL epitope-containing and Th epitope-containing peptides. It also became clear from these experiments that the Th response is essential for the induction of antitumor immunity. The necessity of the Th response was demonstrated in a Moloney mouse leukemia tumor model. Mice were immunized with either a Pam_3CSK_4 conjugate containing a Th epitope, a mixture of free Pam_3CSK_4 and peptide, or peptide alone. Immunization with the conjugate containing the Th epitope alone was enough to protect mice from growing a tumor (Khan *et al.*, 2012, submitted for publication). This finding confirms the essential role that Th cells play in antitumor immunity, as previously described by our group and others (Bennett *et al.*, 1997; Ossendorp *et al.*, 1998, 2000).

4.2. Therapeutic peptide vaccination

About a decade ago, we showed that vaccination with a long HPV16 E7 peptide combined with the DC-activating agent TLR9 ligand (CpG), resulted in a superior induction of E7-specific $CD8^+$ T-cells. Thus, despite the fact that TLRs are expressed on several cell types, direct injection of antigen combined with TLR ligands leads to strong adjuvant effects resulting in effective T-cell priming. The efficacy of the induced HPV-specific T-cell responses was demonstrated by the fact that therapeutic prime–boost vaccination with the long peptide admixed with CpG resulted in the eradication of large established HPV16-expressing tumors. The advantage of using CpG in the vaccine was a strong CTL response induction after only one injection, confirming that TLR ligands are potent adjuvants for priming peptide-specific CTL responses. The fact that the CTL response was abolished in $MHC2^{-/-}$ mice, in the absence of CpG, indicates the importance of the Th response (Zwaveling *et al.*, 2002). Interestingly, in therapeutic vaccination with overlapping 32–35-amino acid-long peptides, together spanning the E6 and E7 protein sequences of cottontail rabbit papilloma virus (CRPV), marked suppression of CRPV-induced wart growth, and abrogation of latent CRPV infection in rabbits was observed (Vambutas *et al.*, 2005).

Also Daftarian *et al.* (2006) showed eradication of palpable HPV16-expressing tumors using a liposome-encapsulated CTL–Th fusion peptide and using a mixture of liposome-encapsulated melanoma-associated CTL and Th peptides (Mansour *et al.*, 2007). Still, peptide vaccines have not been reported to efficiently eradicate established murine tumors in a spontaneous tumor model.

A few years later, a vaccine consisting of overlapping SLPs covering the HPV16 E6 and E7 oncogenic proteins was tested in patients with a premalignant HPV16-induced VIN3 (vulvar intraepithelial neoplasia grade III) lesion. A complete regression was observed in 47% of patients, while an additional 32% of patients showed a partial regression (Kenter *et al.*, 2009). These clinical outcomes inversely correlated with the size of the lesion and the presence of $CD4^+CD25^+$ $FoxP3^+$ T-cells (Welters *et al.*, 2010). However, it proved to be more difficult to obtain similar results with the same SLP vaccine in end-stage cervical cancer patients, although IFNγ-associated T-cell responses were induced. The vaccination itself was shown to be safe. Out of 48 enrolled patients in this phase 1 trial, only one patient showed a complete regression (Kenter *et al.*, 2008). Looking more in depth at the T-cell responses induced in six $HPV16^+$ cervical cancer patients vaccinated with the same SLP vaccine revealed that both activity and number of CTL and Th responses were increased against a broad array of epitopes of E6 and E7 (Welters *et al.*, 2008). Importantly, all six patients showed enhanced IFNγ production. IFNγ is known to play a major role in the expression of TAP, proteasomal components, MHC class I and II (York *et al.*, 1999) and is thus associated with cellular immunity.

The fact that patients with a premalignant stage of disease have a better clinical outcome when treated with these peptide vaccines than end-stage cervical cancer patients may partially be explained by the induction of HPV-specific T regulatory cells (Tregs), downregulation of essential processing and antigen presentation molecules, and failure of effector T-cells to home into cancer tissue in the context of cervical cancer patients. This is not surprising regarding the advanced stage of disease which may be accompanied by an immunocompromised state of the patient and long-term exhaustion of immune responses. A more potent vaccine formulation that is able to induce type 1 T-cell responses is therefore demanded to efficiently treat cancer patients.

5. FUTURE DIRECTIONS

5.1. Synergy between different PRR routes

A natural infection always brings forth a broad array of antigenic ligands, which can be recognized by divergent PRRs. For example, the bacterial cell wall harbors both TLR ligands, such as lipopeptides and lipoproteins, CLR ligands, such as (amino)sugars, as well as NLR ligands, such as muropeptides (MDP). Therefore, it seems plausible to combine multiple PRR ligands (PRR-Ls) in one molecule to even increase the potency of such conjugates.

5.1.1. Cross talk between TLR and NLR

The observation that the administration of TLR4 ligand LPS can induce endotoxic shock in the presence of Nod2 ligands' muropeptides, while muropeptides itself are not able to induce an acute-phase immune response, suggested that cross talk between TLR and NLR signaling exists (Takada and Galanos, 1987). In fact, multiple studies have by now shown a synergistic outcome in cytokine release when monocytes and DCs (Fritz *et al.*, 2005; Tada *et al.*, 2005; Uehara *et al.*, 2005) or B-cells (Petterson *et al.*, 2011) were stimulated with both NLR and TLR ligands. Several theories may explain this effect. First, Takahashi *et al.* (2006) reported increased mRNA expression of Nod1 and Nod2 upon TLR4 stimulation of murine macrophages. In turn, MDP was shown to enhance the expression of the TLR pathway adaptor protein MyD88 (Takada *et al.*, 2002). Also protein–protein interactions have been implicated. TAK1, a signaling protein part of the MAPK signaling cascade downstream of TLR signaling, was also shown to bind the LRR of Nod2, a binding that was necessary for NFκB activation (Chen *et al.*, 2004). The RIP2 protein may play a role in the synergistic effects of NLR and TLR signaling as well as it interacts with both NLR and members of TLR2, 3, and 4 signaling pathways (Meylan and Tschopp, 2005). Combining both TLR and NLR ligands in one vaccine, either conjugated or free, may therefore be an interesting novel vaccine formulation.

5.1.2. Further putative synergism

As indicated in Section 2.2.3, also the RLR and TLR signaling cascades share different components. Importantly, both routes ultimately activate the NFκB, MAPKs, and IRF transcription factors. The NFκB family consists of five dimeric members, which differ in their dimer composition (Kawai and Akira, 2009). Simultaneous TLR, RLR, and NLR triggering may lead to the activation of different NFκB family members, thereby inducing the production of proinflammatory cytokines in a nonredundant way.

Signaling by CLR, for example Dectin-1, is Syk mediated, as indicated in Section 2.2.2. This Syk signaling also leads to activation of NFκB, as well as activation of nuclear factor of activated T-cells (NFAT) and MAPK, which again supports the assumption that divergent PRR signaling cascades may synergize. Dectin-1 was originally defined as a protein associating with TLR2 in macrophages when stimulated with zymosan. This collaboration results in the production of proinflammatory cytokines, such as TNFα, a process that was dependent on the synergistic activation of transcription factors via the TLR2-MyD88 and Dectin-1-Syk pathways (Dennehy *et al.*, 2008). Moreover, Syk signaling was shown to be involved in activation of the NLRP3 inflammasome, as well as in the synthesis of pro-IL-1β (Gross *et al.*, 2009), molecules that are essential in NLR signaling.

The overlapping functions of proteins in these different PRR signaling routes offer many possibilities in producing a synergistically functioning adjuvant for vaccine design.

5.2. Opportunities in chemistry

Since it has become clear, on the one hand, that the covalent conjugation of PRR-Ls to antigenic peptides improves the immunogenicity of the antigen and, on the other hand, the synergistic action of the PRRs of different kind has been observed, combining of different PRR-Ls in a single covalent construct appears to be the next logical step in the development of synthetic vaccines. The compounds designed on the basis of this straightforward idea are depicted schematically in Fig. 7.2 (construct **5**). Covalent joining of different components of a synthetic vaccine in a modular fashion with different nonpeptidic linkers has been reported for Pam_2Cys lipopeptides containing different combinations of MHC class I

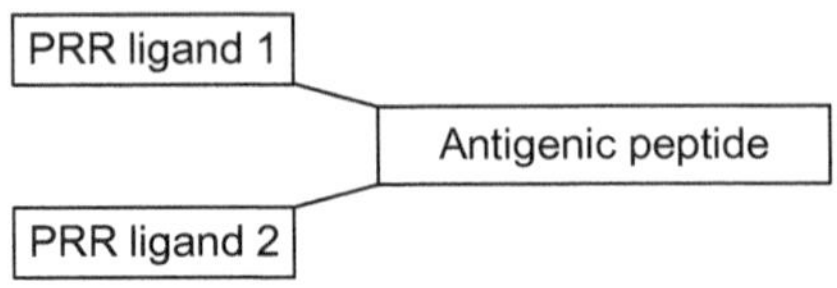

5

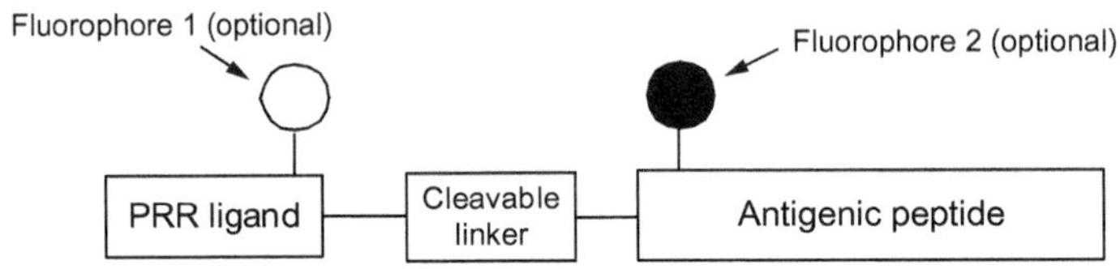

6

FIGURE 7.2 Structures of advanced conjugated vaccines. Construct **5** contains two well-defined PRR ligands attached to an antigenic peptide. Construct **6** is provided with a linker cleavable under the physiological conditions and optional fluorophores.

and class II epitopes (Zeng *et al.*, 2011). Similar Pam_3Cys lipoglycopeptides have been reported (Ingale *et al.*, 2009) that contain a tumor-associated MUC-1 glycopeptide B-epitope and a promiscuous Th-cell epitope. The modules to be joined in these constructs are peptide epitopes (class I, class II), a peptide antigen for antibody recognition, a B-cell epitope, and a TLR-ligand. It has to be recognized that the structure of the target conjugate in the work cited above as well as in our previous studies (Khan *et al.*, 2007) has been primarily dictated by synthetic methods available to produce these compounds. It has been shown, however, that varying the nature and the stability of the linker connecting the different modules in the constructs (Daftarian *et al.*, 2005; Zeng *et al.*, 2011) influences the immunogenicity of the conjugates. The variation, however, has been done largely by trial-and-error, and the outcome seems to depend on the exact nature of the conjugated vaccine under investigation. No generally applicable, unambiguous guideline for the design of such a vaccine can be discerned from the available literature. It can be concluded that the better understanding of the cross-presentation mechanisms and pathway is essential if one wishes to design PRR-L-based conjugated synthetic vaccines rationally. An example of an antigenic conjugate rationally designed to cross-present MHC class I epitope has been described (De Haan *et al.*, 2002), which encompasses MHC class I epitope, SIINFEKL in this instance, chemically conjugated to the receptor binding B subunit of *Escherichia coli* heat-labile toxin (EtxB). A peptide linker containing a sequence facilitating the translocation from the endosome is placed between the endosomal delivery vehicle (EtxB) and the epitope. DCs demonstrated high levels of MHC class I epitope presentation when treated with the construct described above. It is interesting to note that the presentation was dependent on the translocation ability of the linker connecting EtxB and SIINFEKL and on the endosomal cleavage of the linker peptide, presumably by a metalloprotease. Along the lines depicted above, a PRR-L-based conjugate can be designed containing a deliberately introduced enzymatically or chemically cleavable linker placed between the antigenic part of the peptide containing the desired epitopes (class I and class II) and the PRR-L of choice. The choice of the linker would be based on the conditions (pH, redox potential, specific enzymatic activity) in the cellular compartment where the cleavage is desired. Examples of the cleavable linkers include disulfide bond (cleaved under reductive conditions), phosphoramidate (cleavage at low pH), and peptide sequences labile to endosomal proteases known to be involved in the antigen processing (catepsin D or S). The cathepsin labile peptides are known in literature; for example, a cathepsin S substrate of exquisite specificity has been recently described (Lutzner and Kalbacher, 2008) and can be used as the enzymatically cleavable module in the future conjugated vaccines to enable selective liberation of epitopes from the PRR-L in the compartments relevant for antigen processing. Inhibitors of, for example, cathepsin S can be prepared by joining an electrophilic trap to the specific substrate and used to investigate the role of this enzyme in the intracellular processing of the conjugates. The PRR–peptide conjugates endowed with fluorophores, see Fig. 7.2 (construct **6**), can be envisaged to enable the monitoring of the antigen processing events *in vivo* and *in vitro*.

5.3. Toward clinical trials

So far, no conjugates of TLR ligand with synthetic peptides have been tested in a clinical setting. An important criterion before moving into the clinic is the question whether the compound of choice can be produced in a GMP-wise manner. GMP production is standardized, reduces variations, and eases upscaling of production. Generally, the GMP production of conjugates of TLR ligand and a synthetic peptide is relatively straightforward.

After establishing a broad scientific base in both *in vitro* and in rodent models, we aim to conduct a phase 1/2 clinical trial in end-stage cervical cancer patients. These patients will be injected with combined conjugates consisting of TLR ligand and HPV16 E6-derived synthetic long peptides. The study will be designed to determine safety and dosing of these potent molecules with a similar schedule and administration as our earlier clinical studies (see above). Simultaneously, we will characterize the immune response in these patients, with regard to the strength and quality of Th and CTL responses in order to explore the effectiveness of the conjugates. In addition, the presence and induction of HPV-specific Tregs will be included as a monitoring tool because of the potential danger of improperly polarizing the immune response. These clinical studies will reveal the usefulness of this modality of therapeutic vaccination. Obviously, even with improved vaccine formulations, the need of combination therapy with immunomodulatory agents to cure patients with highly aggressive tumors must be explored. Although TLR ligand–antigen conjugates are as such artificial, this type of synthetic vaccine opens possibilities to design the molecules with the vaccine requirements of choice. Our increased knowledge of antigen handling and processing, DC biology, and T-cell immunity will provide unique opportunities for rational design of active vaccination-based immunotherapy of established disease.

REFERENCES

Ahmad-Nejad, P., Hacker, H., *et al.* (2002). Bacterial CpG-DNA and lipopolysaccharides activate Toll-like receptors at distinct cellular compartments. *Eur. J. Immunol.* **32**(7), 1958–1968.

Akira, S., Uematsu, S., *et al.* (2006). Pathogen recognition and innate immunity. *Cell* **124**(4), 783–801.

Anderson, K. V., Jurgens, G., *et al.* (1985). Establishment of dorsal-ventral polarity in the Drosophila embryo: Genetic studies on the role of the Toll gene product. *Cell* **42**(3), 779–789.

Asai, Y., Makimura, Y., *et al.* (2007). Toll-like receptor 2-mediated dendritic cell activation by a *Porphyromonas gingivalis* synthetic lipopeptide. *J. Med. Microbiol.* **56**(Pt 4), 459–465.

Asano, J., Tada, H., *et al.* (2010). Nucleotide oligomerization binding domain-like receptor signaling enhances dendritic cell-mediated cross-priming *in vivo*. *J. Immunol.* **184**(2), 736–745.

Banchereau, J., Briere, F., *et al.* (2000). Immunobiology of dendritic cells. *Annu. Rev. Immunol.* **18,** 767–811.

Baumann, C. L., Aspalter, I. M., *et al.* (2010). CD14 is a coreceptor of Toll-like receptors 7 and 9. *J. Exp. Med.* **207**(12), 2689–2701.

Bennett, S. R., Carbone, F. R., *et al.* (1997). Induction of a CD8+ cytotoxic T lymphocyte response by cross-priming requires cognate CD4+ T cell help. *J. Exp. Med.* **186**(1), 65–70.

Bennett, S. R., Carbone, F. R., *et al.* (1998). Help for cytotoxic-T-cell responses is mediated by CD40 signalling. *Nature* **393**(6684), 478–480.

Bryant, C. E., Spring, D. R., *et al.* (2010). The molecular basis of the host response to lipopolysaccharide. *Nat. Rev. Microbiol.* **8**(1), 8–14.

Buonerba, C., Ferro, M., *et al.* (2011). Sipuleucel-T for prostate cancer: The immunotherapy era has commenced. *Expert Rev. Anticancer Ther.* **11**(1), 25–28.

Chaturvedi, A., and Pierce, S. K. (2009). How location governs toll-like receptor signaling. *Traffic* **10**(6), 621–628.

Chen, C. M., Gong, Y., *et al.* (2004). Reciprocal cross-talk between Nod2 and TAK1 signaling pathways. *J. Biol. Chem.* **279**(24), 25876–25882.

Cho, H. J., Takabayashi, K., *et al.* (2000). Immunostimulatory DNA-based vaccines induce cytotoxic lymphocyte activity by a T-helper cell-independent mechanism. *Nat. Biotechnol.* **18**(5), 509–514.

Daftarian, P., Sharan, R., *et al.* (2005). Novel conjugates of epitope fusion peptides with CpG-ODN display enhanced immunogenicity and HIV recognition. *Vaccine* **23**(26), 3453–3468.

Daftarian, P., Mansour, M., *et al.* (2006). Eradication of established HPV 16-expressing tumors by a single administration of a vaccine composed of a liposome-encapsulated CTL-T helper fusion peptide in a water-in-oil emulsion. *Vaccine* **24**(24), 5235–5244.

De Haan, L., Hearn, A. R., *et al.* (2002). Enhanced delivery of exogenous peptides into the class I antigen processing and presentation pathway. *Infect. Immun.* **70**(6), 3249–3258.

de Jong, A., van Poelgeest, M. I., *et al.* (2004). Human papillomavirus type 16-positive cervical cancer is associated with impaired CD4+ T-cell immunity against early antigens E2 and E6. *Cancer Res.* **64**(15), 5449–5455.

de Vos van Steenwijk, P. J., Heusinkveld, M., *et al.* (2010). An unexpectedly large polyclonal repertoire of HPV-specific T cells is poised for action in patients with cervical cancer. *Cancer Res.* **70**(7), 2707–2717.

Dennehy, K. M., Ferwerda, G., *et al.* (2008). Syk kinase is required for collaborative cytokine production induced through Dectin-1 and Toll-like receptors. *Eur. J. Immunol.* **38**(2), 500–506.

Deres, K., Schild, H., *et al.* (1989). *In vivo* priming of virus-specific cytotoxic T lymphocytes with synthetic lipopeptide vaccine. *Nature* **342**(6249), 561–564.

Feltkamp, M. C., Smits, H. L., *et al.* (1993). Vaccination with cytotoxic T lymphocyte epitope-containing peptide protects against a tumor induced by human papillomavirus type 16-transformed cells. *Eur. J. Immunol.* **23**(9), 2242–2249.

Flinsenberg, T. W., Compeer, E. B., *et al.* (2011). Antigen cross-presentation: Extending recent laboratory findings to therapeutic intervention. *Clin. Exp. Immunol.* **165**(1), 8–18.

Franchi, L., Warner, N., *et al.* (2009). Function of Nod-like receptors in microbial recognition and host defense. *Immunol. Rev.* **227**(1), 106–128.

Frazer, I. H. (2004). Prevention of cervical cancer through papillomavirus vaccination. *Nat. Rev. Immunol.* **4**(1), 46–54.

Fritz, J. H., Girardin, S. E., *et al.* (2005). Synergistic stimulation of human monocytes and dendritic cells by Toll-like receptor 4 and NOD1- and NOD2-activating agonists. *Eur. J. Immunol.* **35**(8), 2459–2470.

Gay, N. J., and Gangloff, M. (2007). Structure and function of Toll receptors and their ligands. *Annu. Rev. Biochem.* **76**, 141–165.

Geiger, J. D., Hutchinson, R. J., *et al.* (2001). Vaccination of pediatric solid tumor patients with tumor lysate-pulsed dendritic cells can expand specific T cells and mediate tumor regression. *Cancer Res.* **61**(23), 8513–8519.

Goodridge, H. S., Shimada, T., *et al.* (2009). Differential use of CARD9 by dectin-1 in macrophages and dendritic cells. *J. Immunol.* **182**(2), 1146–1154.

Gross, O., Poeck, H., *et al.* (2009). Syk kinase signalling couples to the Nlrp3 inflammasome for anti-fungal host defence. *Nature* **459**(7245), 433–436.

Gursel, M., Gursel, I., *et al.* (2006). CXCL16 influences the nature and specificity of CpG-induced immune activation. *J. Immunol.* **177**(3), 1575–1580.

Hedl, M., and Abraham, C. (2011). Distinct roles for Nod2 protein and autocrine interleukin-1 {beta} in muramyl dipeptide-induced mitogen-activated protein kinase activation and cytokine secretion in human macrophages. *J. Biol. Chem.* **286**(30), 26440–26449.

Heit, A., Maurer, T., *et al.* (2003). Cutting edge: Toll-like receptor 9 expression is not required for CpG DNA-aided cross-presentation of DNA-conjugated antigens but essential for cross-priming of CD8 T cells. *J. Immunol.* **170**(6), 2802–2805.

Heit, A., Schmitz, F., *et al.* (2005). Protective CD8 T cell immunity triggered by CpG-protein conjugates competes with the efficacy of live vaccines. *J. Immunol.* **174**(7), 4373–4380.

Hohlich, B. J., Wiesmuller, K. H., *et al.* (2003). Induction of an antigen-specific immune response and partial protection of cattle against challenge infection with foot-and-mouth

disease virus (FMDV) after lipopeptide vaccination with FMDV-specific B-cell epitopes. *J. Gen. Virol.* **84**(Pt 12), 3315–3324.
Ingale, S., Wolfert, M. A., *et al.* (2009). Increasing the antigenicity of synthetic tumor-associated carbohydrate antigens by targeting Toll-like receptors. *Chembiochem* **10**(3), 455–463.
Itoh, K., Watanabe, A., *et al.* (2008). The clathrin-mediated endocytic pathway participates in dsRNA-induced IFN-beta production. *J. Immunol.* **181**(8), 5522–5529.
Jackson, D. C., Lau, Y. F., *et al.* (2004). A totally synthetic vaccine of generic structure that targets Toll-like receptor 2 on dendritic cells and promotes antibody or cytotoxic T cell responses. *Proc. Natl. Acad. Sci. USA* **101**(43), 15440–15445.
Jeannin, P., Bottazzi, B., *et al.* (2005). Complexity and complementarity of outer membrane protein A recognition by cellular and humoral innate immunity receptors. *Immunity* **22**(5), 551–560.
Jin, M. S., and Lee, J. O. (2008). Structures of TLR-ligand complexes. *Curr. Opin. Immunol.* **20**(4), 414–419.
Kast, W. M., Roux, L., *et al.* (1991). Protection against lethal Sendai virus infection by *in vivo* priming of virus-specific cytotoxic T lymphocytes with a free synthetic peptide. *Proc. Natl. Acad. Sci. USA* **88**(6), 2283–2287.
Kawai, T., and Akira, S. (2009). The roles of TLRs, RLRs and NLRs in pathogen recognition. *Int. Immunol.* **21**(4), 317–337.
Kawai, T., and Akira, S. (2010). The role of pattern-recognition receptors in innate immunity: Update on Toll-like receptors. *Nat. Immunol.* **11**(5), 373–384.
Kenter, G. G., Welters, M. J., *et al.* (2008). Phase I immunotherapeutic trial with long peptides spanning the E6 and E7 sequences of high-risk human papillomavirus 16 in end-stage cervical cancer patients shows low toxicity and robust immunogenicity. *Clin. Cancer Res.* **14**(1), 169–177.
Kenter, G. G., Welters, M. J., *et al.* (2009). Vaccination against HPV-16 oncoproteins for vulvar intraepithelial neoplasia. *N. Engl. J. Med.* **361**(19), 1838–1847.
Khan, S., Bijker, M. S., *et al.* (2007). Distinct uptake mechanisms but similar intracellular processing of two different toll-like receptor ligand-peptide conjugates in dendritic cells. *J. Biol. Chem.* **282**(29), 21145–21159.
Khan, S., Weterings, J. J., *et al.* (2009). Chirality of TLR-2 ligand Pam3CysSK4 in fully synthetic peptide conjugates critically influences the induction of specific CD8+ T-cells. *Mol. Immunol.* **46**(6), 1084–1091.
Klinman, D. M., Currie, D., *et al.* (2004). Use of CpG oligodeoxynucleotides as immune adjuvants. *Immunol. Rev.* **199,** 201–216.
Koutsky, L. (1997). Epidemiology of genital human papillomavirus infection. *Am. J. Med.* **102**(5A), 3–8.
Kufer, T. A., and Sansonetti, P. J. (2007). Sensing of bacteria: NOD a lonely job. *Curr. Opin. Microbiol.* **10**(1), 62–69.
Latz, E., Schoenemeyer, A., *et al.* (2004). TLR9 signals after translocating from the ER to CpG DNA in the lysosome. *Nat. Immunol.* **5**(2), 190–198.
Lee, H. K., Dunzendorfer, S., *et al.* (2006). Double-stranded RNA-mediated TLR3 activation is enhanced by CD14. *Immunity* **24**(2), 153–163.
Lemaitre, B., Nicolas, E., *et al.* (1996). The dorsoventral regulatory gene cassette spatzle/Toll/cactus controls the potent antifungal response in Drosophila adults. *Cell* **86**(6), 973–983.
Loo, Y. M., and Gale, M., Jr. (2011). Immune signaling by RIG-I-like receptors. *Immunity* **34** (5), 680–692.
Lutzner, N., and Kalbacher, H. (2008). Quantifying cathepsin S activity in antigen presenting cells using a novel specific substrate. *J. Biol. Chem.* **283**(52), 36185–36194.
Makimura, Y., Asai, Y., *et al.* (2006). Correlation between chemical structure and biological activities of *Porphyromonas gingivalis* synthetic lipopeptide derivatives. *Clin. Exp. Immunol.* **146**(1), 159–168.

Mansour, M., Pohajdak, B., *et al.* (2007). Therapy of established B16-F10 melanoma tumors by a single vaccination of CTL/T helper peptides in VacciMax. *J. Transl. Med.* **5,** 20.
Maurer, T., Heit, A., *et al.* (2002). CpG-DNA aided cross-presentation of soluble antigens by dendritic cells. *Eur. J. Immunol.* **32**(8), 2356–2364.
Melief, C. J., Toes, R. E., *et al.* (2000). Strategies for immunotherapy of cancer. *Adv. Immunol.* **75,** 235–282.
Mellman, I., and Steinman, R. M. (2001). Dendritic cells: Specialized and regulated antigen processing machines. *Cell* **106**(3), 255–258.
Metzger, J., Jung, G., *et al.* (1991). Lipopeptides containing 2-(palmitoylamino)-6,7-bis(palmitoyloxy) heptanoic acid: Synthesis, stereospecific stimulation of B-lymphocytes and macrophages, and adjuvanticity *in vivo* and *in vitro*. *J. Med. Chem.* **34**(7), 1969–1974.
Meylan, E., and Tschopp, J. (2005). The RIP kinases: Crucial integrators of cellular stress. *Trends Biochem. Sci.* **30**(3), 151–159.
Mocsai, A., Ruland, J., *et al.* (2010). The SYK tyrosine kinase: A crucial player in diverse biological functions. *Nat. Rev. Immunol.* **10**(6), 387–402.
Monie, T. P., Bryant, C. E., *et al.* (2009). Activating immunity: Lessons from the TLRs and NLRs. *Trends Biochem. Sci.* **34**(11), 553–561.
Obert, M., Pleuger, H., *et al.* (1998). Protection of mice against SV40 tumours by Pam3Cys, MTP-PE and Pam3Cys conjugated with the SV40 T antigen-derived peptide, K(698)-T (708). *Vaccine* **16**(2–3), 161–169.
Osorio, F., and Reis e Sousa, C. (2011). Myeloid C-type lectin receptors in pathogen recognition and host defense. *Immunity* **34**(5), 651–664.
Ossendorp, F., Mengede, E., *et al.* (1998). Specific T helper cell requirement for optimal induction of cytotoxic T lymphocytes against major histocompatibility complex class II negative tumors. *J. Exp. Med.* **187**(5), 693–702.
Ossendorp, F., Toes, R. E., *et al.* (2000). Importance of CD4(+) T helper cell responses in tumor immunity. *Immunol. Lett.* **74**(1), 75–79.
Ossendorp, F., Fu, N., *et al.* (2005). Differential expression regulation of the alpha and beta subunits of the PA28 proteasome activator in mature dendritic cells. *J. Immunol.* **174**(12), 7815–7822.
Palefsky, J. M. (2000). Human papillomavirus-related tumors. *AIDS* **14**(Suppl 3), S189–S195.
Palefsky, J. M., and Holly, E. A. (2003). Chapter 6: Immunosuppression and co-infection with HIV. *J. Natl. Cancer Inst. Monogr.* (31), 41–46.
Pedicord, V. A., Montalvo, W., *et al.* (2011). Single dose of anti-CTLA-4 enhances CD8+ T-cell memory formation, function, and maintenance. *Proc. Natl. Acad. Sci. USA* **108**(1), 266–271.
Petterson, T., Jendholm, J., *et al.* (2011). Effects of NOD-like receptors in human B lymphocytes and crosstalk between NOD1/NOD2 and Toll-like receptors. *J. Leukoc. Biol.* **89**(2), 177–187.
Poltorak, A., He, X., *et al.* (1998). Defective LPS signaling in C3H/HeJ and C57BL/10ScCr mice: Mutations in Tlr4 gene. *Science* **282**(5396), 2085–2088.
Ribas, A., Camacho, L. H., *et al.* (2010). Multicenter phase II study of matured dendritic cells pulsed with melanoma cell line lysates in patients with advanced melanoma. *J. Transl. Med.* **8,** 89.
Ridge, J. P., Di Rosa, F., *et al.* (1998). A conditioned dendritic cell can be a temporal bridge between a CD4+ T-helper and a T-killer cell. *Nature* **393**(6684), 474–478.
Rosenberg, S. A., Yang, J. C., *et al.* (2004). Cancer immunotherapy: Moving beyond current vaccines. *Nat. Med.* **10**(9), 909–915.
Rosenblatt, J., Glotzbecker, B., *et al.* (2011). PD-1 blockade by CT-011, anti-PD-1 antibody, enhances *ex vivo* T-cell responses to autologous dendritic cell/myeloma fusion vaccine. *J. Immunother.* **34**(5), 409–418.
Sasadeusz, J., Kelly, H., *et al.* (2001). Abnormal cervical cytology in bone marrow transplant recipients. *Bone Marrow Transplant.* **28**(4), 393–397.

Schoenberger, S. P., Toes, R. E., *et al.* (1998). T-cell help for cytotoxic T lymphocytes is mediated by CD40-CD40L interactions. *Nature* **393**(6684), 480–483.
Schultz, E. S., Schuler-Thurner, B., *et al.* (2004). Functional analysis of tumor-specific Th cell responses detected in melanoma patients after dendritic cell-based immunotherapy. *J. Immunol.* **172**(2), 1304–1310.
Schuurhuis, D. H., Laban, S., *et al.* (2000). Immature dendritic cells acquire CD8(+) cytotoxic T lymphocyte priming capacity upon activation by T helper cell-independent or -dependent stimuli. *J. Exp. Med.* **192**(1), 145–150.
Schuurhuis, D. H., Ioan-Facsinay, A., *et al.* (2002). Antigen-antibody immune complexes empower dendritic cells to efficiently prime specific CD8+ CTL responses *in vivo*. *J. Immunol.* **168**(5), 2240–2246.
Segura, E., and Villadangos, J. A. (2009). Antigen presentation by dendritic cells *in vivo*. *Curr. Opin. Immunol.* **21**(1), 105–110.
Shamsul, H. M., Hasebe, A., *et al.* (2010). The Toll-like receptor 2 (TLR2) ligand FSL-1 is internalized via the clathrin-dependent endocytic pathway triggered by CD14 and CD36 but not by TLR2. *Immunology* **130**(2), 262–272.
Shirota, H., Sano, K., *et al.* (2001). Novel roles of CpG oligodeoxynucleotides as a leader for the sampling and presentation of CpG-tagged antigen by dendritic cells. *J. Immunol.* **167** (1), 66–74.
Shortman, K., and Heath, W. R. (2010). The CD8+ dendritic cell subset. *Immunol. Rev.* **234**(1), 18–31.
Speiser, D. E., Lienard, D., *et al.* (2005). Rapid and strong human CD8+ T cell responses to vaccination with peptide, IFA, and CpG oligodeoxynucleotide 7909. *J. Clin. Invest.* **115**(3), 739–746.
Spohn, R., Buwitt-Beckmann, U., *et al.* (2004). Synthetic lipopeptide adjuvants and Toll-like receptor 2—Structure-activity relationships. *Vaccine* **22**(19), 2494–2499.
Steinman, R. M. (2008). Dendritic cells *in vivo*: A key target for a new vaccine science. *Immunity* **29**(3), 319–324.
Tada, H., Aiba, S., *et al.* (2005). Synergistic effect of Nod1 and Nod2 agonists with toll-like receptor agonists on human dendritic cells to generate interleukin-12 and T helper type 1 cells. *Infect. Immun.* **73**(12), 7967–7976.
Takada, H., and Galanos, C. (1987). Enhancement of endotoxin lethality and generation of anaphylactoid reactions by lipopolysaccharides in muramyl-dipeptide-treated mice. *Infect. Immun.* **55**(2), 409–413.
Takada, H., Yokoyama, S., *et al.* (2002). Enhancement of endotoxin activity by muramyldipeptide. *J. Endotoxin Res.* **8**(5), 337–342.
Takahashi, Y., Isuzugawa, K., *et al.* (2006). Up-regulation of NOD1 and NOD2 through TLR4 and TNF-alpha in LPS-treated murine macrophages. *J. Vet. Med. Sci.* **68**(5), 471–478.
Takeuchi, O., and Akira, S. (2008). MDA5/RIG-I and virus recognition. *Curr. Opin. Immunol.* **20**(1), 17–22.
Tighe, H., Takabayashi, K., *et al.* (2000). Conjugation of immunostimulatory DNA to the short ragweed allergen amb a 1 enhances its immunogenicity and reduces its allergenicity. *J. Allergy Clin. Immunol.* **106**(1 Pt 1), 124–134.
Toes, R. E., Blom, R. J., *et al.* (1996a). Enhanced tumor outgrowth after peptide vaccination. Functional deletion of tumor-specific CTL induced by peptide vaccination can lead to the inability to reject tumors. *J. Immunol.* **156**(10), 3911–3918.
Toes, R. E., Offringa, R., *et al.* (1996b). Peptide vaccination can lead to enhanced tumor growth through specific T-cell tolerance induction. *Proc. Natl. Acad. Sci. USA* **93**(15), 7855–7860.
Uehara, A., Yang, S., *et al.* (2005). Muramyldipeptide and diaminopimelic acid-containing desmuramylpeptides in combination with chemically synthesized Toll-like receptor agonists synergistically induced production of interleukin-8 in a NOD2- and NOD1-dependent manner, respectively, in human monocytic cells in culture. *Cell. Microbiol.* **7**(1), 53–61.

Vambutas, A., DeVoti, J., *et al.* (2005). Therapeutic vaccination with papillomavirus E6 and E7 long peptides results in the control of both established virus-induced lesions and latently infected sites in a pre-clinical cottontail rabbit papillomavirus model. *Vaccine* **23**(45), 5271–5280.

van den Broeke, L. T., Daschbach, E., *et al.* (2003). Dendritic cell-induced activation of adaptive and innate antitumor immunity. *J. Immunol.* **171**(11), 5842–5852.

van Montfoort, N., Camps, M. G., *et al.* (2009). Antigen storage compartments in mature dendritic cells facilitate prolonged cytotoxic T lymphocyte cross-priming capacity. *Proc. Natl. Acad. Sci. USA* **106**(16), 6730–6735.

van Poelgeest, M. I., van Seters, M., *et al.* (2005). Detection of human papillomavirus (HPV) 16-specific CD4+ T-cell immunity in patients with persistent HPV16-induced vulvar intraepithelial neoplasia in relation to clinical impact of imiquimod treatment. *Clin. Cancer Res.* **11**(14), 5273–5280.

Welters, M. J., Kenter, G. G., *et al.* (2008). Induction of tumor-specific CD4+ and CD8+ T-cell immunity in cervical cancer patients by a human papillomavirus type 16 E6 and E7 long peptides vaccine. *Clin. Cancer Res.* **14**(1), 178–187.

Welters, M. J., Kenter, G. G., *et al.* (2010). Success or failure of vaccination for HPV16-positive vulvar lesions correlates with kinetics and phenotype of induced T-cell responses. *Proc. Natl. Acad. Sci. USA* **107**(26), 11895–11899.

Weterings, J. J., Khan, S., *et al.* (2006). Synthesis of 2-alkoxy-8-hydroxyadenylpeptides: Towards synthetic epitope-based vaccines. *Bioorg. Med. Chem. Lett.* **16**(12), 3258–3261.

Wille-Reece, U., Wu, C. Y., *et al.* (2005). Immunization with HIV-1 Gag protein conjugated to a TLR7/8 agonist results in the generation of HIV-1 Gag-specific Th1 and CD8+ T cell responses. *J. Immunol.* **174**(12), 7676–7683.

Wu, C. C., Hayashi, T., *et al.* (2007). Immunotherapeutic activity of a conjugate of a Toll-like receptor 7 ligand. *Proc. Natl. Acad. Sci. USA* **104**(10), 3990–3995.

York, I. A., Goldberg, A. L., *et al.* (1999). Proteolysis and class I major histocompatibility complex antigen presentation. *Immunol. Rev.* **172,** 49–66.

Zarour, H. M., and Ferrone, S. (2011). Cancer immunotherapy: Progress and challenges in the clinical setting. *Eur. J. Immunol.* **41**(6), 1510–1515.

Zeng, W., Horrocks, K. J., *et al.* (2011). A modular approach to assembly of totally synthetic self-adjuvanting lipopeptide-based vaccines allows conformational epitope building. *J. Biol. Chem.* **286**(15), 12944–12951.

Zhang, X., Chentoufi, A. A., *et al.* (2009). A genital tract peptide epitope vaccine targeting TLR-2 efficiently induces local and systemic CD8+ T cells and protects against herpes simplex virus type 2 challenge. *Mucosal Immunol.* **2**(2), 129–143.

zur Hausen, H. (2002). Papillomaviruses and cancer: From basic studies to clinical application. *Nat. Rev. Cancer* **2**(5), 342–350.

Zwaveling, S., Ferreira Mota, S. C., *et al.* (2002). Established human papillomavirus type 16-expressing tumors are effectively eradicated following vaccination with long peptides. *J. Immunol.* **169**(1), 350–358.

CHAPTER 8

Behavior and Function of Tissue-Resident Memory T cells

Silvia Ariotti, John B. Haanen, and **Ton N. Schumacher**

Contents

Abstract

Our understanding of memory T cell function in mice and men is to date in large part restricted to the behavior of circulating memory T cells. Emerging evidence, however, suggests that in addition to such systemic memory T cell populations, a separate population of locally confined memory T cells is generated at former sites of antigen encounter. Here, we discuss the potential function of these long-term tissue-resident memory T cells (T_{TRM}), how such local T cell memory can be maintained for prolonged periods of time, and how the induction of long-term tissue-resident memory T cells may potentially be exploited during vaccination.

Division of Immunology, The Netherlands Cancer Institute, Plesmanlaan, Amsterdam, The Netherlands

Advances in Immunology, Volume 114
ISSN 0065-2776, DOI: 10.1016/B978-0-12-396548-6.00008-1

1. INTRODUCTION

The formation of CD8 (cytotoxic) and CD4 (helper) T cell memory results from the encounter and control of infectious pathogens. Upon clearance of infection, the vast majority of the pathogen-specific T lymphocytes that were formed dies, but a small number of these now antigen-experienced T cells remain present in the host, ready to face new attacks from the same pathogen. The CD8 memory T cell pool is generally subdivided into two populations that can be distinguished by their differentiation state and migratory pattern. Lymph nodes harbor a population of memory T cells that express molecules such as CCR7 and CD62L that regulate lymph node access. Following renewed infection, these central memory T cells (T_{CM}) can undergo a renewed burst of proliferation, thereby generating a novel pool of effector T cells. In addition to this population of relatively immature memory T cells that circulate through the lymph nodes, the memory T cell compartment comprises a pool of cells that are more differentiated. These effector memory T cells (T_{EM}) have lost the capacity to enter the lymph nodes through the high endothelial venules and are present in both blood and peripheral tissues (Masopust *et al.*, 2001). Early work by Dudler and colleagues that demonstrated the presence of memory T cells in afferent lymph in sheep suggested a model in which memory T cells that are found in peripheral tissues continuously circulate through the secondary lymphoid organs and blood (Mackay *et al.*, 1990). A more detailed view of the circulation pattern of effector memory T cells was provided by seminal work by the Lefrançois group that examined the redistribution of antigen-specific CD8 memory T cells in mice that were surgically joined, resulting in the formation of a common blood compartment (Klonowski *et al.*, 2004). Analysis of the ratio of T cells derived from either partner in peripheral tissues of these parabiotic mice revealed that memory T cells at sites such as liver, bone marrow, and lung equilibrated within a period of weeks. As such, these data confirmed the model that memory T cells that are found in these tissues are in transit. Interestingly though, CD8 memory T cell populations in brain and also CD8 intestinal intraepithelial lymphocytes (IELs) did not equilibrate for a period of weeks to months. Thus, as based on memory T cell distribution in parabiotic mice, some peripheral tissues appear to contain stable compartments of memory T cells. Recent work has provided firm evidence that such tissue-resident memory T cells should indeed be seen as a separate memory T cell compartment and that the properties of these cells are influenced by the environment in which they reside.

2. REGULATION OF TISSUE-RESIDENT MEMORY T CELLS

2.1. Tissue-resident memory T cell compartments at different sites

Evidence for the presence of a long-term resident memory T cell population has now been provided for at least four tissue sites: sensory ganglia, skin, brain, and the intestinal epithelium. Specifically, (1) Gebhardt and colleagues used transplantation experiments to demonstrate that memory CD8 T cells present within the dorsal root ganglia of HSV-infected mice do not contribute to a subsequent systemic T cell response, whereas recent CD8 T cell immigrants in the very same ganglia do (Gebhardt *et al.*, 2009). (2). Likewise, transplantation of HSV-1 infected skin onto naïve recipients has been used to demonstrate that at least some skin-resident HSV-specific CD8 T cells persist within the tissue of origin for weeks (Gebhardt *et al.*, 2009). Further, in more recent work, this group exploited the immune response of female mice to male minor histocompatibility antigens to create a situation in which circulating memory T cells were rejected, and the fate of skin-resident T cells could thus be evaluated without potential influx of systemic memory T cells as a confounding factor. These experiments demonstrated that, whereas male HSV-specific T cells were no longer detectable in blood less than 2 weeks after transfer, skin-resident male T cells could still be recovered for at least 10 weeks (Gebhardt *et al.*, 2011). (3). CD8 T cells that reside within the brain parenchyma have been observed to remain present for at least 4 months after VSV infection (Wakim *et al.*, 2010). Further, *in situ* CFSE labeling revealed that at least part of this memory T cell population is in disequilibrium with the circulating memory T cell population, and therefore locally confined. (4). Following LCMV infection of mice, memory T cells are found in the intestinal epithelium. Importantly, these cells appear to be long-term residents as based on the fact that FTY treatment—a drug that prevents lymph node egress—does not reduce their numbers, whereas the frequency of T cells with the same antigen-specificity does go down in blood. Likewise, transplantation experiments indicated that no substantial turnover of these CD8 IEL occurred over a period of weeks (Masopust *et al.*, 2010).

A central issue in the experiments in these different models is whether the T cells can truly be considered (resting) memory T cells, or whether the cells may potentially receive continued signals by residual antigen, which could thereby promote their local maintenance. For skin, brain, and the intestinal epithelium, the evidence that T cells can survive locally without such an antigenic trigger appears solid: first, in the case of skin memory T cells, local retention can be observed for bystander T cells (although at somewhat lower numbers; see further), thereby excluding a role for TCR triggering (Gebhardt *et al.*, 2009). Second, resident memory T cells are formed within the intestinal epithelium even when the antigen is provided by the systemic route, thereby making it unlikely that a local antigen depot is maintained within the intestine (Masopust *et al.*, 2010; Wakim *et al.*, 2010). Finally, tissue-resident memory T cells in brain parenchyma have not only been observed following VSV infection, but also upon intracranial injection of peptide-loaded DC, indicating that retention is independent of *de novo* production of antigen during the memory phase (Wakim *et al.*, 2010). The issue of potential TCR triggering is more complicated though in the case of memory T cells that reside in sensory ganglia following HSV infection. HSV is generally assumed to enter into a latent phase following infection of mice, in which the immunodominant structural epitopes recognized by the TCR transgenic mice utilized in adoptive transfer experiments might not be expressed. The fact though that robust viral reactivation can occur under conditions of trauma (Wakim *et al.*, 2008) makes it difficult to exclude a lower level of expression of structural genes under steady state conditions. Indeed, it has been argued that HSV in latently infected ganglia is under continued active surveillance (Khanna *et al.*, 2003). Because of this concern, it will be important to validate observations that are made on T_{TRM} maintenance in latently infected ganglia in other experimental systems in which antigen expression is more readily controlled.

In conclusion, for a number of body sites—including the body sites that form major routes of pathogen entry—tissue-infiltrating memory T cells have been shown to exist as a self-sustaining population that can survive in the local environment and that is separated from its circulating counterpart.

2.2. Molecular mediators of retention

What are the molecular mediators that result in prolonged tissue retention? CD8 memory T cells that reside within peripheral tissues show a number of phenotypic changes that are likely to be associated with T cell retention. As a first (and thus far most well-studied) example, memory T cells that reside within the epidermis (Gebhardt *et al.*, 2009, 2011) and within the brain (Wakim *et al.*, 2010) show a clear-cut expression of the αEβ7 integrin CD103 that is not observed to the same extent on their circulating counterparts. The expression of CD103 by tissue-resident memory CD8 T cells is of interest as CD103 is also expressed by other immune cell types that reside within the epidermis such as epidermal γδT cells, regulatory T cells, and epithelial dendritic APCs (Bedoui *et al.*, 2009; Johansson-Lindbom and Agace, 2007; Lehmann *et al.*, 2002). Further, the key ligand of CD103, E-cadherin, is constitutively expressed on many epithelial tissues (Niessen, 2007), and γδT cells are significantly diminished in the epidermis of CD103-deficient mice (Schon *et al.*, 2002). In support of the hypothesis that CD103 could also be involved in the tissue retention of CD8 memory T cells, prior work has demonstrated that CD103 mediates the adhesion of activated CD8 T cells to cultured human keratinocytes (Pauls *et al.*, 2001).

Several models may be put forward to explain why $CD103^+$ T cells selectively accumulate at peripheral sites. As a first possibility, a small proportion of effector T cells that "happen" to express CD103 may simply be retained once these cells have entered the peripheral tissue. While a contribution of such straightforward local trapping of CD103-expressing cells cannot be excluded in full, it is plausible that more sophisticated mechanisms play a significant role. Prior work has established that CD103 surface expression on CD8 cells is increased upon exposure to TGFβ (Hadley *et al.*, 1997). Intriguingly, TGFβ is produced by dermal cells under steady-state conditions and this production is increased during wound healing when dermal fibroblasts migrate toward the lesion (Freedberg *et al.*, 2001). In addition, TGFβ produced by keratinocytes (Lee *et al.*, 1997) may potentially be sensed by incoming T cells, and either source of TGFβ may thereby induce increased surface expression of CD103. As a second mechanism for regulated expression of CD103, in a series of well-controlled experiments, Bevan and colleagues demonstrated that CD103 expression is primarily observed on CD8 T cells that encounter antigen locally (Wakim *et al.*, 2010). Thus, a feedback loop appears to exist that couples local antigen expression to prolonged phenotypic alterations. Evidence that CD103 expression is linked to the long-term presence of tissue-resident memory T cells was further provided by experiments that demonstrated the reduced presence of memory T cells in brain when CD103 expression was inhibited. While the latter observation seems most consistent with an effect of CD103 on local T cell accumulation by interaction with its ligand, it should be noted that E-cadherin is only expressed within epithelia, and currently there is no evidence that N-cadherin (neural cadherin) forms a ligand for CD103. It is possible that within the brain parenchyma, CD103 binds to other, as yet undefined, ligands.

In addition to its postulated effect on T cell retention, CD103 expression may also influence local T cell memory by other means, and it has been proposed that CD103 triggering that occurs concurrently with antigen recognition could act as a costimulatory signal and direct lytic granule polarization (Le Floc'h *et al.*, 2011). As a side note, KLRG1, another molecule expressed by effector phase T cells also forms a ligand for E- and N-cadherin (Ito *et al.*, 2006). However, at present there is no evidence that this interaction would promote long-term T cell retention, and such a hypothesis would also seem to go against the notion that KLRG1 expression forms one of the hallmarks of short-lived effector cells.

A feature that is shared by memory T cells derived from different tissues is the expression of CD69 (Gebhardt *et al.*, 2009; Laffon *et al.*, 1991;

Ostler *et al.*, 2001; Wang *et al.*, 2002). CD69 is an early leukocyte activation marker that is also expressed on T cells upon TCR triggering. It seems though that CD69 expression on tissue-resident T cells can occur independently of TCR triggering. Specifically, a gradual increase in CD69 expression on donor-derived IEL and lamina propria T cells was observed in parabiosis experiments in which antigen was unlikely to be present (Klonowski *et al.*, 2004). Notably, such CD69 expression was not observed on memory T cells in liver, spleen, and lung tissue, where memory T cells are only transient visitors. These data suggest that, for at least some of the peripheral tissues that harbor long-term residents, a tissue-derived signal leads to the expression of CD69. At present, there is no data that directly address the role of CD69 in the retention of tissue-resident T cells. However, in lymph node T cells, expression of CD69 has been shown to inhibit the function of the Sphingosine-1-Phosphate receptor 1 and thereby reduce T cell migration out of the lymph node in response to a S1P gradient (Shiow *et al.*, 2006). By analogy, it seems plausible that induction of CD69 on T cells that have entered certain peripheral sites could form a mechanism to desensitize the cells to chemotactic triggers that would otherwise promote their exit. In this regard, it is interesting to note that expression of the Aryl hydrocarbon receptor (AhR) has recently been shown to be required for the maintenance of γδ T cells in the epidermis and that AhR-deficient γδ T cells show less frequent expression of CD69 than wild-type γδ T cells (Kadow *et al.*, 2011). These data seem consistent with a model in which CD69 expression by tissue-resident cells is a reflection of their (nonantigen dependent) interaction with the surrounding tissue, thereby influencing T cell maintenance. Finally, it is likely that other molecular mediators exist that influence the local retention of T cells within peripheral tissue, and in case of T_{TRM} that reside in the skin, increased expression of VLA-1 has, for instance, been observed (Gebhardt *et al.*, 2009).

2.3. Local survival and proliferation

As discussed above, resident memory CD8 T cells have been recovered from skin, ganglia, and intestinal epithelium weeks after initial antigen encounter (Gebhardt *et al.*, 2009, 2011; Masopust JEM 2010), and brain-resident T cells have been detected up to 120 days after VSV inoculation (Wakim *et al.*, 2010). Further, cutaneous vaccination with naked DNA has been shown to lead to the presence of memory CD8 T cells at the vaccination site, but not in other skin areas of the same animal for at least 1 year (S. Ariotti *et al.*, unpublished observations). Thus, while no careful analysis of the long-term stability of the tissue-resident T cell population has been performed, the evidence for long-term maintenance is substantial.

As the available data suggest that the tissue-resident population does not depend on *de novo* influx of circulating memory T cells, long-term maintenance must rely either on a very low death rate of the tissue-resident cells or on a sufficient level of proliferation to allow maintenance of the resident T cell pool. Experiments that examined BrdU uptake in brain- and skin-resident memory CD8 T cells during the steady state (i.e., in the absence of antigen) indicate that in both cases the level of homeostatic T cell proliferation is low (Gebhardt *et al.*, 2009; Wakim *et al.*, 2010). Thus, maintenance of the local T cell pool seems to largely rely on the longevity of the T cells at those sites.

A plethora of studies that examined the maintenance of the systemic memory T cell pool has previously shown that this cell population depends on cytokines such as IL-7 and IL-15 for homeostatic proliferation and survival (Becker *et al.*, 2002; Goldrath *et al.*, 2002; Judge *et al.*, 2002). Assuming that tissue-resident memory T cells would display a similar cytokine requirement, how can these cells get access to prosurvival cytokines while deeply buried in peripheral tissues? Intriguingly, IL-15 has been shown to be expressed by a large array of cells, stimulating survival and proliferation in all immune and nonimmune cell types that express the IL-15Rα receptor (Budagian *et al.*, 2006). In the central nervous system, IL-15 mRNA is expressed in microglia, astrocytes, and neural cells, and it is upregulated upon inflammation (Gomez-Nicola *et al.*, 2011). In the skin, keratinocytes express both IL-15 and its receptor, and IL-15 signaling is important in the regulation of keratinocyte turnover (Ruckert *et al.*, 2000). Thus, it is conceivable that effector phase T cells that have infiltrated the peripheral tissue might rely on locally produced IL-15 (and potentially other survival-inducing molecules) for their survival once the infection-induced inflammation has resolved. Some support for this hypothesis is provided by the observation that local amounts of IL-15 correlate with the number and the proliferative status of infiltrating T cells in human hypertrophic skin (Castagnoli *et al.*, 1999). On the other hand, evidence against a dominant role of IL-15 signaling in local T cell maintenance is provided by the observation that CD122 (the IL-2 and IL-15 receptor β chain) expression on brain-resident CD8 T cells is low, as compared to that found on systemic memory CD8 T cells (Wakim *et al.*, 2010). Furthermore, IL-15 appeared dispensable for the maintenance of HSV-specific CD8 T cells in the trigeminal ganglia of previously infected mice, although in the latter case, low-level antigen production is likely to have influenced the cytokine requirements of these cells (Sheridan *et al.*, 2006).

3. POTENTIAL FUNCTIONS OF TISSUE-RESIDENT MEMORY T CELLS

3.1. Requirements for reactivation

The long-term presence of a local CD8 T cell memory pool only seems of value if these T cells could undergo reactivation at that peripheral site. T cell reactivation may then lead either to effector functions (see Section 3.2) or to *in situ* proliferation of the tissue-resident memory CD8 T cells. At present, the only data on the cellular requirements for T_{TRM} reactivation come from work by Carbone and colleagues that examined the proliferation of ganglia-resident memory CD8 T cells following viral reactivation (Wakim *et al.*, 2008). When latently infected ganglia of HSV-1 immune mice that contained HSV-specific memory T cells were transferred into naïve recipients, a drop in the number of tissue-resident CD8 T cells was initially observed, but this was followed by a substantial increase in HSV-specific T cell numbers in the following days. This increase in cell numbers was not observed for control memory T cells residing at the same site, indicating that it was antigen driven. Further, when two latently infected ganglia containing HSV-specific T cells that could be distinguished by allotype markers were cotransplanted, no substantial mingling of the two expanding cell populations was observed, providing strong evidence that T cell proliferation took place *in situ*. Further experiments in this model that addressed the cellular requirements for the observed *in situ* proliferation demonstrated that depletion of $CD4^+$ T cells reduced *in situ* memory CD8 T cell proliferation and demonstrated that MHC class I-restricted antigen presentation by bone marrow-derived APC was also required for optimal expansion. It is important to note that these experiments did not address the acquisition of effector functions and it is possible that these cell functions would not rely on antigen presentation by APCs and/or the presence of CD4 helper cells. This issue is of particular relevance, as there is little evidence that the intestinal epithelium contains resident CD4 memory T cells. Likewise, recent work has demonstrated that following clearance of HSV infection of the skin, CD4 T cells are primarily found in the dermal layer and are not found in substantial numbers within the epidermal layer in which CD8 memory T cells reside (Gebhardt *et al.*, 2011). Based on these observations, it would seem plausible that tissue-resident memory CD8 T cells can exert at least some functions independently of CD4 T cell help at the moment antigen is again encountered. The possible role of local APCs, such as Langerhans cells in the skin, in resident CD8 memory T cell reactivation has to date not been established.

3.2. Evidence for effector activity

What is the evidence for a local function of tissue-resident memory T cells? Recent analysis of the transcription profile of ganglia- and skin-resident memory T cells of HSV-immune mice demonstrated that these two memory T cell populations are not alike (Mintern *et al.*, 2007, JI, AOP). Specifically, transcripts of "T cell effector proteins" such as perforin and granzymes were low in skin-resident memory T cells even though they were abundant during the effector phase. In contrast, tissue-resident cells derived from infected or latent ganglia showed transcription of cytolytic molecules at both time points. These data fit with earlier work in which the activation profile of HSV- and OVA-specific CD8 T cells infiltrating latently infected ganglia was analyzed, and that demonstrated that only HSV-specific memory T cells maintained the production of granzyme B and the expression of CD69 (van Lint *et al.*, 2005). As there is evidence for continued antigen presentation in latently infected ganglia (van Lint *et al.*, 2005), these data suggest that effector T cells that reside in tissues in which antigen has been fully cleared are incapable of immediate activity and first need to restart production of effector phase molecules.

Taking advantage of the fact that skin-resident memory T cells remain confined to areas of former infection, Gebhardt and colleagues devised an experiment to investigate the "added value" of a local memory T cell pool. B cell-deficient mice that had experienced a prior HSV flank infection were depleted of CD4 and/or CD8 cells and then reinfected, both at the site of the primary infection and at the contralateral site, and viral titers were compared (Gebhardt *et al.*, 2009). This experiment demonstrated that secondary HSV infection was cleared faster at the site of prior infection. Further, antibody depletion experiments demonstrated that this superior protection could be attributed to CD4 cells and—to a lesser extent—CD8 cells. Thus, although the mechanisms of viral control have not been established, there is at least some evidence for a value of local T cell memory upon a second encounter of the same pathogen.

For some of the Herpes viruses, such a second encounter at the same site is plausible when reactivation from the latent state occurs (Diefenbach *et al.*, 2008). A question that comes up though is why epidermal memory cells do not in substantial numbers populate—and thereby protect—the entire surface of the skin or intestinal epithelium. As a first potential explanation, CD8 memory T cells may simply not have the opportunity to accumulate at other sites, as tissue entry is guided by local inflammatory signals. In addition, the energetic cost of such organ-wide resident memory may outweigh its potential benefit. Finally, as discussed in Section 4.1, tissue-resident T cell memory is not only beneficial but can also be a cause of pathology.

4. TISSUE-RESIDENT MEMORY T CELLS AND VACCINATION

4.1. Evidence for T_{TRM} in humans

Fixed drug eruption (FDE) is a human skin disorder in which the intake of an inducing drug leads to the formation of erythematous lesions on well-circumscribed areas of the skin. Because the lesions occur in the same skin areas even when the inducing antigen is given after a long-time interval, and as FDE appears to be due to IFNγ-mediated autoimmune destruction of skin keratinocytes, FDE can be considered a form of locally confined immune memory. Interestingly, skin-infiltrating T cells in the patients with FDE have been found in diseased areas up to 4 years after the last antigenic stimulation (Mizukawa *et al.*, 2008), and FDE skin sites are characterized by the presence of CD8 T cells at the basal or suprabasal layer (Hindsen *et al.*, 1987), the site in which antigen-specific skin-resident CD8 memory T cells have recently been found in mice. Further, the T cell receptor repertoire of intra-epidermal T cells in clinically resolved FDE lesions has been shown to be narrow, consistent with the thought that T cells at FDE sites form the long-term memory of an antigen-specific T cell response (Komatsu *et al.*, 1996). In support of this notion, FDE has been observed to occur at sites of prior trauma (Mizukawa and Shiohara, 2002). Finally, consistent with findings in mice, phenotypic analysis of intra-epidermal T cells in the dormant phase revealed that virtually all T cells expressed CD103 and high levels of CD69 (Mizukawa *et al.*, 2002). Further evidence for the presence of a pathogen-specific epidermal memory CD8 T cell compartment in humans comes from the analysis of T cell infiltrates in active and resolved HSV lesions. Whereas during active infection, CD4 and CD8 cells were shown to be intermingled, CD4 cells retreated from the epidermis after resolution of the lesion whereas CD8 cells stayed put (Zhu *et al.*, 2009). It should be noted that in this case, local CD8 numbers appear to go down over a period of months, something that appears to contrast with the longevity of T cells in at least some FDE lesions. Because of this apparent discrepancy, a more detailed analysis of the stability of local T cell memory in humans would certainly be useful.

4.2. Potential value of T_{TRM} in vaccination

Analysis of the ratio of T cells versus virus-infected cells at early time points of infection has led to the model that vaccines that would yield a sufficient number of pathogen-specific T cells at portals of pathogen entry may efficiently limit viral spreading (Li *et al.*, 2009). One potential way by which such a rapid local T cell response may be achieved is through the continuous stimulation of a T_{EM} pool that is capable of circulating through peripheral tissues (Hansen *et al.*, 2011). Alternatively, or in addition, if a tissue-resident T cell pool can be generated by vaccination, this could form a valuable first defense upon pathogen entry. How could one best induce such tissue-resident memory T cell populations in humans?

First, at least in the case of IEL, the development of a T cell response upon systemic vaccination leads to the formation of T_{TRM}. Thus, without any deliberate effort to create a local memory T cell population, such a pool can apparently already be formed. Further, based on the fact that CLA and Integrin alpha4Beta7 expression is also induced on human T cells following conventional vaccination, it seems plausible that vaccination of humans can likewise lead to the formation of a T_{TRM} pool (Masopust *et al.*, 2010).

Second, there is abundant evidence that—at least in mice—the route of vaccination can increase the expression of cell surface markers such as CLA that guide T cell homing to different peripheral sites (Santamaria-Babi, 2004; Warger *et al.*, 2007). Consequently, the strength of the tissue-resident memory T cell response can be expected to be increased when vaccine is delivered at a matched site. In line with this, skin scarification with vaccinia virus was recently shown to generate superior protection against a cutaneous challenge as compared to systemic vaccine delivery (Liu *et al.*, 2010).

Third, comparison of the frequency of long-term memory cells in skin tissue sites that were inflamed at the time of vaccination or that were quiescent suggests that the presence of an inflammatory signal at the time of vaccination contributes substantially to the creation of long-term T cell memory at that site (S. Ariotti *et al.*, unpublished observations). At present, the molecular signals that are required for T cells to gain access and remain at peripheral sites have not been defined. However, when it would be clear which signals are essential, it may theoretically be possible to steer the T cells that are induced by classical vaccination to an epithelial tissue of interest.

Fourth, data from both the Carbone and Bevan labs suggest that T_{TRM} numbers remain higher and CD103 expression is increased when antigen is encountered at the peripheral site, (Gebhardt *et al.*, 2009; Wakim *et al.*, 2010). At present, it has not been established whether the increase in local T cell numbers is primarily due to local T cell proliferation or due to increased retention/survival. However, regardless of the mechanism, these data indicate that optimal generation of a local T cell pool would probably not only require the administration of T cell attracting/retaining signals at a site of interest but may also require the supply of local antigen.

5. CONCLUDING REMARKS

Recent work provides strong evidence for the presence of locally confined T cell memory in peripheral tissues. Based on the fact that this local T cell memory appears to be regulated by defined molecular interactions, such as the induction of CD103, it seems likely that this local memory does not simply form an "immunological scar" of a prior encounter but serves to protect against recurrent infection with the same pathogen or pathogen reactivation. If it proves possible to induce prolonged local memory at defined epithelial surfaces in humans by vaccination, this could be a useful approach to induce a first line of defense against human pathogens such as HIV or HPV.

REFERENCES

Becker, T. C., Wherry, E. J., Boone, D., Murali-Krishna, K., Antia, R., Ma, A., and Ahmed, R. (2002). Interleukin 15 is required for proliferative renewal of virus-specific memory CD8 T cells. *J. Exp. Med.* **195,** 1541–1548.

Bedoui, S., Whitney, P. G., Waithman, J., Eidsmo, L., Wakim, L., Caminschi, I., Allan, R. S., Wojtasiak, M., Shortman, K., Carbone, F. R., Brooks, A. G., and Heath, W. R. (2009). Cross-presentation of viral and self antigens by skin-derived CD103+ dendritic cells. *Nat. Immunol.* **10,** 488–495.

Budagian, V., Bulanova, E., Paus, R., and Bulfone-Paus, S. (2006). IL-15/IL-15 receptor biology: A guided tour through an expanding universe. *Cytokine Growth Factor Rev.* **17,** 259–280.

Castagnoli, C., Trombotto, C., Ariotti, S., Millesimo, M., Ravarino, D., Magliacani, G., Ponzi, A. N., Stella, M., Teich-Alasia, S., Novelli, F., and Musso, T. (1999). Expression and role of IL-15 in post-burn hypertrophic scars. *J. Invest. Dermatol.* **113,** 238–245.

Diefenbach, R. J., Miranda-Saksena, M., Douglas, M. W., and Cunningham, A. L. (2008). Transport and egress of herpes simplex virus in neurons. *Rev. Med. Virol.* **18,** 35–51.

Freedberg, I. M., Tomic-Canic, M., Komine, M., and Blumenberg, M. (2001). Keratins and the keratinocyte activation cycle. *J. Invest. Dermatol.* **116,** 633–640.

Gebhardt, T., Wakim, L. M., Eidsmo, L., Reading, P. C., Heath, W. R., and Carbone, F. R. (2009). Memory T cells in nonlymphoid tissue that provide enhanced local immunity during infection with herpes simplex virus. *Nat. Immunol.* **10,** 524–530.

Gebhardt, T., Whitney, P. G., Zaid, A., Mackay, L. K., Brooks, A. G., Heath, W. R., Carbone, F. R., and Mueller, S. N. (2011). Different patterns of peripheral migration by memory CD4(+) and CD8(+) T cells. *Nature* **477,** 216–219.

Goldrath, A. W., Sivakumar, P. V., Glaccum, M., Kennedy, M. K., Bevan, M. J., Benoist, C., Mathis, D., and Butz, E. A. (2002). Cytokine requirements for acute and basal homeostatic proliferation of naive and memory CD8(+) T cells. *J. Exp. Med.* **195,** 1515–1522.

Gomez-Nicola, D., Valle-Argos, B., Pallas-Bazarra, N., and Nieto-Sampedro, M. (2011). Interleukin-15 regulates proliferation and self-renewal of adult neural stem cells. *Mol. Biol. Cell* **22,** 1960–1970.

Hadley, G. A., Bartlett, S. T., Via, C. S., Rostapshova, E. A., and Moainie, S. (1997). The epithelial cell-specific integrin, CD103 (alpha E integrin), defines a novel subset of alloreactive CD8+ CTL. *J. Immunol.* **159,** 3748–3756.

Hansen, S. G., Ford, J. C., Lewis, M. S., Ventura, A. B., Hughes, C. M., Coyne-Johnson, L., Whizin, N., Oswald, K., Shoemaker, R., Swanson, T., Legasse, A. W., Chiuchiolo, M. J., *et al.* (2011). Profound early control of highly pathogenic SIV by an effector memory T-cell vaccine. *Nature* **473,** 523–527.

Hindsen, M., Christensen, O. B., Gruic, V., and Lofberg, H. (1987). Fixed drug eruption: An immunohistochemical investigation of the acute and healing phase. *Br. J. Dermatol.* **116,** 351–360.

Ito, M., Maruyama, T., Saito, N., Koganei, S., Yamamoto, K., and Matsumoto, N. (2006). Killer cell lectin-like receptor G1 binds three members of the classical cadherin family to inhibit NK cell cytotoxicity. *J. Exp. Med.* **203,** 289–295.

Johansson-Lindbom, B., and Agace, W. W. (2007). Generation of gut-homing T cells and their localization to the small intestinal mucosa. *Immunol. Rev.* **215,** 226–242.

Judge, A. D., Zhang, X., Fujii, H., Surh, C. D., and Sprent, J. (2002). Interleukin 15 controls both proliferation and survival of a subset of memory-phenotype CD8(+) T cells. *J. Exp. Med.* **196,** 935–946.

Kadow, S., Jux, B., Zahner, S. P., Wingerath, B., Chmill, S., Clausen, B. E., Hengstler, J., and Esser, C. (2011). Aryl hydrocarbon receptor is critical for homeostasis of invariant gamma-delta T cells in the murine epidermis. *J. Immunol.* **187,** 3104–3110.

Khanna, K. M., Bonneau, R. H., Kinchington, P. R., and Hendricks, R. L. (2003). Herpes simplex virus-specific memory CD8(+) T cells are selectively activated and retained in latently infected sensory ganglia. *Immunity* **18,** 593–603.

Klonowski, K. D., Williams, K. J., Marzo, A. L., Blair, D. A., Lingenheld, E. G., and Lefrancois, L. (2004). Dynamics of blood-borne CD8 memory T cell migration *in vivo*. *Immunity* **20,** 551–562.

Komatsu, T., Moriya, N., and Shiohara, T. (1996). T cell receptor (TCR) repertoire and function of human epidermal T cells: Restricted TCR V alpha-V beta genes are utilized by T cells residing in the lesional epidermis in fixed drug eruption. *Clin. Exp. Immunol.* **104,** 343–350.

Laffon, A., Garcia-Vicuna, R., Humbria, A., Postigo, A. A., Corbi, A. L., de Landazuri, M. O., and Sanchez-Madrid, F. (1991). Upregulated expression and function of VLA-4 fibronectin receptors on human activated T cells in rheumatoid arthritis. *J. Clin. Invest.* **88,** 546–552.

Le Floc'h, A., Jalil, A., Franciszkiewicz, K., Validire, P., Vergnon, I., and Mami-Chouaib, F. (2011). Minimal engagement of CD103 on cytotoxic T lymphocytes with an E-cadherin-Fc molecule triggers lytic granule polarization via a phospholipase Cgamma-dependent pathway. *Cancer Res.* **71,** 328–338.

Lee, H. S., Kooshesh, F., Sauder, D. N., and Kondo, S. (1997). Modulation of TGF-beta 1 production from human keratinocytes by UVB. *Exp. Dermatol.* **6,** 105–110.

Lehmann, J., Huehn, J., de la Rosa, M., Maszyna, F., Kretschmer, U., Krenn, V., Brunner, M., Scheffold, A., and Hamann, A. (2002). Expression of the integrin alpha Ebeta 7 identifies unique subsets of CD25(+) as well as CD25(−) regulatory T cells. *Proc. Natl. Acad. Sci. USA* **99,** 13031–13036.

Li, Q., Skinner, P. J., Ha, S. J., Duan, L., Mattila, T. L., Hage, A., White, C., Barber, D. L., O'Mara, L., Southern, P. J., Reilly, C. S., Carlis, J. V., *et al.* (2009). Visualizing antigen-specific and infected cells *in situ* predicts outcomes in early viral infection. *Science* **323,** 1726–1729.

Liu, L., Zhong, Q., Tian, T., Dubin, K., Athale, S. K., and Kupper, T. S. (2010). Epidermal injury and infection during poxvirus immunization is crucial for the generation of highly protective T cell-mediated immunity. *Nat. Med.* **16,** 224–227.

Mackay, C. R., Marston, W. L., and Dudler, L. (1990). Naive and memory T cells show distinct pathways of lymphocyte recirculation. *J. Exp. Med.* **171,** 801–817.

Masopust, D., Vezys, V., Marzo, A. L., and Lefrancois, L. (2001). Preferential localization of effector memory cells in nonlymphoid tissue. *Science* **291,** 2413–2417.

Masopust, D., Choo, D., Vezys, V., Wherry, E. J., Duraiswamy, J., Akondy, R., Wang, J., Casey, K. A., Barber, D. L., Kawamura, K. S., Fraser, K. A., Webby, R. J., *et al.* (2010). Dynamic T cell migration program provides resident memory within intestinal epithelium. *J. Exp. Med.* **207,** 553–564.

Mintern, J. D., Guillonneau, C., Carbone, F. R., Doherty, P. C., and Turner, S. J. (2007). Cutting edge: Tissue-resident memory CTL down-regulate cytolytic molecule expression following virus clearance. *J. Immunol.* **179,** 7220–7224.

Mizukawa, Y., and Shiohara, T. (2002). Trauma-localized fixed drug eruption: Involvement of burn scars, insect bites and venipuncture sites. *Dermatology* **205,** 159–161.

Mizukawa, Y., Yamazaki, Y., Teraki, Y., Hayakawa, J., Hayakawa, K., Nuriya, H., Kohara, M., and Shiohara, T. (2002). Direct evidence for interferon-gamma production by effector-memory-type intraepidermal T cells residing at an effector site of immunopathology in fixed drug eruption. *Am. J. Pathol.* **161,** 1337–1347.

Mizukawa, Y., Yamazaki, Y., and Shiohara, T. (2008). *In vivo* dynamics of intraepidermal CD8(+) T cells and CD4(+) T cells during the evolution of fixed drug eruption. *Br. J. Dermatol.* **158,** 1230–1238.

Niessen, C. M. (2007). Tight junctions/adherens junctions: Basic structure and function. *J. Invest. Dermatol.* **127,** 2525–2532.

Ostler, T., Hussell, T., Surh, C. D., Openshaw, P., and Ehl, S. (2001). Long-term persistence and reactivation of T cell memory in the lung of mice infected with respiratory syncytial virus. *Eur. J. Immunol.* **31,** 2574–2582.

Pauls, K., Schon, M., Kubitza, R. C., Homey, B., Wiesenborn, A., Lehmann, P., Ruzicka, T., Parker, C. M., and Schon, M. P. (2001). Role of integrin alphaE(CD103)beta7 for tissue-specific epidermal localization of CD8(+) T lymphocytes. *J. Invest. Dermatol.* **117,** 569–575.

Ruckert, R., Asadullah, K., Seifert, M., Budagian, V. M., Arnold, R., Trombotto, C., Paus, R., and Bulfone-Paus, S. (2000). Inhibition of keratinocyte apoptosis by IL-15: A new parameter in the pathogenesis of psoriasis? *J. Immunol.* **165,** 2240–2250.

Santamaria-Babi, L. F. (2004). CLA(+) T cells in cutaneous diseases. *Eur. J. Dermatol.* **14,** 13–18.

Schon, M. P., Schon, M., Parker, C. M., and Williams, I. R. (2002). Dendritic epidermal T cells (DETC) are diminished in integrin alphaE(CD103)-deficient mice. *J. Invest. Dermatol.* **119,** 190–193.

Sheridan, B. S., Khanna, K. M., Frank, G. M., and Hendricks, R. L. (2006). Latent virus influences the generation and maintenance of CD8(+) T cell memory. *J. Immunol.* **177,** 8356–8364.

Shiow, L. R., Rosen, D. B., Brdickova, N., Xu, Y., An, J., Lanier, L. L., Cyster, J. G., and Matloubian, M. (2006). CD69 acts downstream of interferon-alpha/beta to inhibit S1P1 and lymphocyte egress from lymphoid organs. *Nature* **440,** 540–544.

van Lint, A. L., Kleinert, L., Clarke, S. R., Stock, A., Heath, W. R., and Carbone, F. R. (2005). Latent infection with herpes simplex virus is associated with ongoing CD8(+) T-cell stimulation by parenchymal cells within sensory ganglia. *J. Virol.* **79,** 14843–14851.

Wakim, L. M., Waithman, J., van Rooijen, N., Heath, W. R., and Carbone, F. R. (2008). Dendritic cell-induced memory T cell activation in nonlymphoid tissues. *Science* **319,** 198–202.

Wakim, L. M., Woodward-Davis, A., and Bevan, M. J. (2010). Memory T cells persisting within the brain after local infection show functional adaptations to their tissue of residence. *Proc. Natl. Acad. Sci. USA* **107,** 17872–17879.

Wang, H. C., Zhou, Q., Dragoo, J., and Klein, J. R. (2002). Most murine CD8(+) intestinal intraepithelial lymphocytes are partially but not fully activated T cells. *J. Immunol.* **169,** 4717–4722.

Warger, T., Schild, H., and Rechtsteiner, G. (2007). Initiation of adaptive immune responses by transcutaneous immunization. *Immunol. Lett.* **109,** 13–20.

Zhu, J., Hladik, F., Woodward, A., Klock, A., Peng, T., Johnston, C., Remington, M., Magaret, A., Koelle, D. M., Wald, A., and Corey, L. (2009). Persistence of HIV-1 receptor-positive cells after HSV-2 reactivation is a potential mechanism for increased HIV-1 acquisition. *Nat. Med.* **15,** 886–892.

CHAPTER 9

Rational Design of Vaccines: Learning from Immune Evasion Mechanisms of Persistent Viruses and Tumors

Ramon Arens

Contents

Abstract

The induction of adaptive immunity and prevention of tolerance is a critical component of vaccination and immunotherapy in order to prevent pathogen-related diseases and to eradicate malignant cells. Although many acute infections can be controlled by vaccination, the development of prophylactic and therapeutic vaccines against persistent viruses and tumors remains challenging. The diverse immune evasion strategies used by persistent DNA viruses such as herpesviruses contribute directly to their persistence and escape from immune control. Intriguingly, many tumors have also developed

Department of Immunohematology and Blood Transfusion, Leiden University Medical Center, Albinusdreef 2, Leiden, The Netherlands

Advances in Immunology, Volume 114
ISSN 0065-2776, DOI: 10.1016/B978-0-12-396548-6.00009-3

escape mechanisms to dismantle similar aspects of the host's immune system. Analogous targets of immune evasion mechanisms comprise suppression of antigen presentation and T cell costimulatory pathways, induction of immunosuppressive cytokines, and obstruction of interferon and chemokine functions, which emphasizes them not only as critical elements of T cell activation pathways but also as the potential "Achilles' heels" of the host immune system. The insight that immune evasion by viruses and tumors targets analogous host immune pathways might lead to cross-pollination of the viral and tumor immunology research fields, which could lead to new perspectives and appreciation of the intricacies and subtleties that arise from the merging of these fields. Accordingly, a rational and combinatorial manipulation of immune evasion pathways and their targets should aid in the development of safer and more effective vaccine strategies and immunotherapies for a wide range of infections and malignancies.

1. IMMUNE EVASION BY PERSISTENT VIRUSES AND TUMORS

Vaccination is the most successful and cost-effective of all medical achievements available to public health (Rappuoli *et al.*, 2002; Roush and Murphy, 2007). The morbidity and mortality of pathogen-related diseases such as diphtheria, pertussis, tetanus, polio, measles, mumps, rubella, and smallpox have declined drastically (>95–100%) due to prophylactic vaccines, usually provided during childhood. The success of preventive vaccines in combating these contagious diseases is based on effective induction of B cell memory and long-lasting production of antibodies that are capable of directly inactivating pathogens or by acting through co-operation with other immune cells or complement. $CD8^+$ T cell responses are also key parameters of protective immunity, especially in the case of infection with intracellular bacteria and viruses. Helper $CD4^+$ T cells are important for development of B cell expansion, class switching, and affinity maturation as well as for development of memory $CD8^+$ T cell responses. In addition, direct $CD4^+$ T cell effector activity is important to combat certain persistent infections such as tuberculosis and malaria. Effective eradication of tumor cells typically involves both effector $CD8^+$ and $CD4^+$ T cell responses, but sometimes humoral responses are induced as well. Thus, depending on the nature of the pathogen or tumor type, development of B cell, $CD8^+$ T cell, and/or $CD4^+$ T cell responses is critical to confer protective immunity.

During the past decades, an exceptional increase in novel vaccine development has occurred, with design of vaccines not only for infectious diseases in children but also for infections in healthy adults, pregnant women, and elderly people, and for certain types of cancer. Novel methods of discovery based on genomic analysis and systems biology have been instrumental and provided unique opportunities to select the most appropriate antigens (Rappuoli *et al.*, 2011). Promising new vaccines for different diseases are on their way and the use of synthetic vaccines provides a safer method to overcome certain risks associated with live attenuated pathogens. Despite these hopeful prospects, still numerous devastating pathogen-induced diseases and most types of tumors are currently not vaccine preventable.

An important hurdle toward the goal of protection against persistent pathogens and malignant diseases is their evasion of the host immune system. Whereas RNA viruses like human immunodeficiency virus (HIV), hepatitis C virus, and influenza virus undergo, due to selective pressure of the immune system, extensive antigenic variation leading to immune escape, large DNA viruses such as herpesviruses and poxviruses encode immunomodulatory genes that directly evade the host innate and adaptive immune responses. The long coevolution of these viruses with their host is believed to have contributed to the evolution of a complex pathogen–host coexistence (Lefkowitz *et al.*, 2006; McGeoch *et al.*, 1995). A sign of successful adaptation and involvement of powerful immune evasion mechanisms is that the vast majority of the human population (estimated 60–100%) is infected with at least one herpesvirus of which Epstein–Barr virus (EBV; human herpesvirus 4) and human cytomegalovirus (HCMV; human herpesvirus-5) are considered as the prototypic members of the γ and β herpesfamily, respectively (Cannon *et al.*, 2010). Moreover, herpesviruses establish lifelong infections in healthy individuals and harbor the ability to reinfect (even by the same viral strain) despite the presence of a detectable immune response. Poxviruses cause generally acute infections but, depending on the route of infection and immunocompetence of the host, persistent infection may occur (Brownstein *et al.*, 1991). The prototype of the poxvirus family is vaccinia virus, which has been used as a successful vaccine to eradicate the human pathogen variola virus (the agent of smallpox). Both herpesviruses and poxviruses have proven adept at preventing T cell activation through the actions of dedicated immune evasion proteins. Although the main strategy of large DNA viruses is to encode for proteins that interact directly with molecules of the host immune system, this does not exclude the possibility that mutations in large DNA viruses can develop through immunological pressure. For example, mutations in the mouse CMV (MCMV) m157 gene, which encodes a viral protein that binds the Ly49H NK cell activation receptor, arise through immunological pressure by strong Ly49H-dependent NK cell responses (French *et al.*, 2004; Voigt *et al.*, 2003).

A critical element for developing immunity to tumors is the recognition of tumor-specific antigens and tumor-associated antigens by the host T cells (Boon *et al.*, 2006; Lee *et al.*, 1999; Savage *et al.*, 2008; Schietinger *et al.*, 2008; Willimsky and Blankenstein, 2007). Well-known tumor-specific antigens, caused by somatic mutations, comprise p53, BCR-ABL, and Ras. Identified tumor-associated antigens include differentiation antigens (tyrosinase, MART-1), amplified and/or overexpressed antigens (MDM2, HER-2/neu), and cancer/testis antigens (MAGE and RAGE families) that are expressed by germ cells and cancers, but not normal somatic cells. In addition, certain viruses such as EBV and human papilloma virus (HPV) cause B cell lymphomas and cervical cancer, respectively, and therefore the viral antigens expressed by these tumors can be considered to be tumor antigens as well. It is well established that the immune system harbors protective capacity against tumor cells and that tumor progression is accompanied by evading attack by immune cells (tumor escape) as a result of selective immunological pressure (Dunn *et al.*, 2004; Schreiber *et al.*, 2011). This immunoediting likely occurs from the beginning since mutations in antigen-recognition pathways, for example, are already present in early malignant lesions and are regularly associated with tumor progression (Garrido *et al.*, 2010; Khong and Restifo, 2002). Tumors most likely acquire progressively more escape mechanisms by the interplay with the immune system, but the exact kinetics of this development is currently unclear.

A better understanding of immune evasion mechanisms by viruses and tumors and the development of host immune responses is of interest not only for understanding disease mechanisms but also for prophylactic and therapeutic vaccination strategies against chronic viruses and cancer. To this end, this review focuses on the immune evasion mechanisms used by both viruses and tumors that target remarkably analogous aspects of the host immune system to achieve the same goal: escape destruction by the immune system to continue to exist. In particular, the immune evasion mechanisms by the prototypic members of the herpesvirus and poxvirus families and by cancers will be discussed side by side. Since control of viral infection and tumor rejection typically involves T cell immunity, those immune evasion mechanisms that target antigen-recognition and T cell activation will be addressed. In addition, the therapeutic interventions that counteract immune evasion by viruses and malignant cells will be considered as well as the possibility to exploit the knowledge regarding immune evasion to improve clinical protocols and develop novel vaccine strategies.

2. IMMUNE EVASION OF ANTIGEN PRESENTATION PATHWAYS

The presentation of virus- or tumor-specific peptides in the context of major histocompatibility complex (MHC) molecules is central for the recognition by the T cell receptor (TCR). MHC class I molecules assemble with peptides in the endoplasmic reticulum (ER) and are transported via the Golgi apparatus to the cell surface for recognition by the TCR. The peptides that are loaded in class I molecules generally result from degradation of proteins in the cytosol by the proteasome and subsequent translocation into the ER by the transporter associated with antigen processing (TAP) protein, but also TAP-independent pathways exist. Exogenous proteins that are taken up from their environment can be processed by professional antigen-presenting cells (APCs) such as dendritic cells and loaded onto class II molecules for presentation to $CD4^+$ T cells, and can, as an alternative to presentation of peptides derived from endogenously synthesized proteins, also be loaded to class I molecules to prime $CD8^+$ T cells. The latter route of presenting exogenous antigens via MHC class I molecules is known as cross-presentation and is an important strategy for development of T cell immunity against certain viruses (Heath and Carbone, 2001).

Viral immune evasion proteins target many different steps of the MHC class I and II presentation pathways including inhibition of assembly, transport, and surface expression of MHC molecules, which emphasize the evolutionary pressure exerted by $CD8^+$ and $CD4^+$ T cells during coevolution of viruses with their hosts (Hansen and Bouvier, 2009; Johnson and Hegde, 2002; Ploegh, 1998; Yewdell and Hill, 2002). EBV encodes the latency-associated protein EBNA1, which interferes with the cleaving action of the proteasome, thereby reducing the generation of antigenic peptides (Lautscham *et al.*, 2003). Other EBV-encoded proteins that interfere with class I presentation include BNLF2a, which inhibits peptide-binding functions of TAP (Hislop *et al.*, 2007), and BILF1, a viral G-protein-coupled receptor (vGPCR) that physically associates with MHC class I molecules to enhance their degradation via lysosomes (Zuo *et al.*, 2009). The murine γ-herpesvirus 68 (MHV68) mK3 protein is an E3 ubiquitin ligase that catalyzes the ubiquitination of cytoplasmic domains of MHC class I resulting in rapid proteasomal degradation of MHC class I molecules, and in addition mK3 also degrades TAP (Boname *et al.*, 2004; Lybarger *et al.*, 2003). CMVs also use a multilayered approach to downmodulate expression levels of MHC class I molecules on infected cells. The HCMV proteins US2 and US11 dislocate MHC class I molecules by targeting them for proteasomal degradation (like mK3), whereas HCMV US6 interferes with translocation of peptides over the ER membrane by binding with TAP (like BNLF2a). An alternative strategy to reduce display of peptide-presenting MHC class I complexes at the surface of infected cells involves the retention of class I in the ER by the HCMV US3 protein, which is related in function to m152/gp40 encoded by MCMV. Other immune evasion proteins of MCMV that interfere with class I presentation are m04/gp34, which binds directly to peptide-loaded MHC class I complexes at the cell surface, and m06/gp48, which binds class I molecules in the cytosol and redirects them to lysosomes for degradation. In addition to encoding immunomodulatory proteins, herpesviruses also encode microRNAs (miRNAs; Grey *et al.*, 2008). Recently, it was shown that one of these miRNAs, miR-US4-1, specifically downregulates the aminopeptidase ERAP1, an enzyme that trims epitopes to fit into MHC class I molecules (Kim *et al.*, 2011). Poxviruses encode inhibitors of MHC class I-restricted antigen presentation as well. For example, cowpox virus, which is closely related to vaccinia virus, encodes the CPX V012 protein that interferes with TAP-mediated peptide transport (analogous to US6) and encodes CPX V203 that retains class I in the ER (resembling the mechanisms of US3 and m152/gp40) (Alzhanova *et al.*, 2009; Byun *et al.*, 2009).

Viruses have also evolved mechanisms to inhibit the MHC class II presentation pathways (Hegde *et al.*, 2003; Johnson and Hegde, 2002). The EBV lytic-phase protein gp42 associates with class II molecules at various stages of their maturation, leading to impaired $CD4^+$ T cell recognition (Ressing *et al.*, 2005). The HCMV proteins US2 and US3, which downmodulate class I expression, also cause inhibition of MHC class II presentation, thereby restraining endogenous presentation of viral antigens to $CD4^+$ T cells. Whereas US2 induces proteasome-mediated degradation of the α-subunits of DR and DM (Tomazin *et al.*, 1999), US3 binds to class II αβ dimers in the ER and prevents their association with the invariant chain (Hegde *et al.*, 2002). Vaccinia virus diminishes MHC class II presentation by directly interfering with peptide binding to class II molecules, likely involving the A35 gene product (Li *et al.*, 2005; Rehm *et al.*, 2010).

The *in vivo* relevance of some of these immunoevasins that interfere with antigen presentation has been demonstrated using mutant viruses lacking the respective gene(s). MHV68 lacking mK3 had normal viral replication, but the number of latently infected spleen cells was reduced and the frequency of virus-specific $CD8^+$ T cells was increased, indicating that mK3 functionally evades $CD8^+$ T cell activation and killing during latency (Stevenson *et al.*, 2002). In experimental CMV models, the homologs of human CMV (i.e., US2, US3, US6, and US11) were shown to be dispensable for primary infection, persistence of the virus, and development of specific T cell responses (Gold *et al.*, 2004; Hansen *et al.*, 2010; Munks *et al.*, 2007) but essential for successful reinfection of a CMV-immune host (Hansen *et al.*, 2010).

The ability to escape from the antitumor adaptive immune response is often associated with downregulation of the cell surface expression of MHC class I and II molecules. The number of reports on loss of MHC molecule expression on human and mouse tumors is overwhelming and this has been reported to take place in most tumor types (Garrido *et al.*, 2010; Seliger, 2008). The underlying molecular mechanisms have largely been unraveled and constitute irreversible structural defects such as loss of heterozygosity (LOH) and point mutations at the MHC class I and β_2-microglobulin locus, but often also reversible regulatory defects occur due to transcriptional downregulation and hypermethylation of MHC molecules or TAP. Accumulating evidence indicates that the defects leading to selection and outgrowth of tumor variants with low or absent MHC molecule expression are caused by immunoediting of an active immune system (Schreiber *et al.*, 2011).

An important consequence of low levels of viral and tumor antigens (despite being immunogenic) is the induction of T cell tolerance or anergy (i.e., loss of the ability to respond to antigen) to these antigens. Induction of T cell anergy can also be caused by low levels of costimulatory signals and by a shortage of metabolic factors such as tryptophan or a combination of these (Chappert and Schwartz, 2010). On the other hand, virally infected cells or tumor cells with low or absent MHC class I expression can cause NK cell activation, as many NK cell receptors are activated by "missing self" class I interactions (Karre, 2008). However, the balance of both activating and inhibitory signals is determining the actual outcome for proper NK cell-mediated immune responses. Also, the loss of certain MHC alleles by LOH can be accompanied by expression of other ones, such as certain nonclassical MHC class I molecules like HLA-G, that can compensate for the loss of classical MHC class I molecules and can interact with inhibitory rather than activating NK cell receptors on T cells and NK cells (Agaugue *et al.*, 2011; Campoli and Ferrone, 2008).

3. IMMUNE EVASION OF COSTIMULATORY PATHWAYS

For optimal T cell expansion and differentiation, not only recognition of antigen by the TCR (signal 1) is crucial but also additional signals from costimulatory receptors (signal 2), which are usually delivered by costimulatory ligands expressed on activated APCs. Besides amplifying TCR-mediated signals, cosignals also induce distinct properties such as cell survival and effector functions like cytokine secretion or cytotoxicity. In particular, members of the immunoglobulin-like CD28-B7 costimulatory family and the costimulatory members of the tumor necrosis factor receptor (TNFR) superfamily, that is, CD27, OX40 (CD134), and 4-1BB (CD137), are important during both early and late phases of adaptive immune responses (Croft, 2003; Greenwald *et al.*, 2005; Watts, 2005).

The costimulatory receptors CD27 and CD28 are constitutively expressed on T cells, whereas OX40 and 4-1BB are temporally upregulated upon TCR activation. Feedback on the positive costimulatory system is provided by induction of the inhibitory receptors CTLA-4 and PD-1, which are structurally related to CD28. Whereas CTLA-4 binds the same ligands as CD28 (i.e., B7.1/CD80 and B7.2/CD86), PD1 has two unique ligands (i.e., PDL1/B7H1 and PDL2/B7DC). The complexity of T cell costimulation lies not only in differential signaling properties of costimulatory receptors but also in the fact that expression of costimulatory receptors and ligands is influenced by the type of inflammatory environment and is regulated in a spatiotemporal manner, likely to both initiate and sustain the T cell response and promote long-lived immunity (Croft, 2003; Greenwald *et al.*, 2005; Watts, 2005).

CMVs have developed strategies to downmodulate expression of numerous costimulatory molecules on the surface of infected APCs, which functionally restrict these cells (Andrews *et al.*, 2001; Benedict *et al.*, 2008; Moutaftsi *et al.*, 2002). For MCMV, the particular gene products causing the downmodulation of the ligands for CD28 have been identified: m138 induces the downregulation of B7.1 via direct targeting resulting in mislocalization of B7.1 into lysosomal compartments (Mintern *et al.*, 2006), while m147.5 specifically mediates the downregulation of B7.2 (Loewendorf *et al.*, 2004). The *in vivo* role of these viral genes has been interrogated by the generation of m138/m147.5-deficient CMVs, which elicit improved $CD4^+$ T cell responses and decreased viral persistence, indicating a direct role for immune evasion of B7-mediated signaling in establishing the host–virus equilibrium (Arens *et al.*, 2011). The TNFR family member CD40 provides important signals for DC maturation, and hence T cell activation (van Kooten and Banchereau, 2000). Like the CMV mutants that lack the ability to downmodulate B7.1/B7.2, CMV mutants lacking the gene responsible for CD40 downmodulation, m155 (Loewendorf *et al.*, 2011), elicit enhanced $CD4^+$ T cell responses, stressing the importance of this T cell subset to control CMV. The HCMV UL144 gene encodes a structural homolog of TNFR member herpesvirus entry mediator (Benedict *et al.*, 1999). UL144 gene polymorphisms found in clinical isolates of HCMV are associated with viremia and clinical manifestations, indicating that UL144 possesses functional immune evasion properties (Arav-Boger *et al.*, 2002; Waters *et al.*, 2010). Intriguingly, expression of the negative costimulatory molecule PDL1 is not downmodulated by CMV but is maintained at a high level on CMV-infected DCs, which causes a net inhibitory signal for T cell activation (Benedict *et al.*, 2008).

Tumor cells often overexpress inhibitory and downregulate costimulatory molecules to escape the immune system as well. The inhibitory molecule PDL1 is highly expressed on many different types of tumors and is linked to repression of tumor immunity by providing coinhibitory signals to $PD\text{-}1^+$ T cells (Seliger *et al.*, 2008a). The closely related B7H4 molecule, which also induces inhibitory signals, is expressed by tumor cells of various origin (Zou and Chen, 2008). In gastric cancer and melanoma patients, high tumor B7H4 expression is associated with poor patient survival, likely due to inhibition of tumor-specific T cell responses

(Jiang *et al.*, 2010; Quandt *et al.*, 2011). In ovarian cancer, B7H4 is found to be expressed not only by the tumor cells but also by FoxP3^{+} regulatory (suppressor) T cells (Tregs) and on an associated subset of suppressive macrophages, which jointly smother tumor-specific T cell immunity (Kryczek *et al.*, 2006, 2007).

Indirect evidence that tumors can downmodulate the positive costimulatory B7 molecules as an immune evasion mechanism comes from studies in which enhanced B7.1 cell surface expression on tumors correlated with tumor eradication accompanied with enhanced T cell responses and in which the lack of B7.1 expression contributes to tumor progression (Thomas and Wen, 2006). The ligand of CD27, CD70, has been shown to be epigenetically downregulated via DNA hypermethylation within its promoter region during breast cancer cell progression (Yu *et al.*, 2010). Aberrant overexpression of CD70 also occurs, for example, in the case of certain malignant gliomas and leukemic B cells and is accompanied with elevated soluble forms of its receptor CD27, which likely hampers T cell immunity (Ranheim *et al.*, 1995; van Oers *et al.*, 1993; Wischhusen *et al.*, 2002).

4. IMMUNE EVASION AND THE INTERFERON SYSTEM

Interferons (IFNs), named after their ability to interfere with virus replication (Isaacs and Lindenmann, 1957), are key cytokines secreted in response to viruses that inhibit several steps of virus replication in the host. Both type I (α and β) and type II (γ) IFNs act on many cells, but the most profound effects are on cells of the immune system that mediate innate and adaptive immune responses. IFNs signal through broadly expressed IFN-specific cell surface receptors activating the JAK (Janus kinase)/STAT (signal transducers and activators of transcription) signal transduction pathways, which lead to synthesis of hundreds of gene products including enzymes, signaling proteins, chemokines, antigen presentation proteins, transcription factors, heat shock proteins, and apoptotic proteins (Sen, 2001). Type I IFN-induced transcription is rapid and transient (continues for several hours) but has pleiotropic effects on many aspects of cell physiology, including cell growth, cell motility, and apoptosis. IFN-γ, made by natural killer (NK) cells and T cells, is produced later and may promote cell proliferation or apoptosis depending on the cell type and the presence of secondary signals produced by viral or bacterial infections. IFN-γ is the major immunomodulator and primary activator of macrophages and has an important role in the development of Th1 CD4^{+} T helper and CD8^{+} T cell responses. Both type I and II IFNs play positive roles in antigen presentation by inducing expression of MHC proteins and augmenting the expression of proteins responsible for generating antigenic peptides. Eventually, the rate of IFN-induced transcription subsides to basal levels through mechanisms that include receptor downregulation, action of suppressors of cytokine signaling (SOCS) family members on the JAK tyrosine kinases, and the dephosphorylation and degradation of STATs. Experiments with various knockout mice missing functional IFN genes or genes encoding proteins required for IFN signaling firmly established that without the IFN system natural viral infections including those with herpesviruses and poxviruses are more virulent.

Viruses have evolved sophisticated mechanisms to evade one or more steps of the IFN system including IFN synthesis, receptor binding, signaling pathways, induction of IFN-stimulated genes, and functioning of the encoded proteins (Defilippis, 2007). The HCMV immediate-early 2 (IE2) gene product IE86 can effectively block the expression of IFN-β (Taylor and Bresnahan, 2005, 2006). The HCMV 72-kDa immediate-early-1 protein (IE1-72kDa) confers partial resistance to the antiviral activity of type I IFNs by forming a physical complex with STAT proteins in nuclei of infected cells (Huh *et al.*, 2008; Krauss *et al.*, 2009; Paulus *et al.*, 2006). MCMV uses a similar strategy via the M27 gene encoding a 79-kDa protein that blocks type I and II IFN responses via binding to STAT2 (Zimmermann *et al.*, 2005). Another shared strategy among human and MCMV is specific targeting of an important IFN-induced protein, the serine–threonine protein kinase, PKR. The TSR1/IRS1 genes of HCMV belonging to the US22 family encode proteins that block the PKR pathway in infected cells (Child *et al.*, 2004), and in the case of MCMV, the US22 family genes m142 and m143 inhibit PKR activation in a mutually dependent manner (Budt *et al.*, 2009; Child and Geballe, 2009; Valchanova *et al.*, 2006). The IFN-inducible host cell protein viperin is directly induced by HCMV and, through recruitment by the viral mitochondria-localized inhibitor of apoptosis protein, relocalizes to the mitochondria where it disrupts cellular metabolism (i.e., reducing adenosine triphosphate (ATP) levels) and alters the cytoskeleton, which in turn, enhances viral replication (Seo *et al.*, 2011). Vaccinia virus encodes the B18R protein that acts as a decoy receptor by binding to IFN-α/β (Symons *et al.*, 1995), while the B8R protein of vaccinia virus binds directly to IFN-γ. The importance to block IFN for this poxvirus is further illustrated by the vaccinia virus K3L and E3L proteins. E3L binds double-stranded RNA structures, thereby inhibiting activation of PKR, and K3L functions as a decoy for the translation initiation factor eIF-2, the natural substrate of PKR (Smith *et al.*, 1997). Thus viruses use different strategies to evade IFN signaling and the action of selective IFN-induced proteins.

IFNs have emerged as the central coordinators of the immune-mediated control of tumors as demonstrated by the sensitivity to tumor formation of mice deficient for one of the associated genes (cytokines, receptors, or signal transducers) (Dunn *et al.*, 2006). Evasion of the IFN system by cancers has been reported to comprise partial or permanent resistance to IFNs via downmodulation of the receptor (Billard *et al.*, 1986), constitutive expression of SOCS (Komyod *et al.*, 2007), or dysregulation of STATs due to epigenetic modification events in the tumor cell (Rodriguez *et al.*, 2007; Seliger *et al.*, 2008b; Xi *et al.*, 2006). Constitutive STAT3 activation, which is frequently observed in tumors, causes decreased production of functionally competent DCs and additionally the accumulation of inhibitory DCs and inhibitory myeloid cells, leading to inhibition of (antigen-specific) T cell responses (Lee *et al.*, 2011).

5. IMMUNE EVASION AND INDUCTION OF INHIBITORY CYTOKINES

Interleukins are a family of secreted cytokines produced by a wide variety of cells including NK cells, T cells, B cells, dendritic cells, and macrophages and primarily act as mediators between leukocytes to induce activation and differentiation processes. For example, IL-12 promotes proinflammatory Th1 responses while IL-4 induces Th2 responses. Other interleukins, such as IL-10, have been shown to function primarily as an inhibitory and anti-inflammatory cytokine. The immunoregulation by IL-10 is accomplished by negatively affecting MHC and costimulatory molecule expression and inflammatory cytokine and chemokine secretion of APCs, resulting in inferior differentiation and function of these cells (Sabat *et al.*, 2010; Wilke *et al.*, 2011). In addition, IL-10 has a direct suppressive action on T cells and is associated with the suppressive effects and development of Tregs and suppressive myeloid cells (e.g., myeloid-derived suppressor cells and M2 macrophages). Thus, both direct and indirect actions of IL-10 suppress T cell-mediated immunity.

The first reported herpesvirus cytokine, encoded by the BCRF1 gene of EBV, was a viral IL-10 (vIL-10), and because of the highly similar sequence homology of BCRF1 with mouse and human IL-10, it was suggested that during evolution, EBV or its predecessor acquired this gene from the host (Moore *et al.*, 1990; Vieira *et al.*, 1991). EBV vIL-10 impairs the antigen-presenting function of monocytes/macrophages by inhibiting the upregulation of class II and B7 molecules, which possibly avoids detection of the virus-infected cells (de Waal *et al.*, 1991; Salek-Ardakani *et al.*, 2002). Later reports showed that HCMV also encodes an IL-10 homolog (cmvIL-10) (Kotenko *et al.*, 2000), which can bind to the human IL-10 receptor. Besides affecting antigen presentation and costimulation, the viral IL-10 proteins are thought to additionally affect immune evasion by shifting the host Th1 inflammatory response toward Th2 responses and through suppression of monocyte/macrophage function.

In the case of tumor escape, tumor-induced IL-10 production has been implicated to be involved in the induction of T cell anergy via the inhibitory effects on APCs. However, although IL-10 is predominantly immunosuppressive for T cell responses, especially during viral infections, in the tumor microenvironment, it may also be stimulatory for $CD8^+$ T cells (Wilke *et al.*, 2011), which warrants caution for the use of IL-10 blocking reagents for clinical application against cancer.

Another secreted cytokine with suppressive capacity is transforming growth factor beta (TGF-β), which is produced by most cells in the body including immune cells, epithelial cells, and endothelial cells (Blobe *et al.*, 2000). One of the actions of TGF-β is that it inhibits T cell proliferation. At the same time, TGF-β functions as a positive differentiation factor for $FoxP3^+$ Tregs and a negative differentiation factor for Th1 and Th2 cells (Li and Flavell, 2008).

During EBV infection, TGF-β can induce reactivation of latently infected cells by activating the expression of the viral BZLF1 gene involving the Smad transcription factors that mediate the signaling of the TGF-β intracellular pathway, but TGF-β is likely produced by other immune cells rather than by the infected cell itself (Iempridee *et al.*, 2011; Liang *et al.*, 2002). HCMV is a potent inducer of TGF-β secretion by infected cells, likely via transcriptional mechanisms involving the IE genes, which enhance viral replication (Michelson *et al.*, 1994).

Tumor cells usually have increased secretion of TGF-β and at the same time can circumvent the autocrine proliferation inhibiting actions of TGF-β by mutations in parts of the TGF-β signaling pathway (Blobe *et al.*, 2000; Massague, 2008; Meulmeester and Ten Dijke, 2011). These increased TGF-β levels do not only have immunosuppressive effects that contribute to tumor progression like the suppression of infiltrating effector T cells and conversion of these cells into Tregs, which produce TGF-β as well. TGF-β also stimulates angiogenesis and invasiveness of the tumor cells by modulating adhesive properties and increasing the deposition of extracellular matrix proteins. The source of TGF-β that induces tolerance of T cells in a tumor setting can also be derived from conventional T cells rather than tumor cells or Tregs (Donkor *et al.*, 2011). Thus, induction of TGF-β production by tumor cells, conventional T cells, or Tregs is an effective mechanism for malignant cells to evade the host immune system.

6. IMMUNE EVASION AND CHEMOKINES

Chemokines comprise a large family of small chemotactic cytokines that interact with G-protein-coupled receptors and direct the migration of innate and adaptive immune cells into sites of inflammation and infection. Based on the presence and relative positioning of N-terminal cysteine residues, chemokines are divided into four classes: CXC, CC, C, and CX3C (Zlotnik and Yoshie, 2000).

The importance of chemokines is well illustrated by the many mechanisms that herpesviruses and poxviruses have evolved to disrupt chemokine function (Seet and McFadden, 2002). The EBV-encoded BILF1 is a constitutively active (ligand independent) vGPCR that, besides inhibiting MHC class I presentation, forms complexes with human CXCR4 (Beisser *et al.*, 2005; Nijmeijer *et al.*, 2010; Paulsen *et al.*, 2005). This functionally attenuates CXCL12 (SDF-1)-induced CXCR4 signaling, which may be favorable for EBV by allowing virally infected B cells to home and/or remain at sites that are most optimal for viral replication and dissemination. Latent membrane protein-1 (LMP-1) encoded by EBV selectively induces production of CCL17 (TARC) and CCL22 (MDC), which attract $CCR4^+$ Tregs that on their turn may help EBV-infected B cells to evade the host immune attack (Nakayama *et al.*, 2004; Takegawa *et al.*, 2008). The MHV-68 M3 gene encodes a herpesvirus chemokine binding protein that binds a broad range of chemokines (Parry *et al.*, 2000; van Berkel *et al.*, 2000) and functionally inhibits inflammatory responses in a central nervous system model of MHV-68 (van Berkel *et al.*, 2002). The ORF74 of MHV-68 encodes a vGPCR homologous to CXCR2 (IL-8Rβ) and has been reported to play a role in viral reactivation from latency (Lee *et al.*, 2003; Moorman *et al.*, 2003).

The HCMV genes UL146 and UL147 encode the two CXC chemokines vCXCL1 and vCXCL2 (Penfold *et al.*, 1999). Studies on vCXCL1 showed that this cytokine specifically targets CXCR2 and with a lower affinity also CXCR1 (IL-8Rα) as an agonist, which could be involved in attracting $CXCR1^+CXCR2^+$ neutrophils to sites of viral infection as a way to use this cell type as a vehicle for dissemination (Luttichau, 2010). US28 is a constitutively active chemokine receptor encoded by HCMV that binds several chemokines, including CCL2 (MCP-1), CCL3 (MIP-1α), CCL4 (MIP-1β), CCL5 (RANTES), and CX3CL1 (Kledal *et al.*, 1998; Kuhn *et al.*, 1995). Transgenic mice expressing US28 in intestinal epithelial cells develop accelerated intestinal neoplasia likely due to glycogen synthase 3β inhibition leading to accumulation of β-catenin protein and increased expression of Wnt target genes involved in the control of the cell proliferation (Bongers *et al.*, 2010). This suggests that CMV infection may facilitate intestinal tumor development in humans and may be one of the reasons for the accumulating evidence for an association of CMV with cancer development (Michaelis *et al.*, 2009; Soderberg-Naucler, 2006). HCMV also encodes less promiscuous chemokine binding receptors, such as pUL21.5 protein, a soluble CC chemokine receptor that functions as a decoy to selectively bind CCL5, which is expressed by activated T cells and stimulates migration of monocytes and T cells (Wang *et al.*, 2004). Other viral chemokine receptor homologs encoded by HCMV are US27,

UL33, and UL78 (Maussang *et al.*, 2009). *In vitro* and *in vivo* studies (using rat and MCMV models) indicated that these genes contribute to virus replication, but their particular role in immune evasion remains to be elucidated (Beisser *et al.*, 1998; Davis-Poynter *et al.*, 1997; Kaptein *et al.*, 2003; O'Connor and Shenk, 2011; Oliveira and Shenk, 2001). The m131/129 gene product of MCMV, a CC chemokine homolog, contributes to viral dissemination in an NK- and T cell-dependent manner (Fleming *et al.*, 1999). In addition to expressing virus-encoded chemokine receptors and chemokine analogues, herpesviruses also encode proteins that function to block the expression of chemokines. The HCMV gene product IE86 that blocks the expression of IFN-β also blocks transcription of the chemokines CCL3, CCL5, CCL8 (MCP-2), CXCL9 (MIG), and CXCL8 (also known as IL-8) (Taylor and Bresnahan, 2006). Vaccinia virus and other orthopoxviruses (cowpox and camelpox) express a secreted chemokine binding protein (vCKBP) that binds CC, but not CXC or C, chemokines with high affinity, and inhibits chemokine-induced signaling and chemotaxis (Alcami *et al.*, 1998).

Also in the field of tumor immunology, reports have been published showing the modulation of chemokine function as an immune escape mechanism. Mouse and human melanomas express the chemokine CCL21 (6Ckine, SLC), which recruits $CCR7^+$ lymphoid tissue inducer cells that reorganize the tumor stroma and supports the recruitment of suppressive cell populations (i.e., $FoxP3^+$ Tregs, myeloid-derived suppressor cells, M2 macrophages), thereby facilitating tumor progression (Shields *et al.*, 2010). CCL28 (MEC) secretion by ovarian cancer cells promotes tumor tolerance and angiogenesis via recruitment of Tregs as well (Facciabene *et al.*, 2011). CXCL8, which has proangiogenic properties, is frequently overexpressed in many tumors and has functional implications for tumor progression and metastasis (Mestas *et al.*, 2005; Singh *et al.*, 2010). In this respect, it is interesting to note that CXCL8 is a transcriptional target of the oncogene Ras, revealing one of the mechanisms of the cancer promoting properties associated with Ras oncogenes (Sparmann and Bar-Sagi, 2004). Moreover, inactivation of the tumor suppressor gene ING4 in brain tumors leads to increased CXCL8 expression, which promotes tumor angiogenesis and growth (Garkavtsev *et al.*, 2004). Another example is found in CCL2, a chemokine that attracts and activates mononuclear cells. CCL2 secreted by tumor cells and/or the tumor microenvironment enhances the tumor malignancy either by acting directly on the tumor cells, which enhances their metastatic properties, or by attracting leukocyte cell types with suppressive actions (e.g., Tregs) for antitumor T cell activities (Conti and Rollins, 2004; Soria and Ben-Baruch, 2008). Besides expressing chemokines which attract, for example, Tregs, certain tumor cells can also express chemokine receptors. For example, T cell leukemia/lymphoma cells express CCR4 on the cell surface, which is associated with poor prognosis (Ishida and Ueda, 2011). Thus, tumor cells exploit chemokines and their receptors to attract immunosuppressive cells and/or to mediate angiogenesis in order to promote tumor progression.

7. COPING WITH IMMUNE EVASION: IMPLICATIONS FOR RATIONAL DESIGN OF VACCINES AND IMMUNOTHERAPY

Elucidation of the mechanisms underlying immune evasion strategies of persistent viruses and tumors has revealed fundamental cell biological and immunological processes. A striking occurrence is that these immune evasion mechanisms by viruses and tumors target essentially the same host T cell activation systems such as peptide–MHC–TCR interactions, costimulation signals, and cytokine/chemokine pathways (Table 9.1). Although not discussed here, a similar analogy between persistent viruses and tumors can be found for other targets of immune evasion mechanism such as NK cell activation, complement activation, and apoptosis pathways. From a virus/tumor perspective, the development of analogous strategic targets emphasizes that these are critical aspects of the host immune system that need to be overcome to become persistent and thrive. *Vice versa*, from a host perspective, it is essential to prevail over immune evasion by persistent viruses and cancer to effectively contain disease. Although immune evasion by viruses and tumors target equivalent pathways of host immune responses, the evolution of the acquired evasion mechanisms is fundamentally different and operates in a different way. Whereas persistent large DNA viruses encode immunomodulatory proteins, tumor cells acquire somatic or epigenetic mutations leading to selective outgrowth.

Another remarkable analogy between persistent viruses and tumors lies in the fact that both follow a similar course of three sequential phases. Persistent viral infections start with an acute phase in which the virus replicates and the innate and adaptive immune responses develop to control the virus. This is followed by a persistent phase during which the virus becomes latent, and especially in cases of immunosuppression or senescence, this can be followed by reactivation of the virus with sometimes pathogenic consequences. Likewise, the cancer immunoediting process proceeds through an elimination phase during which the innate and adaptive immunity eradicates developing tumors, an equilibrium phase in which surviving tumors are kept in check but not destroyed by immunological mechanisms, and an escape phase in which as a result of immune evasion mechanisms tumor cells emerge leading to tumor progression and clinical disease (Dunn *et al.*, 2004; Schreiber *et al.*, 2011). Perhaps, a consequence of the aforementioned similarities is that the dynamics of the T cell response and the phenotypical and/or functional

TABLE 9.1 Analogous targets of immune evasion by persistent viruses and tumors

Viral immune evasion	Tumor immune evasion
Antigen presentation pathways	
Downmodulation of MHC molecules by immunomodulatory proteins and/or microRNAs	Downmodulation of MHC molecules by irreversible alterations (LOH, somatic mutations) and reversible defects by epigenetic modifications
Costimulatory pathways	
Upregulation of coinhibitory molecules (e.g., PDL1) Downmodulation of costimulatory molecules by immunomodulatory genes (e.g., B7.1)	Upregulation of coinhibitory molecules (e.g., PDL1) Downmodulation of costimulatory molecules by epigenetic modifications (e.g., CD70) Aberrant expression of costimulatory molecules
Interferon system	
Inhibiting IFN signaling by immunomodulatory proteins that hamper IFN synthesis, receptor binding, signaling pathways, induction of IFN-stimulated genes, and functioning of the encoded proteins	Inhibiting IFN signaling by downmodulation of the IFN receptor, constitutive expression of SOCS, and dysregulation of STATs
Inhibitory cytokines	
Expression of viral IL10 Induction of TGF-β	Induction of IL-10 Induction of TGF-β accompanied by mutations in parts of the TGF-β signaling pathway
Chemokine function	
Interference of chemokine function by immunomodulatory proteins	Induction of chemokines (to attract immunosuppressive immune cells)

characteristics of responding T cells during persistent/chronic infection and cancer are comparable as well (Kim and Ahmed, 2010).

The lack of effective treatment for many devastating infections and cancers urges the rational design of novel prophylactic and therapeutic vaccines and immunotherapies. Many current vaccination strategies and methods based on synthetic peptides, DNA-encoding tumor antigens, recombinant proteins, antigen-loaded DCs, and adoptive transfer of *in vitro* generated T cells focus on the enhancement of antigen-specific T cell responses. Even though a high frequency of specific T cells is critical, it does not guarantee therapeutic efficacy by itself, as their function could be repressed or virally infected cells/tumors could become resistant to immune attack. Therefore, the effectiveness of such strategies could be increased by simultaneous counter targeting of immune evasion, which might also reduce the generation of immune escape variants.

A straightforward approach to counteract downmodulation of MHC molecules is the replacement of the defective genes with, for example, viral vectors encoding TAP (Alimonti *et al.*, 2000), but a major drawback of this approach is the local delivery of the gene, especially when the tumor is situated in internal organs (Lampen and van Hall, 2011). Epigenetic modulators, such as histone methylase or deacetylase inhibitors, can be used as tools to restore the epigenetic repression of tumor antigens (Khan and Tomasi, 2008; Setiadi *et al.*, 2008). Alternatively, IFNs can restore MHC molecule expression caused by reversible (but not structural) alterations and thereby improve, for example, $CD8^+$ T cell-mediated lysis of tumors (Carretero *et al.*, 2008; Seliger *et al.*, 2008b). In addition, IFNs induce other immune-stimulating properties that further could improve their therapeutic use. Among chronic viral diseases, type I IFNs are clinically used to treat chronic active hepatitis caused by hepatitis B/C viruses, and IFN-α is used for treating genital warts caused by HPV, but it may have therapeutic efficacy for other persistent infections as well. The lack of costimulatory molecules on tumor cells or APCs can be overcome by ligation with agonistic monoclonal antibodies, such as those against the TNFR family members CD27, OX40, 4-1BB, and CD40, which have already proven their efficacy in preclinical investigations and recently also in clinical settings (French *et al.*, 1999, 2007; Gray *et al.*, 2008; Jensen *et al.*, 2010; Khalil and Vonderheide, 2007). As an alternative, antibodies that block the function of inhibitory receptors (e.g., CTLA-4 and PD-1) can be used therapeutically (Jin *et al.*, 2011; Kaufmann and Walker, 2009; Korman *et al.*, 2006). Likewise, the suppressive actions of IL-10 and TGF-β can be neutralized by antibodies as well (Korpal and Kang, 2010; Wilson and Brooks, 2011).

The insight that immune evasion by viruses and tumors targets analogous host immune pathways might lead to cross-pollination of the viral and tumor immunology research fields, which could lead to new viewpoints and appreciation of the intricacies and subtleties that arise from the merging of these fields. In this respect, it is also interesting to note that the study and identification of microbial immunomodulatory proteins may also lead to their usage as therapeutic agents and/or as targets of immunotherapy. An interesting example is the use of viral TAP inhibitors to induce T cells recognizing an alternative peptide repertoire carried by tumor cells with antigen processing defects (van Hall *et al.*, 2006).

Exploiting the capacity of attenuated large DNA viruses to vaccinate immune hosts and to induce and maintain strong memory T cell immunity might be rewarding in case of building up protective immunity for viruses as well as cancer (Kwak *et al.*, 2003). The potential of this approach for protection against highly active chronic viruses has recently been demonstrated in an experimental monkey CMV model, in which CMV-based vectors inducing huge effector-memory T cell responses could reduce the risk of progressive infection following repeated exposure to simian immunodeficiency virus (SIV), a virus related to HIV that infects monkeys (Hansen *et al.*, 2009, 2011). Conventional vaccines, such as DNA vaccines and adenovirus-based vaccines that predominantly induce central-memory T cells, could not provide protection to SIV.

8. FUTURE PROSPECTS

A major challenge for immunologists and vaccinologists is not only the enhancement of specific adaptive immune responses (and prevention of tolerance and/or autoimmunity) but also to counterattack immune evasion by viruses and tumors. Although we know much about the immune system and the evasion of this ancient defense system for the benefit of persistent viruses and tumors, more understanding of the basic mechanisms of immune evasion is required and is an ongoing line of research. Immune evasion by persistent viruses and tumors occurs at multiple levels of the T cell response including interference with antigen presentation pathways, costimulation, cytokine, and chemokine signaling. Moreover, the signaling pathways used by different costimulatory molecules and cytokines are often partially overlapping, thus providing the opportunity for cross talk among them and causing either synergistic or antagonistic results. Such cross talk is physiologically significant because more than one costimulatory receptor or cytokine is induced during viral infection and cancer. As a result, cells are often exposed to mixtures of signals *in vivo*, and the resultant patterns of gene expression are dictated by the simultaneous actions of multiple signaling pathways leading to different spectra of cellular actions. Thus, our detailed knowledge on the role of individual molecules is not matched by similar understanding of how multiple signals are integrated. At the same time, we do know that multiple aspects of the immune system are targeted by viruses and tumors but that the current immunotherapeutic strategies usually target a single pathway. Therefore, most likely disruption of immune evasion by combined therapeutic (vaccine) strategies is more optimal to counterattack virus propagation or tumor outgrowth than stand-alone therapies. Combinatorial treatments will presumably also diminish the likelihood of emerging viral mutants and malignant cells that become resistant.

Therefore, insight in synergistic mechanisms is essential and should also be approached experimentally and clinically. This is a challenging issue and not only requires a major systematic effort to make meaningful progress but also entails the need to overcome the willingness of pharmaceutical companies and legal authorities for easing the approval of combinatorial therapies.

ACKNOWLEDGMENTS

The author would like to acknowledge S. van der Burg, T. van Hall, F. Ossendorp, and E. van Leeuwen and members of the Tumor Immunology group for critical reading of the chapter and discussion. Financial support is received from a Marie Curie Fellowship.

REFERENCES

Agaugue, S., Carosella, E. D., and Rouas-Freiss, N. (2011). Role of HLA-G in tumor escape through expansion of myeloid-derived suppressor cells and cytokinic balance in favor of Th2 versus Th1/Th17. *Blood* **117,** 7021–7031.

Alcami, A., Symons, J. A., Collins, P. D., Williams, T. J., and Smith, G. L. (1998). Blockade of chemokine activity by a soluble chemokine binding protein from vaccinia virus. *J. Immunol.* **160,** 624–633.

Alimonti, J., Zhang, Q. J., Gabathuler, R., Reid, G., Chen, S. S., and Jefferies, W. A. (2000). TAP expression provides a general method for improving the recognition of malignant cells in vivo. *Nat. Biotechnol.* **18,** 515–520.

Alzhanova, D., Edwards, D. M., Hammarlund, E., Scholz, I. G., Horst, D., Wagner, M. J., Upton, C., Wiertz, E. J., Slifka, M. K., and Fruh, K. (2009). Cowpox virus inhibits the transporter associated with antigen processing to evade T cell recognition. *Cell Host Microbe* **6,** 433–445.

Andrews, D. M., Andoniou, C. E., Granucci, F., Ricciardi-Castagnoli, P., and Degli-Esposti, M. A. (2001). Infection of dendritic cells by murine cytomegalovirus induces functional paralysis. *Nat. Immunol.* **2,** 1077–1084.

Arav-Boger, R., Willoughby, R. E., Pass, R. F., Zong, J. C., Jang, W. J., Alcendor, D., and Hayward, G. S. (2002). Polymorphisms of the cytomegalovirus (CMV)-encoded tumor necrosis factor-alpha and beta-chemokine receptors in congenital CMV disease. *J. Infect. Dis.* **186,** 1057–1064.

Arens, R., Loewendorf, A., Her, M. J., Schneider-Ohrum, K., Shellam, G. R., Janssen, E., Ware, C. F., Schoenberger, S. P., and Benedict, C. A. (2011). B7-mediated costimulation of CD4 T cells constrains cytomegalovirus persistence. *J. Virol.* **85,** 390–396.

Beisser, P. S., Vink, C., van Dam, J. G., Grauls, G., Vanherle, S. J., and Bruggeman, C. A. (1998). The R33 G protein-coupled receptor gene of rat cytomegalovirus plays an essential role in the pathogenesis of viral infection. *J. Virol.* **72,** 2352–2363.

Beisser, P. S., Verzijl, D., Gruijthuijsen, Y. K., Beuken, E., Smit, M. J., Leurs, R., Bruggeman, C. A., and Vink, C. (2005). The Epstein-Barr virus BILF1 gene encodes a G protein-coupled receptor that inhibits phosphorylation of RNA-dependent protein kinase. *J. Virol.* **79,** 441–449.

Benedict, C. A., Butrovich, K. D., Lurain, N. S., Corbeil, J., Rooney, I., Schneider, P., Tschopp, J., and Ware, C. F. (1999). Cutting edge: A novel viral TNF receptor superfamily member in virulent strains of human cytomegalovirus. *J. Immunol.* **162,** 6967–6970.

Benedict, C. A., Loewendorf, A., Garcia, Z., Blazar, B. R., and Janssen, E. M. (2008). Dendritic cell programming by cytomegalovirus stunts naive T cell responses via the PD-L1/PD-1 pathway. *J. Immunol.* **180,** 4836–4847.

Billard, C., Sigaux, F., Castaigne, S., Valensi, F., Flandrin, G., Degos, L., Falcoff, E., and Aguet, M. (1986). Treatment of hairy cell leukemia with recombinant alpha interferon: II. In vivo down-regulation of alpha interferon receptors on tumor cells. *Blood* **67,** 821–826.

Blobe, G. C., Schiemann, W. P., and Lodish, H. F. (2000). Role of transforming growth factor beta in human disease. *N. Engl. J. Med.* **342,** 1350–1358.

Boname, J. M., de Lima, B. D., Lehner, P. J., and Stevenson, P. G. (2004). Viral degradation of the MHC class I peptide loading complex. *Immunity* **20,** 305–317.

Bongers, G., Maussang, D., Muniz, L. R., Noriega, V. M., Fraile-Ramos, A., Barker, N., Marchesi, F., Thirunarayanan, N., Vischer, H. F., Qin, L., Mayer, L., Harpaz, N., *et al.* (2010). The cytomegalovirus-encoded chemokine receptor US28 promotes intestinal neoplasia in transgenic mice. *J. Clin. Invest.* **120,** 3969–3978.

Boon, T., Coulie, P. G., Van den Eynde, B. J., and van der Bruggen, P. (2006). Human T cell responses against melanoma. *Annu. Rev. Immunol.* **24,** 175–208.

Brownstein, D. G., Bhatt, P. N., Gras, L., and Jacoby, R. O. (1991). Chromosomal locations and gonadal dependence of genes that mediate resistance to ectromelia (mousepox) virus-induced mortality. *J. Virol.* **65,** 1946–1951.

Budt, M., Niederstadt, L., Valchanova, R. S., Jonjic, S., and Brune, W. (2009). Specific inhibition of the PKR-mediated antiviral response by the murine cytomegalovirus proteins m142 and m143. *J. Virol.* **83,** 1260–1270.

Byun, M., Verweij, M. C., Pickup, D. J., Wiertz, E. J., Hansen, T. H., and Yokoyama, W. M. (2009). Two mechanistically distinct immune evasion proteins of cowpox virus combine to avoid antiviral CD8 T cells. *Cell Host Microbe* **6,** 422–432.

Campoli, M., and Ferrone, S. (2008). HLA antigen changes in malignant cells: Epigenetic mechanisms and biologic significance. *Oncogene* **27,** 5869–5885.

Cannon, M. J., Schmid, D. S., and Hyde, T. B. (2010). Review of cytomegalovirus seroprevalence and demographic characteristics associated with infection. *Rev. Med. Virol.* **20,** 202–213.

Carretero, R., Romero, J. M., Ruiz-Cabello, F., Maleno, I., Rodriguez, F., Camacho, F. M., Real, L. M., Garrido, F., and Cabrera, T. (2008). Analysis of HLA class I expression in progressing and regressing metastatic melanoma lesions after immunotherapy. *Immunogenetics* **60,** 439–447.

Chappert, P., and Schwartz, R. H. (2010). Induction of T cell anergy: Integration of environmental cues and infectious tolerance. *Curr. Opin. Immunol.* **22,** 552–559.

Child, S. J., and Geballe, A. P. (2009). Binding and relocalization of protein kinase R by murine cytomegalovirus. *J. Virol.* **83,** 1790–1799.

Child, S. J., Hakki, M., De Niro, K. L., and Geballe, A. P. (2004). Evasion of cellular antiviral responses by human cytomegalovirus TRS1 and IRS1. *J. Virol.* **78,** 197–205.

Conti, I., and Rollins, B. J. (2004). CCL2 (monocyte chemoattractant protein-1) and cancer. *Semin. Cancer Biol.* **14,** 149–154.

Croft, M. (2003). Co-stimulatory members of the TNFR family: Keys to effective T-cell immunity? *Nat. Rev. Immunol.* **3,** 609–620.

Davis-Poynter, N. J., Lynch, D. M., Vally, H., Shellam, G. R., Rawlinson, W. D., Barrell, B. G., and Farrell, H. E. (1997). Identification and characterization of a G protein-coupled receptor homolog encoded by murine cytomegalovirus. *J. Virol.* **71,** 1521–1529.

de Waal, M. R., Haanen, J., Spits, H., Roncarolo, M. G., te Velde, A., Figdor, C., Johnson, K., Kastelein, R., Yssel, H., and de Vries, J. E. (1991). Interleukin 10 (IL-10) and viral IL-10 strongly reduce antigen-specific human T cell proliferation by diminishing the antigen-presenting capacity of monocytes via downregulation of class II major histocompatibility complex expression. *J. Exp. Med.* **174,** 915–924.

Defilippis, V. R. (2007). Induction and evasion of the type I interferon response by cytomegaloviruses. *Adv. Exp. Med. Biol.* **598,** 309–324.

Donkor, M. K., Sarkar, A., Savage, P. A., Franklin, R. A., Johnson, L. K., Jungbluth, A. A., Allison, J. P., and Li, M. O. (2011). T cell surveillance of oncogene-induced prostate cancer is impeded by T cell-derived TGF-beta1 cytokine. *Immunity* **35,** 123–134.

Dunn, G. P., Old, L. J., and Schreiber, R. D. (2004). The three Es of cancer immunoediting. *Annu. Rev. Immunol.* **22,** 329–360.

Dunn, G. P., Koebel, C. M., and Schreiber, R. D. (2006). Interferons, immunity and cancer immunoediting. *Nat. Rev. Immunol.* **6,** 836–848.

Facciabene, A., Peng, X., Hagemann, I. S., Balint, K., Barchetti, A., Wang, L. P., Gimotty, P. A., Gilks, C. B., Lal, P., Zhang, L., and Coukos, G. (2011). Tumour hypoxia promotes tolerance and angiogenesis via CCL28 and T(reg) cells. *Nature* **475,** 226–230.

Fleming, P., Davis-Poynter, N., Degli-Esposti, M., Densley, E., Papadimitriou, J., Shellam, G., and Farrell, H. (1999). The murine cytomegalovirus chemokine homolog, m131/129, is a determinant of viral pathogenicity. *J. Virol.* **73,** 6800–6809.

French, R. R., Chan, H. T., Tutt, A. L., and Glennie, M. J. (1999). CD40 antibody evokes a cytotoxic T-cell response that eradicates lymphoma and bypasses T-cell help. *Nat. Med.* **5,** 548–553.

French, A. R., Pingel, J. T., Wagner, M., Bubic, I., Yang, L., Kim, S., Koszinowski, U., Jonjic, S., and Yokoyama, W. M. (2004). Escape of mutant double-stranded DNA virus from innate immune control. *Immunity* **20,** 747–756.

French, R. R., Taraban, V. Y., Crowther, G. R., Rowley, T. F., Gray, J. C., Johnson, P. W., Tutt, A. L., Al-Shamkhani, A., and Glennie, M. J. (2007). Eradication of lymphoma by CD8 T cells following anti-CD40 monoclonal antibody therapy is critically dependent on CD27 costimulation. *Blood* **109,** 4810–4815.

Garkavtsev, I., Kozin, S. V., Chernova, O., Xu, L., Winkler, F., Brown, E., Barnett, G. H., and Jain, R. K. (2004). The candidate tumour suppressor protein ING4 regulates brain tumour growth and angiogenesis. *Nature* **428,** 328–332.

Garrido, F., Cabrera, T., and Aptsiauri, N. (2010). "Hard" and "soft" lesions underlying the HLA class I alterations in cancer cells: Implications for immunotherapy. *Int. J. Cancer* **127,** 249–256.

Gold, M. C., Munks, M. W., Wagner, M., McMahon, C. W., Kelly, A., Kavanagh, D. G., Slifka, M. K., Koszinowski, U. H., Raulet, D. H., and Hill, A. B. (2004). Murine cytomegalovirus interference with antigen presentation has little effect on the size or the effector memory phenotype of the CD8 T cell response. *J. Immunol.* **172,** 6944–6953.

Gray, J. C., French, R. R., James, S., Al-Shamkhani, A., Johnson, P. W., and Glennie, M. J. (2008). Optimising anti-tumour CD8 T-cell responses using combinations of immunomodulatory antibodies. *Eur. J. Immunol.* **38,** 2499–2511.

Greenwald, R. J., Freeman, G. J., and Sharpe, A. H. (2005). The B7 family revisited. *Annu. Rev. Immunol.* **23,** 515–548.

Grey, F., Hook, L., and Nelson, J. (2008). The functions of herpesvirus-encoded microRNAs. *Med. Microbiol. Immunol.* **197,** 261–267.

Hansen, T. H., and Bouvier, M. (2009). MHC class I antigen presentation: Learning from viral evasion strategies. *Nat. Rev. Immunol.* **9,** 503–513.

Hansen, S. G., Vieville, C., Whizin, N., Coyne-Johnson, L., Siess, D. C., Drummond, D. D., Legasse, A. W., Axthelm, M. K., Oswald, K., Trubey, C. M., Piatak, M., Jr., Lifson, J. D., *et al.* (2009). Effector memory T cell responses are associated with protection of rhesus monkeys from mucosal simian immunodeficiency virus challenge. *Nat. Med.* **15,** 293–299.

Hansen, S. G., Powers, C. J., Richards, R., Ventura, A. B., Ford, J. C., Siess, D., Axthelm, M. K., Nelson, J. A., Jarvis, M. A., Picker, L. J., and Fruh, K. (2010). Evasion of CD8+ T cells is critical for superinfection by cytomegalovirus. *Science* **328,** 102–106.

Hansen, S. G., Ford, J. C., Lewis, M. S., Ventura, A. B., Hughes, C. M., Coyne-Johnson, L., Whizin, N., Oswald, K., Shoemaker, R., Swanson, T., Legasse, A. W., Chiuchiolo, M. J., *et al.* (2011). Profound early control of highly pathogenic SIV by an effector memory T-cell vaccine. *Nature* **473,** 523–527.
Heath, W. R., and Carbone, F. R. (2001). Cross-presentation in viral immunity and self-tolerance. *Nat. Rev. Immunol.* **1,** 126–134.
Hegde, N. R., Tomazin, R. A., Wisner, T. W., Dunn, C., Boname, J. M., Lewinsohn, D. M., and Johnson, D. C. (2002). Inhibition of HLA-DR assembly, transport, and loading by human cytomegalovirus glycoprotein US3: A novel mechanism for evading major histocompatibility complex class II antigen presentation. *J. Virol.* **76,** 10929–10941.
Hegde, N. R., Chevalier, M. S., and Johnson, D. C. (2003). Viral inhibition of MHC class II antigen presentation. *Trends Immunol.* **24,** 278–285.
Hislop, A. D., Ressing, M. E., van Leeuwen, D., Pudney, V. A., Horst, D., Koppers-Lalic, D., Croft, N. P., Neefjes, J. J., Rickinson, A. B., and Wiertz, E. J. (2007). A CD8+ T cell immune evasion protein specific to Epstein-Barr virus and its close relatives in Old World primates. *J. Exp. Med.* **204,** 1863–1873.
Huh, Y. H., Kim, Y. E., Kim, E. T., Park, J. J., Song, M. J., Zhu, H., Hayward, G. S., and Ahn, J. H. (2008). Binding STAT2 by the acidic domain of human cytomegalovirus IE1 promotes viral growth and is negatively regulated by SUMO. *J. Virol.* **82,** 10444–10454.
Iempridee, T., Das, S., Xu, I., and Mertz, J. E. (2011). Transforming growth factor beta-induced reactivation of Epstein-Barr virus involves multiple Smad-binding elements cooperatively activating expression of the latent-lytic switch BZLF1 gene. *J. Virol.* **85,** 7836–7848.
Isaacs, A., and Lindenmann, J. (1957). Virus interference. I. The interferon. *Proc. R. Soc. Lond. B Biol. Sci.* **147,** 258–267.
Ishida, T., and Ueda, R. (2011). Immunopathogenesis of lymphoma: Focus on CCR4. *Cancer Sci.* **102,** 44–50.
Jensen, S. M., Maston, L. D., Gough, M. J., Ruby, C. E., Redmond, W. L., Crittenden, M., Li, Y., Puri, S., Poehlein, C. H., Morris, N., Kovacsovics-Bankowski, M., Moudgil, T., *et al.* (2010). Signaling through OX40 enhances antitumor immunity. *Semin. Oncol.* **37,** 524–532.
Jiang, J., Zhu, Y., Wu, C., Shen, Y., Wei, W., Chen, L., Zheng, X., Sun, J., Lu, B., and Zhang, X. (2010). Tumor expression of B7-H4 predicts poor survival of patients suffering from gastric cancer. *Cancer Immunol. Immunother.* **59,** 1707–1714.
Jin, H. T., Ahmed, R., and Okazaki, T. (2011). Role of PD-1 in regulating T-cell immunity. *Curr. Top. Microbiol. Immunol.* **350,** 17–37.
Johnson, D. C., and Hegde, N. R. (2002). Inhibition of the MHC class II antigen presentation pathway by human cytomegalovirus. *Curr. Top. Microbiol. Immunol.* **269,** 101–115.
Kaptein, S. J., Beisser, P. S., Gruijthuijsen, Y. K., Savelkouls, K. G., van Cleef, K. W., Beuken, E., Grauls, G. E., Bruggeman, C. A., and Vink, C. (2003). The rat cytomegalovirus R78 G protein-coupled receptor gene is required for production of infectious virus in the spleen. *J. Gen. Virol.* **84,** 2517–2530.
Karre, K. (2008). Natural killer cell recognition of missing self. *Nat. Immunol.* **9,** 477–480.
Kaufmann, D. E., and Walker, B. D. (2009). PD-1 and CTLA-4 inhibitory cosignaling pathways in HIV infection and the potential for therapeutic intervention. *J. Immunol.* **182,** 5891–5897.
Khalil, M., and Vonderheide, R. H. (2007). Anti-CD40 agonist antibodies: Preclinical and clinical experience. *Update Cancer Ther.* **2,** 61–65.
Khan, A. N., and Tomasi, T. B. (2008). Histone deacetylase regulation of immune gene expression in tumor cells. *Immunol. Res.* **40,** 164–178.
Khong, H. T., and Restifo, N. P. (2002). Natural selection of tumor variants in the generation of "tumor escape" phenotypes. *Nat. Immunol.* **3,** 999–1005.

Kim, P. S., and Ahmed, R. (2010). Features of responding T cells in cancer and chronic infection. *Curr. Opin. Immunol.* **22,** 223–230.

Kim, S., Lee, S., Shin, J., Kim, Y., Evnouchidou, I., Kim, D., Kim, Y. K., Kim, Y. E., Ahn, J. H., Riddell, S. R., Stratikos, E., Kim, V. N., *et al.* (2011). Human cytomegalovirus microRNA miR-US4-1 inhibits CD8(+) T cell responses by targeting the aminopeptidase ERAP1. *Nat. Immunol.* **12,** 984–991.

Kledal, T. N., Rosenkilde, M. M., and Schwartz, T. W. (1998). Selective recognition of the membrane-bound CX3C chemokine, fractalkine, by the human cytomegalovirus-encoded broad-spectrum receptor US28. *FEBS Lett.* **441,** 209–214.

Komyod, W., Bohm, M., Metze, D., Heinrich, P. C., and Behrmann, I. (2007). Constitutive suppressor of cytokine signaling 3 expression confers a growth advantage to a human melanoma cell line. *Mol. Cancer Res.* **5,** 271–281.

Korman, A. J., Peggs, K. S., and Allison, J. P. (2006). Checkpoint blockade in cancer immunotherapy. *Adv. Immunol.* **90,** 297–339.

Korpal, M., and Kang, Y. (2010). Targeting the transforming growth factor-beta signalling pathway in metastatic cancer. *Eur. J. Cancer* **46,** 1232–1240.

Kotenko, S. V., Saccani, S., Izotova, L. S., Mirochnitchenko, O. V., and Pestka, S. (2000). Human cytomegalovirus harbors its own unique IL-10 homolog (cmvIL-10). *Proc. Natl. Acad. Sci. USA* **97,** 1695–1700.

Krauss, S., Kaps, J., Czech, N., Paulus, C., and Nevels, M. (2009). Physical requirements and functional consequences of complex formation between the cytomegalovirus IE1 protein and human STAT2. *J. Virol.* **83,** 12854–12870.

Kryczek, I., Zou, L., Rodriguez, P., Zhu, G., Wei, S., Mottram, P., Brumlik, M., Cheng, P., Curiel, T., Myers, L., Lackner, A., Alvarez, X., *et al.* (2006). B7-H4 expression identifies a novel suppressive macrophage population in human ovarian carcinoma. *J. Exp. Med.* **203,** 871–881.

Kryczek, I., Wei, S., Zhu, G., Myers, L., Mottram, P., Cheng, P., Chen, L., Coukos, G., and Zou, W. (2007). Relationship between B7-H4, regulatory T cells, and patient outcome in human ovarian carcinoma. *Cancer Res.* **67,** 8900–8905.

Kuhn, D. E., Beall, C. J., and Kolattukudy, P. E. (1995). The cytomegalovirus US28 protein binds multiple CC chemokines with high affinity. *Biochem. Biophys. Res. Commun.* **211,** 325–330.

Kwak, H., Horig, H., and Kaufman, H. L. (2003). Poxviruses as vectors for cancer immunotherapy. *Curr. Opin. Drug Discov. Devel.* **6,** 161–168.

Lampen, M. H., and van Hall, T. (2011). Strategies to counteract MHC-I defects in tumors. *Curr. Opin. Immunol.* **23,** 293–298.

Lautscham, G., Rickinson, A., and Blake, N. (2003). TAP-independent antigen presentation on MHC class I molecules: Lessons from Epstein-Barr virus. *Microbes Infect.* **5,** 291–299.

Lee, P. P., Yee, C., Savage, P. A., Fong, L., Brockstedt, D., Weber, J. S., Johnson, D., Swetter, S., Thompson, J., Greenberg, P. D., Roederer, M., and Davis, M. M. (1999). Characterization of circulating T cells specific for tumor-associated antigens in melanoma patients. *Nat. Med.* **5,** 677–685.

Lee, B. J., Koszinowski, U. H., Sarawar, S. R., and Adler, H. (2003). A gammaherpesvirus G protein-coupled receptor homologue is required for increased viral replication in response to chemokines and efficient reactivation from latency. *J. Immunol.* **170,** 243–251.

Lee, H., Pal, S. K., Reckamp, K., Figlin, R. A., and Yu, H. (2011). STAT3: A target to enhance antitumor immune response. *Curr. Top. Microbiol. Immunol.* **344,** 41–59.

Lefkowitz, E. J., Wang, C., and Upton, C. (2006). Poxviruses: Past, present and future. *Virus Res.* **117,** 105–118.

Li, M. O., and Flavell, R. A. (2008). TGF-beta: A master of all T cell trades. *Cell* **134,** 392–404.

Li, P., Wang, N., Zhou, D., Yee, C. S., Chang, C. H., Brutkiewicz, R. R., and Blum, J. S. (2005). Disruption of MHC class II-restricted antigen presentation by vaccinia virus. *J. Immunol.* **175,** 6481–6488.

Liang, C. L., Chen, J. L., Hsu, Y. P., Ou, J. T., and Chang, Y. S. (2002). Epstein-Barr virus BZLF1 gene is activated by transforming growth factor-beta through cooperativity of Smads and c-Jun/c-Fos proteins. *J. Biol. Chem.* **277,** 23345–23357.

Loewendorf, A., Kruger, C., Borst, E. M., Wagner, M., Just, U., and Messerle, M. (2004). Identification of a mouse cytomegalovirus gene selectively targeting CD86 expression on antigen-presenting cells. *J. Virol.* **78,** 13062–13071.

Loewendorf, A. I., Steinbrueck, L., Peter, C., Busche, A., Benedict, C. A., and Kay-Jackson, P. C. (2011). The mouse cytomegalovirus glycoprotein m155 inhibits CD40 expression and restricts CD4 T cell responses. *J. Virol.* **85,** 5208–5212.

Luttichau, H. R. (2010). The cytomegalovirus UL146 gene product vCXCL1 targets both CXCR1 and CXCR2 as an agonist. *J. Biol. Chem.* **285,** 9137–9146.

Lybarger, L., Wang, X., Harris, M. R., Virgin, H. W., and Hansen, T. H. (2003). Virus subversion of the MHC class I peptide-loading complex. *Immunity* **18,** 121–130.

Massague, J. (2008). TGFbeta in Cancer. *Cell* **134,** 215–230.

Maussang, D., Vischer, H. F., Leurs, R., and Smit, M. J. (2009). Herpesvirus-encoded G protein-coupled receptors as modulators of cellular function. *Mol. Pharmacol.* **76,** 692–701.

McGeoch, D. J., Cook, S., Dolan, A., Jamieson, F. E., and Telford, E. A. (1995). Molecular phylogeny and evolutionary timescale for the family of mammalian herpesviruses. *J. Mol. Biol.* **247,** 443–458.

Mestas, J., Burdick, M. D., Reckamp, K., Pantuck, A., Figlin, R. A., and Strieter, R. M. (2005). The role of CXCR2/CXCR2 ligand biological axis in renal cell carcinoma. *J. Immunol.* **175,** 5351–5357.

Meulmeester, E., and Ten Dijke, P. (2011). The dynamic roles of TGF-beta in cancer. *J. Pathol.* **223,** 205–218.

Michaelis, M., Doerr, H. W., and Cinatl, J. (2009). The story of human cytomegalovirus and cancer: Increasing evidence and open questions. *Neoplasia* **11,** 1–9.

Michelson, S., Alcami, J., Kim, S. J., Danielpour, D., Bachelerie, F., Picard, L., Bessia, C., Paya, C., and Virelizier, J. L. (1994). Human cytomegalovirus infection induces transcription and secretion of transforming growth factor beta 1. *J. Virol.* **68,** 5730–5737.

Mintern, J. D., Klemm, E. J., Wagner, M., Paquet, M. E., Napier, M. D., Kim, Y. M., Koszinowski, U. H., and Ploegh, H. L. (2006). Viral interference with B7-1 costimulation: A new role for murine cytomegalovirus fc receptor-1. *J. Immunol.* **177,** 8422–8431.

Moore, K. W., Vieira, P., Fiorentino, D. F., Trounstine, M. L., Khan, T. A., and Mosmann, T. R. (1990). Homology of cytokine synthesis inhibitory factor (IL-10) to the Epstein-Barr virus gene BCRFI. *Science* **248,** 1230–1234.

Moorman, N. J., Virgin, H. W., and Speck, S. H. (2003). Disruption of the gene encoding the gammaHV68 v-GPCR leads to decreased efficiency of reactivation from latency. *Virology* **307,** 179–190.

Moutaftsi, M., Mehl, A. M., Borysiewicz, L. K., and Tabi, Z. (2002). Human cytomegalovirus inhibits maturation and impairs function of monocyte-derived dendritic cells. *Blood* **99,** 2913–2921.

Munks, M. W., Pinto, A. K., Doom, C. M., and Hill, A. B. (2007). Viral interference with antigen presentation does not alter acute or chronic CD8 T cell immunodominance in murine cytomegalovirus infection. *J. Immunol.* **178,** 7235–7241.

Nakayama, T., Hieshima, K., Nagakubo, D., Sato, E., Nakayama, M., Kawa, K., and Yoshie, O. (2004). Selective induction of Th2-attracting chemokines CCL17 and CCL22 in human B cells by latent membrane protein 1 of Epstein-Barr virus. *J. Virol.* **78,** 1665–1674.

Nijmeijer, S., Leurs, R., Smit, M. J., and Vischer, H. F. (2010). The Epstein-Barr virus-encoded G protein-coupled receptor BILF1 hetero-oligomerizes with human CXCR4, scavenges Galphai proteins, and constitutively impairs CXCR4 functioning. *J. Biol. Chem.* **285,** 29632–29641.

O'Connor, C. M., and Shenk, T. (2011). Human cytomegalovirus pUS27 G protein-coupled receptor homologue is required for efficient spread by the extracellular route but not for direct cell-to-cell spread. *J. Virol.* **85,** 3700–3707.

Oliveira, S. A., and Shenk, T. E. (2001). Murine cytomegalovirus M78 protein, a G protein-coupled receptor homologue, is a constituent of the virion and facilitates accumulation of immediate-early viral mRNA. *Proc. Natl. Acad. Sci. USA* **98,** 3237–3242.

Parry, C. M., Simas, J. P., Smith, V. P., Stewart, C. A., Minson, A. C., Efstathiou, S., and Alcami, A. (2000). A broad spectrum secreted chemokine binding protein encoded by a herpesvirus. *J. Exp. Med.* **191,** 573–578.

Paulsen, S. J., Rosenkilde, M. M., Eugen-Olsen, J., and Kledal, T. N. (2005). Epstein-Barr virus-encoded BILF1 is a constitutively active G protein-coupled receptor. *J. Virol.* **79,** 536–546.

Paulus, C., Krauss, S., and Nevels, M. (2006). A human cytomegalovirus antagonist of type I IFN-dependent signal transducer and activator of transcription signaling. *Proc. Natl. Acad. Sci. USA* **103,** 3840–3845.

Penfold, M. E., Dairaghi, D. J., Duke, G. M., Saederup, N., Mocarski, E. S., Kemble, G. W., and Schall, T. J. (1999). Cytomegalovirus encodes a potent alpha chemokine. *Proc. Natl. Acad. Sci. USA* **96,** 9839–9844.

Ploegh, H. L. (1998). Viral strategies of immune evasion. *Science* **280,** 248–253.

Quandt, D., Fiedler, E., Boettcher, D., Marsch, W. C., and Seliger, B. (2011). B7-h4 expression in human melanoma: Its association with patients' survival and antitumor immune response. *Clin. Cancer Res.* **17,** 3100–3111.

Ranheim, E. A., Cantwell, M. J., and Kipps, T. J. (1995). Expression of CD27 and its ligand, CD70, on chronic lymphocytic leukemia B cells. *Blood* **85,** 3556–3565.

Rappuoli, R., Miller, H. I., and Falkow, S. (2002). Medicine. The intangible value of vaccination. *Science* **297,** 937–939.

Rappuoli, R., Black, S., and Lambert, P. H. (2011). Vaccine discovery and translation of new vaccine technology. *Lancet* **378,** 360–368.

Rehm, K. E., Connor, R. F., Jones, G. J., Yimbu, K., and Roper, R. L. (2010). Vaccinia virus A35R inhibits MHC class II antigen presentation. *Virology* **397,** 176–186.

Ressing, M. E., van Leeuwen, D., Verreck, F. A., Keating, S., Gomez, R., Franken, K. L., Ottenhoff, T. H., Spriggs, M., Schumacher, T. N., Hutt-Fletcher, L. M., Rowe, M., and Wiertz, E. J. (2005). Epstein-Barr virus gp42 is posttranslationally modified to produce soluble gp42 that mediates HLA class II immune evasion. *J. Virol.* **79,** 841–852.

Rodriguez, T., Mendez, R., Del, C. A., Jimenez, P., Aptsiauri, N., Garrido, F., and Ruiz-Cabello, F. (2007). Distinct mechanisms of loss of IFN-gamma mediated HLA class I inducibility in two melanoma cell lines. *BMC Cancer* **7,** 34.

Roush, S. W., and Murphy, T. V. (2007). Historical comparisons of morbidity and mortality for vaccine-preventable diseases in the United States. *JAMA* **298,** 2155–2163.

Sabat, R., Grutz, G., Warszawska, K., Kirsch, S., Witte, E., Wolk, K., and Geginat, J. (2010). Biology of interleukin-10. *Cytokine Growth Factor Rev.* **21,** 331–344.

Salek-Ardakani, S., Arrand, J. R., and Mackett, M. (2002). Epstein-Barr virus encoded interleukin-10 inhibits HLA-class I, ICAM-1, and B7 expression on human monocytes: Implications for immune evasion by EBV. *Virology* **304,** 342–351.

Savage, P. A., Vosseller, K., Kang, C., Larimore, K., Riedel, E., Wojnoonski, K., Jungbluth, A. A., and Allison, J. P. (2008). Recognition of a ubiquitous self antigen by prostate cancer-infiltrating CD8+ T lymphocytes. *Science* **319,** 215–220.

Schietinger, A., Philip, M., and Schreiber, H. (2008). Specificity in cancer immunotherapy. *Semin. Immunol.* **20,** 276–285.

Schreiber, R. D., Old, L. J., and Smyth, M. J. (2011). Cancer immunoediting: Integrating immunity's roles in cancer suppression and promotion. *Science* **331,** 1565–1570.

Seet, B. T., and McFadden, G. (2002). Viral chemokine-binding proteins. *J. Leukoc. Biol.* **72,** 24–34.

Seliger, B. (2008). Molecular mechanisms of MHC class I abnormalities and APM components in human tumors. *Cancer Immunol. Immunother.* **57,** 1719–1726.
Seliger, B., Marincola, F. M., Ferrone, S., and Abken, H. (2008a). The complex role of B7 molecules in tumor immunology. *Trends Mol. Med.* **14,** 550–559.
Seliger, B., Ruiz-Cabello, F., and Garrido, F. (2008b). IFN inducibility of major histocompatibility antigens in tumors. *Adv. Cancer Res.* **101,** 249–276.
Sen, G. C. (2001). Viruses and interferons. *Annu. Rev. Microbiol.* **55,** 255–281.
Seo, J. Y., Yaneva, R., Hinson, E. R., and Cresswell, P. (2011). Human cytomegalovirus directly induces the antiviral protein viperin to enhance infectivity. *Science* **332,** 1093–1097.
Setiadi, A. F., Omilusik, K., David, M. D., Seipp, R. P., Hartikainen, J., Gopaul, R., Choi, K. B., and Jefferies, W. A. (2008). Epigenetic enhancement of antigen processing and presentation promotes immune recognition of tumors. *Cancer Res.* **68,** 9601–9607.
Shields, J. D., Kourtis, I. C., Tomei, A. A., Roberts, J. M., and Swartz, M. A. (2010). Induction of lymphoidlike stroma and immune escape by tumors that express the chemokine CCL21. *Science* **328,** 749–752.
Singh, S., Singh, A. P., Sharma, B., Owen, L. B., and Singh, R. K. (2010). CXCL8 and its cognate receptors in melanoma progression and metastasis. *Future Oncol.* **6,** 111–116.
Smith, G. L., Symons, J. A., Khanna, A., Vanderplasschen, A., and Alcami, A. (1997). Vaccinia virus immune evasion. *Immunol. Rev.* **159,** 137–154.
Soderberg-Naucler, C. (2006). Does cytomegalovirus play a causative role in the development of various inflammatory diseases and cancer? *J. Intern. Med.* **259,** 219–246.
Soria, G., and Ben-Baruch, A. (2008). The inflammatory chemokines CCL2 and CCL5 in breast cancer. *Cancer Lett.* **267,** 271–285.
Sparmann, A., and Bar-Sagi, D. (2004). Ras-induced interleukin-8 expression plays a critical role in tumor growth and angiogenesis. *Cancer Cell* **6,** 447–458.
Stevenson, P. G., May, J. S., Smith, X. G., Marques, S., Adler, H., Koszinowski, U. H., Simas, J. P., and Efstathiou, S. (2002). K3-mediated evasion of CD8(+) T cells aids amplification of a latent gamma-herpesvirus. *Nat. Immunol.* **3,** 733–740.
Symons, J. A., Alcami, A., and Smith, G. L. (1995). Vaccinia virus encodes a soluble type I interferon receptor of novel structure and broad species specificity. *Cell* **81,** 551–560.
Takegawa, S., Jin, Z., Nakayama, T., Oyama, T., Hieshima, K., Nagakubo, D., Shirakawa, A. K., Tsuzuki, T., Nakamura, S., and Yoshie, O. (2008). Expression of CCL17 and CCL22 by latent membrane protein 1-positive tumor cells in age-related Epstein-Barr virus-associated B-cell lymphoproliferative disorder. *Cancer Sci.* **99,** 296–302.
Taylor, R. T., and Bresnahan, W. A. (2005). Human cytomegalovirus immediate-early 2 gene expression blocks virus-induced beta interferon production. *J. Virol.* **79,** 3873–3877.
Taylor, R. T., and Bresnahan, W. A. (2006). Human cytomegalovirus immediate-early 2 protein IE86 blocks virus-induced chemokine expression. *J. Virol.* **80,** 920–928.
Thomas, G. R., and Wen, J. (2006). Endogenous expression of CD80 co-stimulatory molecule facilitates in vivo tumor regression of oral squamous carcinoma. *Anticancer Res.* **26,** 4093–4101.
Tomazin, R., Boname, J., Hegde, N. R., Lewinsohn, D. M., Altschuler, Y., Jones, T. R., Cresswell, P., Nelson, J. A., Riddell, S. R., and Johnson, D. C. (1999). Cytomegalovirus US2 destroys two components of the MHC class II pathway, preventing recognition by CD4+ T cells. *Nat. Med.* **5,** 1039–1043.
Valchanova, R. S., Picard-Maureau, M., Budt, M., and Brune, W. (2006). Murine cytomegalovirus m142 and m143 are both required to block protein kinase R-mediated shutdown of protein synthesis. *J. Virol.* **80,** 10181–10190.
van Berkel, V., Barrett, J., Tiffany, H. L., Fremont, D. H., Murphy, P. M., McFadden, G., Speck, S. H., and Virgin, H. W., IV (2000). Identification of a gammaherpesvirus selective chemokine binding protein that inhibits chemokine action. *J. Virol.* **74,** 6741–6747.
van Berkel, V., Levine, B., Kapadia, S. B., Goldman, J. E., Speck, S. H., and Virgin, H. W. (2002). Critical role for a high-affinity chemokine-binding protein in gamma-herpesvirus-induced lethal meningitis. *J. Clin. Invest.* **109,** 905–914.

van Hall, T., Wolpert, E. Z., van Veelen, P., Laban, S., van der Veer, M., Roseboom, M., Bres, S., Grufman, P., de Ru, A., Meiring, H., de Jong, A., Franken, K., *et al.* (2006). Selective cytotoxic T-lymphocyte targeting of tumor immune escape variants. *Nat. Med.* **12,** 417–424.

van Kooten, C., and Banchereau, J. (2000). CD40-CD40 ligand. *J. Leukoc. Biol.* **67,** 2–17.

van Oers, M. H., Pals, S. T., Evers, L. M., van der Schoot, C. E., Koopman, G., Bonfrer, J. M., Hintzen, R. Q., von dem Borne, A. E., and van Lier, R. A. (1993). Expression and release of CD27 in human B-cell malignancies. *Blood* **82,** 3430–3436.

Vieira, P., de Waal-Malefyt, R., Dang, M. N., Johnson, K. E., Kastelein, R., Fiorentino, D. F., deVries, J. E., Roncarolo, M. G., Mosmann, T. R., and Moore, K. W. (1991). Isolation and expression of human cytokine synthesis inhibitory factor cDNA clones: Homology to Epstein-Barr virus open reading frame BCRFI. *Proc. Natl. Acad. Sci. USA* **88,** 1172–1176.

Voigt, V., Forbes, C. A., Tonkin, J. N., Degli-Esposti, M. A., Smith, H. R., Yokoyama, W. M., and Scalzo, A. A. (2003). Murine cytomegalovirus m157 mutation and variation leads to immune evasion of natural killer cells. *Proc. Natl. Acad. Sci. USA* **100,** 13483–13488.

Wang, D., Bresnahan, W., and Shenk, T. (2004). Human cytomegalovirus encodes a highly specific RANTES decoy receptor. *Proc. Natl. Acad. Sci. USA* **101,** 16642–16647.

Waters, A., Hassan, J., De, G. C., Kissoon, G., Knowles, S., Molloy, E., Connell, J., and Hall, W. W. (2010). Human cytomegalovirus UL144 is associated with viremia and infant development sequelae in congenital infection. *J. Clin. Microbiol.* **48,** 3956–3962.

Watts, T. H. (2005). TNF/TNFR family members in costimulation of T cell responses. *Annu. Rev. Immunol.* **23,** 23–68.

Wilke, C. M., Wei, S., Wang, L., Kryczek, I., Kao, J., and Zou, W. (2011). Dual biological effects of the cytokines interleukin-10 and interferon-gamma. *Cancer Immunol. Immunother.* **60,** 1529–1541.

Willimsky, G., and Blankenstein, T. (2007). The adaptive immune response to sporadic cancer. *Immunol. Rev.* **220,** 102–112.

Wilson, E. B., and Brooks, D. G. (2011). The role of IL-10 in regulating immunity to persistent viral infections. *Curr. Top. Microbiol. Immunol.* **350,** 39–65.

Wischhusen, J., Jung, G., Radovanovic, I., Beier, C., Steinbach, J. P., Rimner, A., Huang, H., Schulz, J. B., Ohgaki, H., Aguzzi, A., Rammensee, H. G., and Weller, M. (2002). Identification of CD70-mediated apoptosis of immune effector cells as a novel immune escape pathway of human glioblastoma. *Cancer Res.* **62,** 2592–2599.

Xi, S., Dyer, K. F., Kimak, M., Zhang, Q., Gooding, W. E., Chaillet, J. R., Chai, R. L., Ferrell, R. E., Zamboni, B., Hunt, J., and Grandis, J. R. (2006). Decreased STAT1 expression by promoter methylation in squamous cell carcinogenesis. *J. Natl. Cancer Inst.* **98,** 181–189.

Yewdell, J. W., and Hill, A. B. (2002). Viral interference with antigen presentation. *Nat. Immunol.* **3,** 1019–1025.

Yu, S. E., Park, S. H., and Jang, Y. K. (2010). Epigenetic silencing of TNFSF7 (CD70) by DNA methylation during progression to breast cancer. *Mol. Cells* **29,** 217–221.

Zimmermann, A., Trilling, M., Wagner, M., Wilborn, M., Bubic, I., Jonjic, S., Koszinowski, U., and Hengel, H. (2005). A cytomegaloviral protein reveals a dual role for STAT2 in IFN-{gamma} signaling and antiviral responses. *J. Exp. Med.* **201,** 1543–1553.

Zlotnik, A., and Yoshie, O. (2000). Chemokines: A new classification system and their role in immunity. *Immunity* **12,** 121–127.

Zou, W., and Chen, L. (2008). Inhibitory B7-family molecules in the tumour microenvironment. *Nat. Rev. Immunol.* **8,** 467–477.

Zuo, J., Currin, A., Griffin, B. D., Shannon-Lowe, C., Thomas, W. A., Ressing, M. E., Wiertz, E. J., and Rowe, M. (2009). The Epstein-Barr virus G-protein-coupled receptor contributes to immune evasion by targeting MHC class I molecules for degradation. *PLoS Pathog.* **5,** e1000255.

INDEX

Note: Page numbers followed by "*f*" indicate figures, and "*t*" indicate tables.

CONTENTS OF RECENT VOLUMES

Volume 88

Volume 89

Volume 90

Volume 91

Volume 92

Volume 93

Volume 94

Volume 95

Volume 96

Volume 97

Volume 98

Volume 99

Volume 100

Volume 101

Volume 102

Volume 103

Volume 104

Volume 105

Volume 106

Volume 107

Volume 108

Volume 109

Volume 110

Volume 111

Sabyasachi Das, Masayuki Hirano, Chelsea McCallister, Rea Tako, and Nikolas Nikolaidis

Pax5: A Master Regulator of B Cell Development and Leukemogenesis
Jasna Medvedovic, Anja Ebert, Hiromi Tagoh, and Meinrad Busslinger

Index

Volume 112

Stability of Regulatory T-cell Lineage
Shohei Hori

Thymic and Peripheral Differentiation of Regulatory T Cells
Hyang-Mi Lee, Jhoanne Lynne Bautista, and Chyi-Song Hsieh

Regulatory T Cells in Infection
Rick M. Maizels and Katherine A. Smith

Biological Functions of Regulatory T Cells
Ethan M. Shevach

Extrathymic Generation of Regulatory T Cells—Chances and Challenges for Prevention of Autoimmune Disease
Carolin Daniel, and Harald von Boehmer

Index

Volume 113

Studies with *Listeria monocytogenes* Lead the Way
Emil R. Unanue and Javier A. Carrero

Interactions of *Listeria monocytogenes* with the Autophagy System of Host Cells
Grace Y. Lam, Mark A. Czuczman, Darren E. Higgins and John H. Brumell

Virulence Factors That Modulate the Cell Biology of *Listeria* Infection and the Host Response
Serge Mostowy and Pascale Cossart

Dendritic Cells in *Listeria monocytogenes* Infection
Brian T. Edelson

Probing CD8 T Cell Responses with *Listeria monocytogenes* Infection
Stephanie A. Condotta, Martin J. Richer, Vladimir P. Badovinac and John T. Harty

Listeria monocytogenes and Its Products as Agents for Cancer Immunotherapy
Patrick Guirnalda, Laurence Wood and Yvonne Paterson

Monocyte-Mediated Immune Defense Against Murine *Listeria monocytogenes* Infection
Natalya V. Serbina, Chao Shi and Eric G. Pamer

Innate Immune Pathways Triggered by *Listeria monocytogenes* and Their Role in the Induction of Cell-Mediated Immunity
Chelsea E. Witte, Kristina A. Archer, Chris S. Rae, John-Demian Sauer, Josh J. Woodward and Daniel A. Portnoy

Mechanisms and Immunological Effects of Lymphocyte Apoptosis Caused by *Listeria monocytogenes*
Javier A. Carrero, and Emil R. Unanue

Index

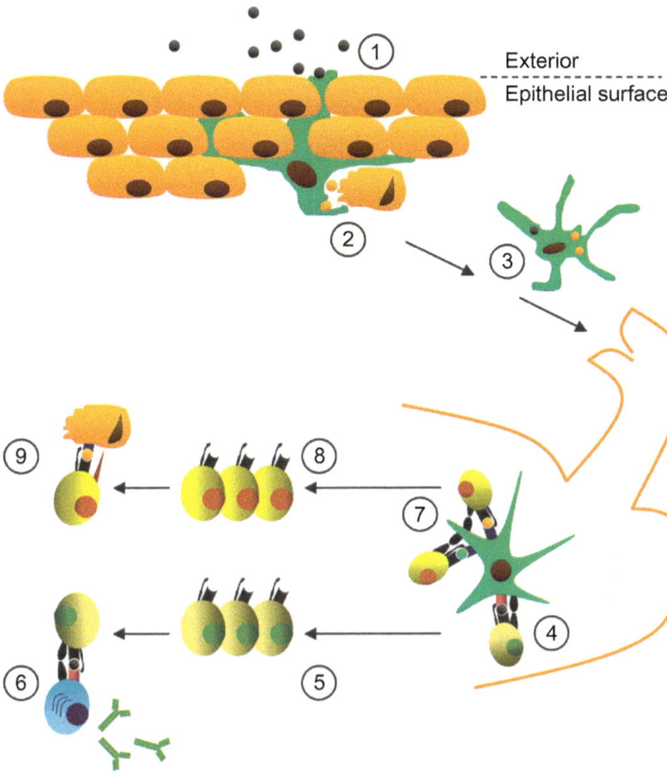

Chapter 1, Figure 1.1 (See page 7 of this volume.)

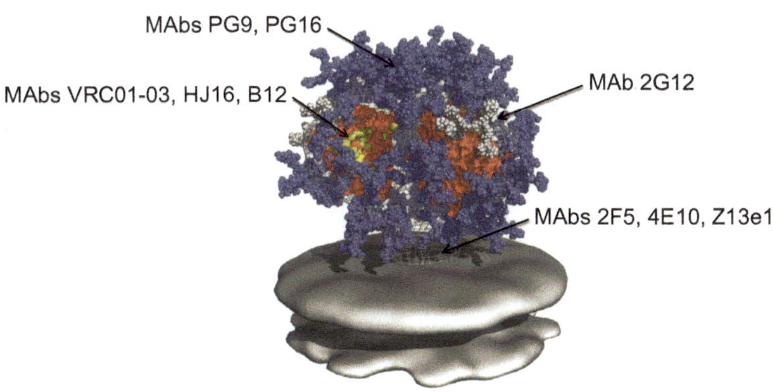

Chapter 2, Figure 2.1 (See page 36 of this volume.)

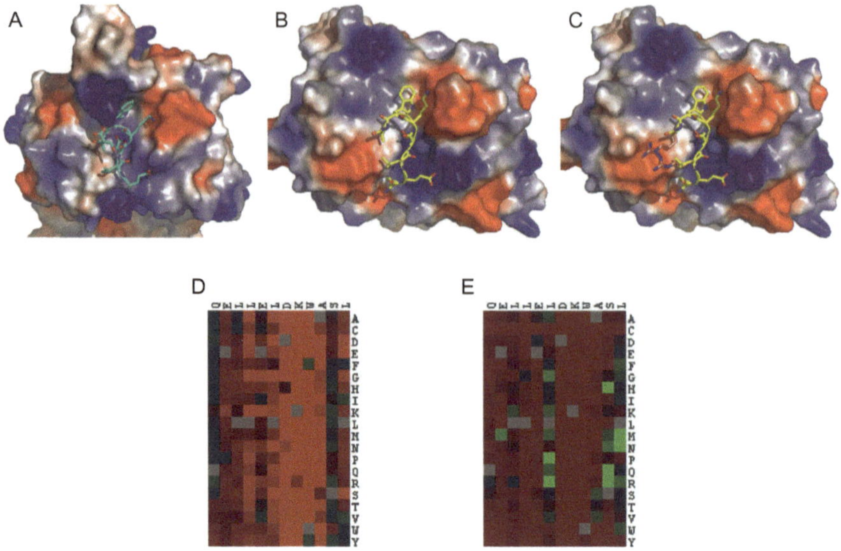

Chapter 2, Figure 2.2 (See page 45 of this volume.)

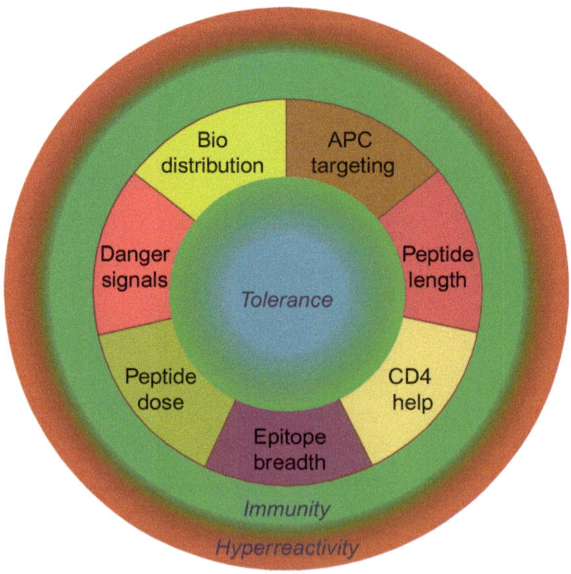

Chapter 3, Figure 3.1 (See page 69 of this volume.)

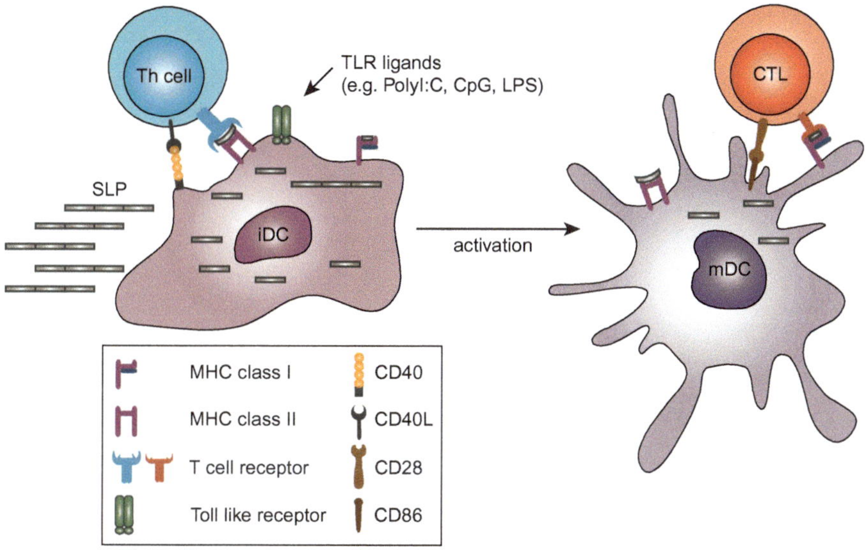

Chapter 4, Figure 4.1 (See page 84 of this volume.)

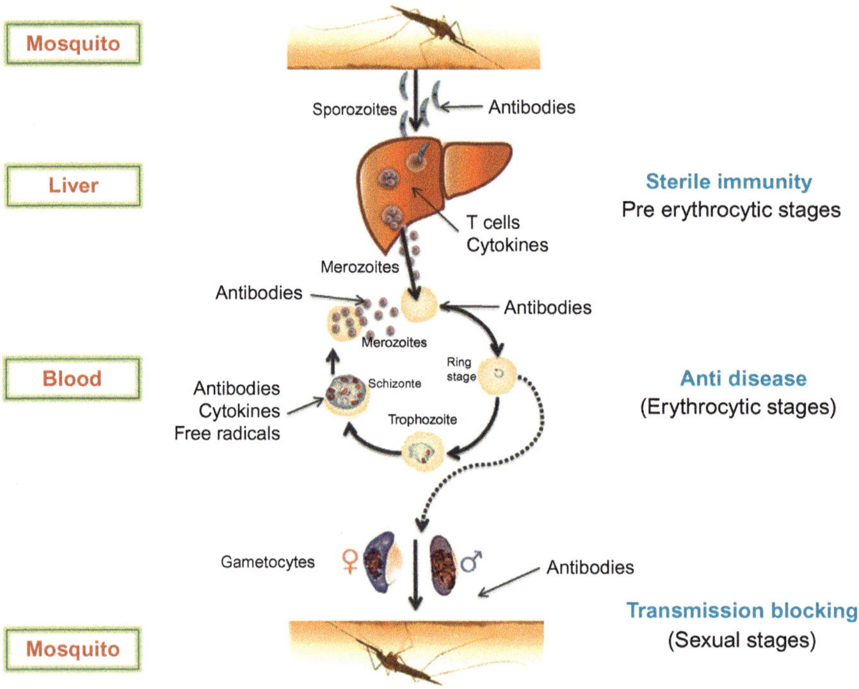

Chapter 5, Figure 5.1 (See page 110 of this volume.)

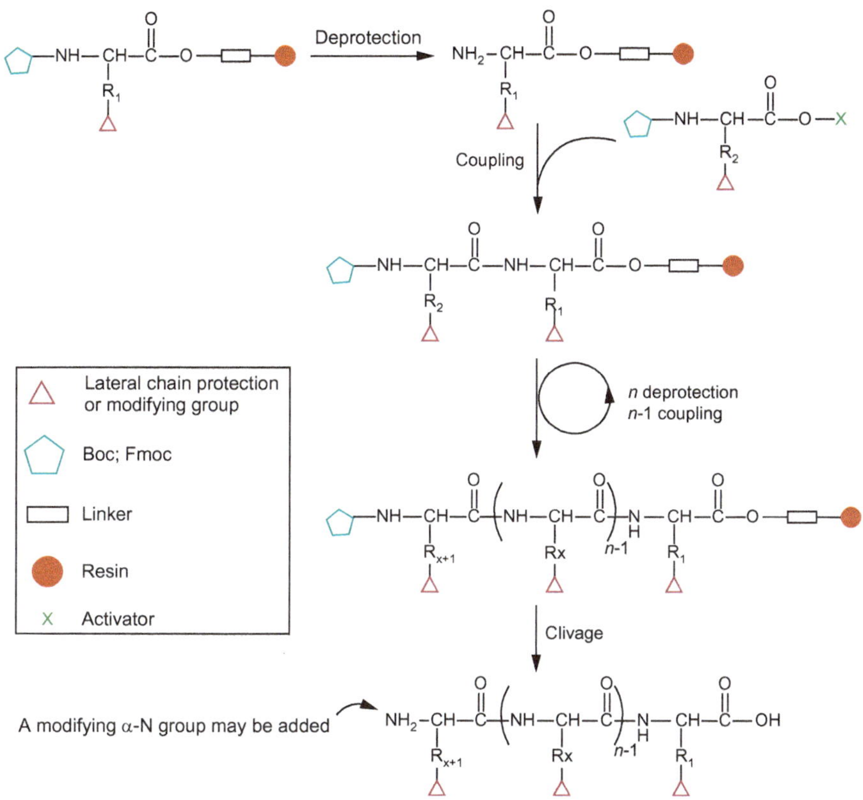

Chapter 5, Figure 5.2 (See page 114 of this volume.)

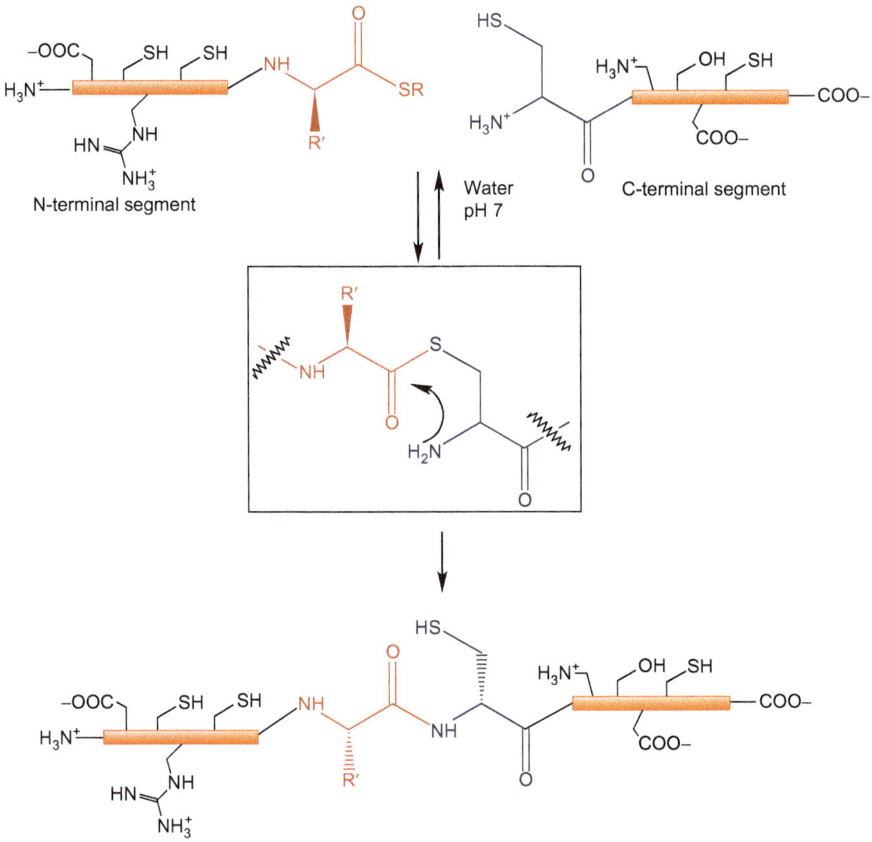

Chapter 5, Figure 5.3 (See page 119 of this volume.)

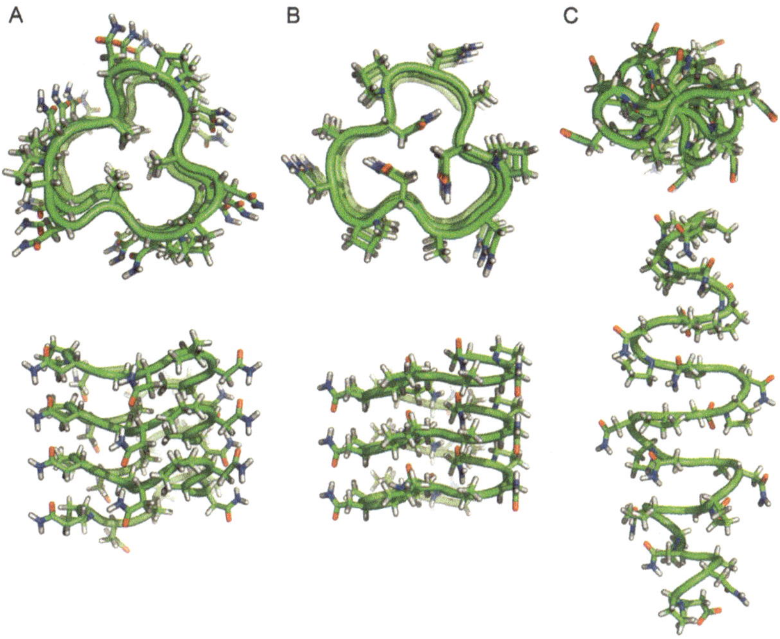

Chapter 5, Figure 5.4 (See page 123 of this volume.)

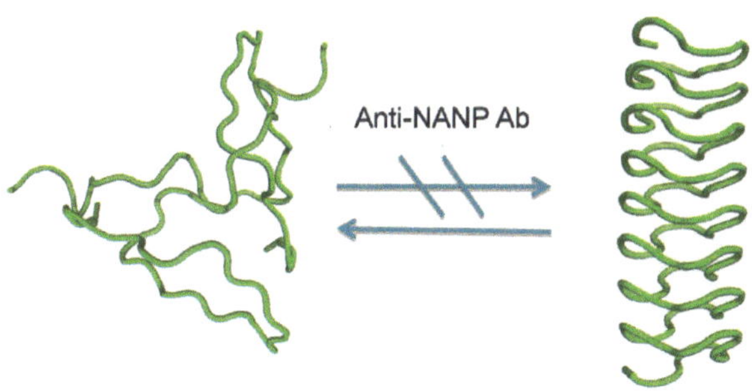

Chapter 5, Figure 5.5 (See page 124 of this volume.)

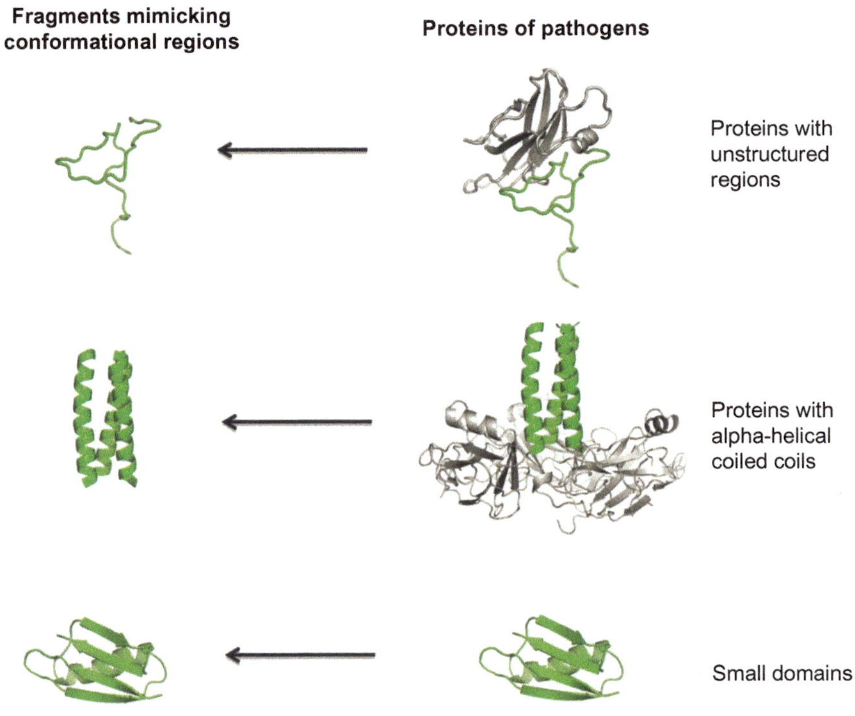

Chapter 5, Figure 5.6 (See page 135 of this volume.)

FSC
www.fsc.org
MIX
Papier | Fördert
gute Waldnutzung
FSC® C083411

Kolibri 360 GmbH
Ferdinand-Jühlke-Straße 7
99095 Erfurt, Deutschland
produktsicherheit@kolibri360.de